An Expanding World
Volume 26

Biological Consequences of the European Expansion, 1450–1800

AN EXPANDING WORLD
The European Impact on World History, 1450–1800

General Editor: A.J.R. Russell-Wood

Please note titles may change prior to publication

An Expanding World
The European Impact on World History 1450–1800

Volume 26

Biological Consequences of European Expansion, 1450–1800

edited by
Kenneth F. Kiple
and Stephen V. Beck

Ashgate
VARIORUM

Published in the **Variorum Expanding World Series** by

Ashgate Publishing Limited	Ashgate Publishing Company
Gower House, Croft Road	Old Post Road
Aldershot, Hampshire GU11 3HR	Brookfield, Vermont 05036–9704
Great Britain	USA

ISBN 0–86078–518–1

British Library CIP data
        Biological Consequences of the European Expansion, 1450–1800.
        (An Expanding World: The European Impact on World History,
        1450–1800: Vol. 26). 1. Communicable diseases–Transmission–
        History. 2. Medical geography. 3. Imperialism–Health aspects.
        I. Kiple, Kenneth F., 1939–　. II. Beck, Stephen V.
        614. 5' 0903

US Library of Congress CIP data
        Biological Consequences of the European Expansion, 1450–1800,
        edited by Kenneth F. Kiple and Stephen V. Beck.
        p.cm. – (An Expanding World: The European Impact on World
        History, 1450–1800: Vol. 26). Includes bibliographical references.
        1. Epidemics–History. 2. Europe–Territorial expansion.
        3. Diseases and history–America. 4. Diseases and history–Europe.
        5. Indians–First contact with Europeans.
        I. Kiple, Kenneth F., 1939–　. II. Beck, Stephen V. III. Series.
        RA649.B54 . 1997   96–52045
        614.4'9–dc21   CIP

This book is printed on acid free paper.

Printed and bound by Biddles Short Run Books, King's Lynn

AN EXPANDING WORLD 26

Contents

Acknowledgements

The chapters in this volume are taken from the sources listed below, for which the editor and publishers wish to thank their authors, original publishers or other copyright holders for permission to use their material as follows:

Chapter 1: Brenda J. Baker and George J. Armelagos, 'The Origin and Antiquity of Syphilis: Paleopathological Diagnosis and Interpretation', *Current Anthropology* XXIX, no. 5 (Chicago, IL, 1988), pp. 703–737. Copyright © 1988 by The University of Chicago Press.

Chapter 2: Noble David Cook, 'Disease and the Depopulation of Hispaniola, 1492–1518', *Colonial Latin American Review* II, nos. 1–2 (San Diego, CA, 1993), pp. 213–245. Copyright © 1993 by San Diego State University Press.

Chapter 3: Donald Joralemon, 'New World Depopulation and the Case of Disease', *Journal of Anthropological Research* XXXVIII, no. 1 (Albuquerque, NM, 1982), pp. 108–127. Copyright © 1982 by The University of New Mexico.

Chapter 4: Alfred W. Crosby, 'Conquistador y Pestilencia: The First New World Pandemic and the Fall of the Great Indian Empires', *Hispanic American Historical Review* XLVII, no. 3 (Durham, NC, 1967), pp. 321–337. Copyright © 1967 by Duke University Press.

Chapter 5: Henry F. Dobyns, 'An Outline of Andean Epidemic History to 1720', *Bulletin of the History of Medicine* XXXVII, no. 6. (Baltimore, MD, 1963), pp. 493–515. Copyright © 1963 by The Johns Hopkins University Press.

Chapter 6: Philip D. Curtin, 'Epidemiology and the Slave Trade', *Political Science Quarterly* LXXXIII, no. 2 (New York, 1968), pp. 190–216. Copyright © 1968 by *Political Science Quarterly*. Reprinted by permission of the Academy of Political Science, New York.

Chapter 7: Francisco Guerra, The Influence of Disease on Race, Logistics and Colonization in the Antilles', *Journal of Tropical Medicine and Hygiene* LXIX (Oxford, 1966), pp. 23–35. Copyright © 1966 by Blackwell Science Ltd.

Chapter 8: Karen Ordahl Kupperman, 'Fear of Hot Climates in the Anglo-American Colonial Experience', *William and Mary Quarterly* (3rd Series) XLI, no. 2 (Williamsburg, VA, 1984), pp. 213–240. Copyright © 1984 by the Institute of Early American History and Culture. Reprinted by permission of the author and the Omohundro Institute of Early American History and Culture.

Chapter 9: Darrett B. Rutman and Anita H. Rutman, 'Of Agues and Fevers: Malaria in the Early Chesapeake', *William and Mary Quarterly* (3rd Series) XXXIII, no. 1 (Williamsburg, VA, 1976), pp. 31–60. Copyright © by the Institute of Early American History and Culture. Reprinted by permission of the author and the Omohundro Institute of Early American History and Culture.

Chapter 10: John Duffy, 'Smallpox and the Indians in the American Colonies', *Bulletin of the History of Medicine* XXV, no. 4 (Baltimore, MD, 1951), pp. 324–341. Copyright © 1951 by The Johns Hopkins University Press.

Chapter 11: Sherburne F. Cook, 'The Significance of Disease in the Extinction of the New England Indians', *Human Biology* XLV, no. 3 (Detroit, MI, 1973), pp. 485–508. Copyright © 1973 by Wayne State University Press. Reprinted by permission of Wayne State University Press.

Chapter 12: Judy Campbell, 'Smallpox in Aboriginal Australia, 1829–1831', *Australian Historical Studies* XX, no. 81 (Parkville, Victoria, 1983), pp. 536–556. Copyright © 1983 by Judy Campbell. Reprinted by permission of the University of Melbourne.

Chapter 13: David E. Stannard, 'Disease and Infertility: A New Look at the Demographic Collapse of Native Populations in the Wake of Western Contact', *Journal of American Studies* XXIV, no. 3 (Cambridge, 1990), pp. 325–350. Copyright © 1990 by Cambridge University Press.

Chapter 14: E.L. Jones, 'Creative Disruptions in American Agriculture, 1620–1820', *Agricultural History* XLVIII, no. 4 (Berkeley, CA, 1974), pp. 510–528. Copyright © 1974 by the University of California Press. Reprinted by permission of the University of California Press.

Chapter 15: William L. Langer, 'Europe's Initial Population Explosion', *The American Historical Review* LXIX, no. 1 (Washington, DC, 1963), pp. 1–17. Copyright © 1963 by The American Historical Association.

Every effort has been made to trace all the copyright holders, but if any have been inadvertently overlooked the publishers will be pleased to make the necessary arrangement at the first opportunity.

Kenneth Kiple would like to thank the Faculty Research Committee of Bowling Green State University for a Basic Grant Award (BA 9307) during the years 1993/ 94 which permitted free time for this and other projects.

In addition, both Kenneth Kiple and Stephen Beck are grateful to the Policy History Programme at Bowling Green State University, which, supported by a Challenge Grant for the Ohio State Board of Regents, has also afforded them the free time and resources to complete this volume.

Finally, the editors would both like to thank Alfred Crosby and Noble David Cook for their reading of the introduction and suggestions for its improvement. Their thanks also goes to Ralph Shlomowitz for his suggestions on the literature of Oceania.

General Editor's Preface

A.J.R. Russell-Wood

An Expanding World: The European Impact on World History, 1450–1800 is designed to meet two objectives: first, each volume covers a specific aspect of the European initiative and reaction across time and space; second, the series represents a superb overview and compendium of knowledge and is an invaluable reference source on the European presence beyond Europe in the early modern period, interaction with non-Europeans, and experiences of peoples of other continents, religions, and races in relation to Europe and Europeans. The series reflects revisionist interpretations and new approaches to what has been called 'the expansion of Europe' and whose historiography traditionally bore the hallmarks of a narrowly Eurocentric perspective, focus on the achievements of individual nations, and characterization of the European presence as one of dominance, conquest, and control. Fragmentation characterized much of this literature: fragmentation by national groups, by geography, and by chronology.

The volumes of *An Expanding World* seek to transcend nationalist histories and to examine on the global stage rather than in discrete regions important selected facets of the European presence overseas. One result has been to bring to the fore the multicontinental, multi-oceanic and multinational dimension of the European activities. A further outcome is compensatory in the emphasis placed on the cross-cultural context of European activities and on how collaboration and cooperation between peoples transcended real or perceived boundaries of religion, nationality, race, and language and were no less important aspects of the European experience in Africa, Asia, the Americas, and Australia than the highly publicized confrontational, bellicose, and exploitative dimensions. Recent scholarship has not only led to greater understanding of peoples, cultures, and institutions of Africa, Asia, the Americas, and Australasia with whom Europeans interacted and the complexity of such interactions and transactions, but also of relations between Europeans of different nationalities and religious persuasions.

The initial five volumes reflect the changing historiography and set the stage for volumes encompassing the broad themes of technology and science, trade and commerce, exploitation as reflected in agriculture and the extractive industries and through systems of forced and coerced labour, government of empire, and society and culture in European colonies and settlements overseas. Final volumes examine the image of Europe and Europeans as 'the other' and the impact of the wider world on European *mentalités* and mores.

An international team of editors was selected to reflect a diversity of educational backgrounds, nationalities, and scholars at different stages of their professional careers. Few would claim to be 'world historians', but each is a recognized authority in his or her field and has the demonstrated capacity to ask the significant questions and provide a conceptual framework for the selection of articles which combine analysis with interpretation. Editors were exhorted to place their specific subjects within a global context and over the *longue durée*. I have been delighted by the enthusiasm with which they took up this intellectual challenge, their courage in venturing beyond their immediate research fields to look over the fences into the gardens of their academic neighbours, and the collegiality which has led to a generous informal exchange of information. Editors were posed the daunting task of surveying a rich historical literature and selecting those essays which they regarded as significant contributions to an understanding of the specific field or representative of the historiography. They were asked to give priority to articles in scholarly journals; essays from conference volumes and *Festschriften* were acceptable; excluded (with some few exceptions) were excerpts from recent monographs or paperback volumes. After much discussion and agonizing, the decision was taken to incorporate essays only in English, French, and Spanish. This has led to the exclusion of the extensive scholarly literature in Danish, Dutch, German and Portuguese. The ramifications of these decisions and how these have had an impact on the representative quality of selections of articles have varied, depending on the theme, and have been addressed by editors in their introductions.

The introduction to each volume enables readers to assess the importance of the topic *per se* and place this in the broader context of European activities overseas. It acquaints readers with broad trends in the historiography and alerts them to controversies and conflicting interpretations. Editors clarify the conceptual framework for each volume and explain the rationale for the selection of articles and how they relate to each other. Introductions permit volume editors to assess the impact on their treatments of discrete topics of constraints of language, format, and chronology, assess the completeness of the journal literature, and address *lacunae*. A further charge to editors was to describe and evaluate the importance of change over time, explain differences attributable to differing geographical, cultural, institutional, and economic circumstances and suggest the potential for cross-cultural, comparative, and interdisciplinary approaches. The addition of notes and bibliographies enhances the scholarly value of the introductions and suggests avenues for further enquiry.

I should like to express my thanks to the volume editors for their willing participation, enthusiasm, sage counsel, invaluable suggestions, and good judgment. Evidence of the timeliness and importance of the series was illustrated by the decision, based on extensive consultation with the scholarly community, to expand a series, which had originally been projected not to exceed eight volumes, to more than thirty volumes. It was John Smedley's initiative which gave rise to discussions as to the viability and need for such a series and he has overseen the publishing, publicity, and marketing of *An Expanding World*. As

General Editor, my task was greatly facilitated by the assistance of Dr Mark Steele who was initially responsible for the 'operations' component of the series as it got under way, latterly this assistance has been provided by staff at Variorum.

The Department of History,
The Johns Hopkins University

Introduction

Kenneth F. Kiple and Stephen V. Beck

Medical statistics have shown, in treating on the different races of mankind the dangers of changing one's position on the globe...

G. Pouchet (1864)[1]

Wherever the European has trod, death seems to pursue the aboriginal.

Charles Darwin (1836)[2]

This volume deals with some of the biological, and especially the medical and demographic consequences of the expansion of Europe. But its essays concentrate heavily on the American theatre of that expansion for the very good reason that the catastrophic die off of the American Indians after 1492 has proved to be a compelling topic of research for historians, and much has been written about it.[3]

In Africa, by contrast, it was the Europeans who were susceptible to disease, and there was relatively little they could do about the problem until the nineteenth century.[4] In Asia, although the Europeans brought syphilis to that part of the world, there was no dramatic melting away of populations. In fact, historically Europe came out a decided second-best in disease exchanges with Asia. The latter was the source of bubonic plague beginning in the fourteenth century, and Asiatic

---

[1] G. Pouchet, *The Plurality of the Human Race*, 2nd edn., tr. and ed. H.J. Beavau (London, 1864), p. 92.

[2] Charles Darwin, *The Voyages of the Beagle* (New York, 1909), p. 459.

[3] It was during the 1940s that modern historians and other scholars began to take notice of the role of disease in the European conquest of the Americas. Two early studies are P.M. Ashburn's *The Ranks of Death: A Medical History of the Conquest of America* (New York, 1947), and Sherburne F. Cook's *The Conflict between the California Indian and White Civilization* (Berkeley, 1943). Cook and his colleague, Woodrow W. Borah, continued to work in this and related fields throughout their careers. More recent discussions of the subject are provided in David E. Stannard's *American Holocaust: The Conquest of the New World* (New York, 1992), and Alfred W. Crosby's *The Columbian Exchange: Biological and Cultural Consequences of 1492* (Westport, Conn., 1972). Broader discussions of the history of biological and epidemiological exchanges among peoples may be found in Crosby's *Ecological Imperialism: The Biological Expansion of Europe, 900–1900* (New York, 1986), and William H. McNeill's *Plagues and Peoples* (New York, 1977).

[4] K.G. Davies's 'The Living and the Dead: White Mortality in West Africa, 1684–1732', in eds., Stanley L. Engerman and Eugene D. Genovese, *Race and Slavery in the Western Hemisphere: Quantitative Studies* (Princeton, 1975), pp. 83–98, and Philip D. Curtin's *Death by Migration* (New York, 1989), illustrate the high 'relocation cost' to Europeans, meaning the price in disease and death, of moving into Africa and other tropical areas of the world before the later nineteenth century. As Curtin's findings indicate, after that time, medical advances and a better overall understanding of man's relationship with his environment combined to reduce this cost.

cholera in the nineteenth century – both plagues whose careers bracket our time period but fall outside of it.[5]

Thus it is the case that, outside of the Americas, it was only the new worlds of the Pacific and Oceania that experienced demographic disaster in the face of the biological Pandora's box opened by the Europeans as they knitted together the globe.

Although it was written in the Bible that 'God hath made of one blood all nations to dwell on the face of the earth' (St Paul, Acts 17:26), the suspicion must have arisen, as the European expansion got under way, that God had not intended the 'nations' in question to change their geographical position on that earth. The technology that carried the expedition of Vasco da Gama around the Cape and across the Indian Ocean to reach Calicut in May of 1498 had made it possible for humans to spend long months at sea. But during the lengthy outbound voyage, and again during the return to Lisbon, a mysterious disease broke out among the seamen which caused hands and feet to swell, gums to grow over the teeth, old wounds to open, and men to die.[6]

The disease was scurvy – brought on by months of vitamin C deprivation. It had doubtless been seen before by Europeans, but only rarely, under circumstances such as those produced by prolonged sieges. Yet prolonged sea voyages without fresh foods provided an even better milieu for the blossoming of scurvy and from this point forward, as Europeans increasingly took to the oceans of the world for exploration, for conquest, and for the defense of the spoils of conquest, the disease became an implacable scourge of seamen, killing more than a million of them by the nineteenth century – many more than those killed by all the naval battles, storms, and shipwrecks of the intervening centuries put together.[7]

---

[5] Philip Ziegler's *The Black Death* (New York, 1969) is still a good introduction to the history of bubonic plague in Europe. For cholera, see Dhiman Barua and William Burrows, eds., *Cholera* (Philadelphia, 1974), and Reinhard S. Speck, 'Cholera,' in ed. Kenneth F. Kiple, *The Cambridge World History of Human Disease* (new York, 1993), pp. 642–9. McNeill, in *Plagues and Peoples*, discusses these pandemics as well. In connection with such major disease exchanges, it is worth noting here McNeill's concept of regional 'disease pools' which may differ greatly from one another. Thus, over time, various peoples have developed varying 'pools' of immunities to disease, which may prove inadequate in the face of new or repeated introductions of diseases from disparate regions. But despite occasional catastrophes resulting from disease exchanges among the regions of the Old World, the frequency and longevity of contacts among them ensured that their peoples had many immunities in common, which were not shared by the more isolated peoples of the New Worlds.

[6] Da Gama's description of the disease is quoted in Kenneth J. Carpenter, *The History of Scurvy and Vitamin C* (Cambridge, 1986), pp. 1–2.

[7] This discussion is based on Carpenter, *History of Scurvy*, pp. 1–76, and R.E. Hughes, 'Scurvy', in ed. Kenneth F. Kiple, *The Cambridge World History of Food and Nutrition* (forthcoming).

Meanwhile, other evidence indicating the perils of venturing to remote lands had been unfolding in Europe. In their ventures down and around the African coastline, the Portuguese had contracted *falciparum* malaria, the most dangerous of the malaria types, and brought it back to Iberia, whereupon it practically depopulated much of the Tagus valley.[8] But an even more dramatic outcome of venturing far from home began to emerge as the fifteenth century came to a close. It seemed that Columbus had scarcely returned from his first voyage to the Americas when another, apparently new, disease burst upon the Europeans in their own homelands. It may be that syphilis had been around Europe in a less malignant form for eons. But it would seem that venereal syphilis, at least in epidemic form, made its European debut in Spain, or Italy, or France in 1493 or 1494 before it erupted in late 1495 among the soldiers of both France and Spain during the Italian Wars.[9]

Because that epidemic began during the French siege of Naples, syphilis was known initially as the 'disease of Naples'. Yet after the French retreat, the disbanding of their multinational army saw the rapid spread of syphilis across Europe, whereupon it became known as the 'French disease' by everyone except, of course, the French. Early in the sixteenth century, however, a Spanish physician suggested that the sailors of Columbus had contracted the disease in the Caribbean during his first voyage and brought it back to Europe, thus giving rise to the Columbian theory of the origin of epidemic venereal syphilis.[10]

There is no question that syphilis in Europe acted like a new disease among inexperienced peoples. It followed a classic pattern of raging among them with extraordinary virulence during much of the sixteenth century, only to become increasingly less malignant afterwards – so much so that by the eighteenth century it was routinely confused with gonorrhea. But despite its apparently exotic nature there were contemporary physicians who stated flatly that they had treated syphilis prior to 1492, albeit in a less severe form.[11]

---

[8] Ralph Linton, *The Tree of Culture* (New York, 1955), p. 27.

[9] The following summary of the early history of syphilis and the debate over its origins is based on Crosby's discussion in *The Columbian Exchange*, pp. 122–64. For further details of the spread of the disease in Europe, and a survey of early writings on the subject, see J. Johnston Abraham, 'The Early History of Syphilis', *British Journal of Surgery* XXXII, no. 126 (1944), pp. 225–37.

[10] Crosby, in *The Columbian Exchange*, pp. 144–7, seemingly favours the Columbian theory, albeit with appropriate disclaimers, and Saul Jarcho briefly states a case for it in 'Some Observations on Disease in Prehistoric North America', *Bulletin of the History of Medicine* XXXVIII (1964), pp. 11–15. In addition, it has been speculated that some New World sculpture suggests the pre-Columbian presence of syphilis or a similar disease; see Abner I. Weisman, 'Syphilis: Was It Endemic in Pre-Columbian America or Was It Brought Here from Europe?', *Bulletin of the New York Academy of Medicine* XLII, no. 4 (1966), pp. 284–300.

[11] A case for the Old World origin of syphilis is presented in Charles Clayton Dennie's *The Gift of Columbus* (Kansas City, 1936), pp. 13–35 and *passim*. For another discussion of the

These two apparently irreconcilable theories of the origin of syphilis in Europe had the field to themselves until the twentieth century, with the Columbian theory clearly the front runner. But syphilis is only one of the treponemal diseases, and other theories emerged following the realization that the causative agents of all of them – pinta, non-venereal syphilis, yaws, and syphilis – were indistinguish-able under the microscope.[12]

Among these theories was the so-called 'unitarian' concept of the treponemata, first proposed by E.H. Hudson in 1946 and subsequently restated and defended a number of times. It held that all of the treponemal diseases, although differing in symptoms, are caused by the same organism which is transmitted differently in different climates. The venereal transmission of syphilis simply represented the adaptation of the treponemata to cooler climates with adult to adult transmission. In tropical climates where the pathogens of pinta and yaws could exist outside the body, they travelled from skin to skin (usually from child to child). In the case of non-venereal syphilis, in hot dry climates, the agents moved via mucosal tissue, as, for example, when children used the same eating utensils or when people kissed.[13]

The unitarian theory does not exclude the Columbian theory, but it has mostly been viewed as supporting the notion of an Old World development of syphilis. In an exploration of the problem of 'The Origin and Antiquity of Syphilis' (Chapter 1), Brenda J. Baker and George J. Armelagos exhaustively review these and other theories in the light of current historical and anthropological evidence. On the basis of skeletal evidence they conclude that non-venereal syphilis was in the Americas prior to 1492 and suggest this was the fountain of what became an Old World plague after that date. But how non-venereal syphilis in the New World became epidemic venereal syphilis in the Old still awaits full explanation.[14]

Yet even if it turns out that contact with the Americas did mean syphilis first for Europe, and then for the rest of the globe as wandering Europeans spread it

---

disease's Old World origins, see C.J. Hackett, 'On the Origin of the Human Treponematoses (Pinta, Yaws, Endemic Syphilis, and Venereal Syphilis)', *Bulletin of the World Health Organization* XXIX (1963), 7–41.

[12] Crosby, *Columbian Exchange*, pp. 123, 141–4.

[13] E.H. Hudson, 'Treponematosis', in ed. Henry A. Christian, *The Oxford Textbook of Medicine*, 8 vols. (Oxford, 1949), Vol. 5, pp. 9–121. Hudson further postulated that the slave trade's forced migration of millions of Africans to other regions of the globe helped to spread *Treponema pallidum* beyond its putative homeland. In cooler, 'more civilized' environments, the importation of Africans carrying non-venereal treponemal infections may have created 'foci for the local propagation of venereal syphilis'. For this discussion, see Hudson, 'Treponematosis and African Slavery', *British Journal of Venereal Diseases* XL (1964), pp. 43–52.

[14] For further discussion of the history of syphilis, see Jon Arrizabalaga's 'Syphilis', and Kenneth F. Kiple's 'Syphilis, Nonvenereal', both in ed. Kenneth F. Kiple, *Cambridge World History of Human Disease*, 1025–1035.

about, this was small revenge for the pathogenic holocaust inadvertently unleashed on New World peoples by Old World pathogens.[15] A crossfire of debate continues over questions concerning the die off of the Native Americans after 1492, not least over questions having to do with the magnitude of that die off. But lively arguments have also taken place over how much blame Iberian procedures, policies, and just plain greed must share with epidemiological factors; and over the extent to which the first Americans were 'virgin soil' peoples for Old World diseases: and even over exactly who the first Americans were and how they became so 'liable' to the pathogens that reached them from Europe and from Africa.[16]

Firm answers have proven elusive. Most probably there were no fewer than 50 million 'Indians' in the Americas when Columbus first set food on Hispaniola and no more than 100 million.[17] Perhaps, as conventional wisdom would have

---

[15] Early accounts of the matter may be found in Bartolome de las Casas, *Historia de las Indias*, 3 vols. (Mexico City, 1951); Gonzalo Fernandez de Oviedo, *Historia general y natural de las Indias, islas, y tierra firme del mar oceano ...*, 4 vols. (Madrid, 1851–5); and Antonio de Herrera y Tordesillas, *Historia general de los hechos de los Castellanos en las islas y tirra firme en el mar oceano*, 17 vols. (Buenos Aires, 1945).

[16] These debates are not confined to questions of factual detail or interpretational nuance; some of the most fundamental findings within the field have been challenged. For a recent provocative critique, see Francis J. Brooks, 'Revising the Conquest of Mexico: Smallpox, Sources, and Populations', *Journal of Interdisciplinary History* XXIV, no. 1 (1993), pp. 1–29. Brooks suggests that the accepted account of the role of disease in the Spanish conquest of Mexico is largely 'false, epidemiologically improbable, historiographically suspect, [and] logically dubious'. Such criticism performs the highly desirable function of helping to synthesize recent research, and of forcing scholars to remain aware of conclusions needing further refinement.

[17] Population estimates for the Western Hemisphere in 1492 have ranged from 8.4 million to well over 100 million persons. Douglas H. Ubelaker's, 'Prehistoric New World Population Size: Historical Review and Current Appraisal of North American Estimates', *American Journal of Physical Anthropology* LXV, no. 3, part II (1976), pp. 661–5, and David Henige's, 'Native American Population at Contact: Discursive Strategies and Standards of Proof in the Debate', *Latin American Population History Bulletin* (1992), pp. 2–23, provide a good overview of much of the scholarship in this area. Many, but not all, scholars have become inclined to accept higher estimates than formerly.

Various aspects of the population debate in recent decades may be followed by referring to essays by Francisco Guerra and M.C. Sanchez Tellez, 'Missionary Reports from Mexico (1550–1563): Estimates on Native Population Decline', *Latin American Population History Bulletin* XXV (1994), pp. 23–5; Michael E. Smith, 'Hernan Cortes on the Size of Aztec Cities', *Latin American Population History Bulletin* XXV (1994), pp. 25–7; Henry F. Dobyns, 'Building Stones and Paper: Evidence of Native American Historical Numbers', *Latin American Population History Bulletin* XXIV (1993), pp. 11–19; Woodrow Borah, Thomas Whitmore, Peter Gerhard, Francisco Guerra, and David Henige (Contributors), 'Debate: 16th-century Demographic Collapse', *Latin American Population History Bulletin* XXIII (1993), pp. 16–23; Thomas M. Whitmore, 'Sixteenth-Century Population Decline in the Basin of Mexico: A Systems Simulation', *Latin American Population History Bulletin* XX (1991), pp. 2–18; Henry F. Dobyns, Dean R. Snow and Kim M. Lanphear, and David Henige (Contributors), 'Commentary on Native American Demography', *Ethnohistory* XXXVI, no. 3 (1989), pp. 285–307; Marshall T. Newman, 'Aboriginal New World Epidemiology

it, the first Americans crossed in many waves from Siberia to Alaska via the land bridge of the Bering Straits, exposed during the last Ice Age. Or perhaps, as has recently been proposed based on genetic data, at least some arrived by sea from Polynesia.[18] But either way, they would have reached the New World before the Old began its Neolithic Revolution. The invention of agriculture, the domestication of animals, and the stimulus such activities provided for urban life, combined to form the Old World crucible for many of the most important epidemic diseases of humankind.[19]

This is not to suggest that the Americas were a disease-free Eden prior to 1492. Although they lagged substantially behind the Old World, New World peoples did mount their own Neolithic revolution that, in fostering sedentarism, doubtless encouraged the proliferation of water-borne diseases such as hepatitis and polio, as well as a variety of intestinal parasites. Present also were encephalitis, arthritis, pinta, and tuberculosis, as well as some uniquely American infections such as Chagas' Disease and American leishmaniasis. But until the Europeans and the Africans arrived, the first Americans had been spared a veritable gauntlet of epidemic diseases that, many have suggested, may have reduced their numbers by a staggering ninety percent.[20]

---

and Medical Care, and the Impact of Old World Disease Imports', *American Journal of Physical Anthropology* LXV, no. 3, part II (1976), pp. 667–72; Wilbur R. Jacobs, 'The Trip of an Iceberg: Pre-Columbian Indian Demography and Some Implications for Revisionism', *William and Mary Quarterly* (3rd series) XXXI, no. 1 (1974), pp. 123–32; Woodrow Borah and Sherburne F. Cook, 'Conquest and Population: A Demographic Approach to Mexican History', *Proceedings of the American Philosophical Society* CXIII, no. 2 (1969), pp. 177–83; and Henry F. Dobyns, 'Estimating Aboriginal American Population: An Appraisal of Techniques with a New Hemispheric Estimate', *Current Anthropology* VII (1966), pp. 395–416.

In addition to the journal literature, a few books have made important contributions to an understanding of aspects of New World demographic history. The most recent is the second edition of William M. Denevan's *The Native Population of the Americas in 1492* (Madison, Wis., 1992). Another recent work, if more generalized, is editor David Hurst Thomas's *Columbian Consequences*, 3 vols. (Washington, 1989–1991). Henry F. Dobyns's *Their Number Become Thinned* (Knoxville, 1983) is a more in-depth study. A seminal, if controversial, study of the question is provided by Sherburne F. Cook and Woodrow Borah in *Essays in Population History: Mexico and the Caribbean*, 3 vols. (Berkeley, 1971-9).

[18] Geneticist Douglas C. Wallace's studies of mitochondrial DNA indicate that native Siberians lack a 'peculiar mutation' which some American Indians, Southeast Asians, and Polynesians share. See Jerry E. Bishop, 'Strands of Time: A Geneticist's Work on DNA Bears Fruit for Anthropologists', *The Wall Street Journal* (November 10, 1993), A1, A8.

[19] McNeill, *Plagues and Peoples*, pp. 31–68.

[20] Crosby, *Ecological Imperialism*, pp. 197–8; McNeill, *Plagues and Peoples*, pp. 176–8; Stannard, *American Holocaust*, X, pp. 53–4; Alfred W. Crosby, 'Virgin Soil Epidemics as a Factor in the Aboriginal Depopulation in America', *William and Mary Quarterly* (3rd Series) XXX, no. 2 (1976), pp. 289–99; Sherburne F. Cook, 'The Incidence and Significance of Disease Among the Aztecs and Related Tribes', *Hispanic American Historical Review* XXVI, no. 3 (1946), pp. 320–35; and Jane E. Buikstra, 'Diseases of the Pre-Columbian Americas', Marvin J. Allison,

For the Tainos of the Caribbean the slaughter began in 1493 when an epidemic swept Hispaniola and radiated out from there to other islands. Swine influenza has been put forward as a candidate, in part at least because the disease attacked the Europeans as well as the Indians and, as we are still periodically reminded, few, if any, develop a steadfast immunity to its rapidly mutating pathogens. Even Columbus became ill, but he recovered and there is little question that the disease, whatever it was, treated the Indians considerably more harshly than the Europeans.[21]

Assuming that the disease among the Indians was the result of Spanish migration, another candidate for this first American epidemic is typhus, a new disease for Europeans, which had slipped into Spain from Cyprus. During the recent war in Granada, Spain's final – and successful – effort to oust the Muslims from the Iberian Peninsula, typhus had killed five times more Spanish soldiers than the enemy. Even if typhus was not the first of the Old World illnesses to reach the New World, there is plenty of evidence to indicate its Caribbean presence during the early years of exploration and conquest.[22] In addition, given the many reports of sickness among the Tainos, it seems clear that numerous other illnesses were intruding as well, and Noble David Cook indicates something of the initial onslaught of European disease in the Americas by looking at 'disease and the Depopulation of Hispaniola, 1492–1518' (Chapter 2).

In shifting our focus from the Caribbean to the mainland, smallpox, which reached the Americas by at least 1518, has been credited with spearheading the conquest of Mexico for Cortez, and that of the Andean regions for the Pizarros.[23] Some of the smallpox, however, may have been measles, which was also a proven scourge of inexperienced peoples as the suddenly not so isolated Japanese had discovered centuries earlier. And in the wake of these diseases from Europe came

---

'Chagas' Disease', and Marvin J. Allison, 'Leishmaniasis', all in ed. Kenneth F. Kiple, *Cambridge World History of Human Disease*, pp. 305–17, 636–8, 832–4.

[21] Francisco Guerra, 'The Earliest American Epidemic: The Influenza of 1493', *Social Science History* XII, no. 3 (1988), pp. 305–25. Influenza also may well have been among the early killers accompanying the conquerors of Central America; see F. Webster McBryde, 'Influenza in America during the Sixteenth Century (Guatemala: 1523, 1559–62, 1576)', *Bulletin of the History of Medicine* VIII, no. 2 (1940), pp. 296–302.

[22] Hans Zinsser, *Rats, Lice, and History* (Boston, 1963), pp. 241–6, 253–7; Kenneth F. Kiple, *The Caribbean Slave: A Biological History* (Cambridge, 1984), pp. 145–6, 173; Crosby, *Columbian Exchange*, p. 42.

[23] It has been suggested, however, that a *virulent* smallpox strain may not have been endemic in Europe at this time, 'raising questions ... about the provenance of the lethal strain and the genetic susceptibility of its isolated [New World] target population'. Ann G. Carmichael and Arthur M. Silverstein, 'Smallpox in Europe before the Seventeenth Century: Virulent Killer or Benign Disease?', *Journal of the History of Medicine and Allied Sciences* LXII, no. 2 (1987), pp. 147–68. This may also be held to throw some doubt on the identification of the pathogens involved in early American epidemics.

countless others – among them diphtheria, chicken pox, scarlet fever, whooping cough, typhoid, mumps, pneumonia, anthrax, even bubonic plague.[24] Donald Joralemon reviews the question of 'New World Depopulation and the Case of Disease' (Chapter 3), and makes that case without assigning responsibility or blame. In his words, 'The tragedy appears to be a necessary outcome of human interaction across biological boundaries'.[25]

Alfred Crosby would doubtless agree. His seminal essay, 'Conquistador y Pestilencia: The First New World Pandemic and the Fall of the Great Indian Empires' (Chapter 4), was crucial in educating historians about the vital role that smallpox played in the Spanish conquest of Mexico and Peru. In this essay, and in his subsequent book on *The Columbian Exchange: Biological and Cultural Consequences of 1492*, Crosby, perhaps wisely, refrained from attempting to measure quantitatively the demographic catastrophe such diseases wreaked on New World Indians, and one of the aims of Henry F. Dobyns, in a book entitled *Their Number Become Thinned*, was to determine the numerical magnitude of that tragedy in a portion of the Americas. This effort has established Dobyns as one of the 'high counters' in the words of David Henige.[26]

In this book, Dobyns was building on much of his earlier work, beginning with his controversial but ground-breaking essay on 'An Outline of Andean Epidemic History to 1720' (Chapter 5). As the reader will soon note, the article is not bound by its title, but ranges over much of Spain's American empire in assigning dates to the major epidemic events.

Unhappily, the pathogens that prevailed in Europe were not the only new microbes invading the Americas. If the diseases brought by the Iberians made conquest easy, they complicated colonization by destroying so many of those that had been counted upon to do the labour. But Spaniards in Hispaniola noticed that the few blacks among them were far hardier and much more disease-resistant than the natives. These first blacks were *ladinos*, born in Iberia, and thus with

---

[24] Crosby, *Columbian Exchange*, p. 42ff.; McNeill, *Plagues and Peoples*, pp. 1–2; Dobyns, *Their Number Become Thinned*, p. 11; W. Wayne Farris, 'Diseases of the Premodern Period in Japan', Ann Ramenofsky, 'Diseases of the Americas, 1492–1700', and Kenneth F. Kiple, 'Disease Ecologies of the Caribbean', all in ed. Kenneth F. Kiple, *Cambridge World History Of Human Disease*, pp. 376–85, 317–28, 497–504. In addition, it seems probable that some of these epidemics swept across parts of North America ahead of the Spanish advance. See, for example, Daniel T. Reff, 'Old World Diseases and the Dynamics of Indian and Jesuit Relations in Northwestern New Spain, 1520–1660', in ed. N. Ross Crumrine and Phil C. Weigand *Ejidos and Regions of Refuge in Northwestern Mexico* (Tucson, 1987), pp. 85–94; and John C. Ewers, 'The Influence of Epidemics on the Indian Populations and Cultures of Texas', *Plains Anthropologist* XVIII (1973), pp. 104–115.

[25] Joraleman, p. 90 of this volume.

[26] Crosby, *Columbian Exchange*, p. 39; Dobyns, *Their Number Become Thinned*, p. 4 and *passim*; Henige, 'Native American Population at Contact', *passim*.

the same disease experience (and immunities) as their masters. But they were too few, and a slave trade directly from Africa was underway by 1518. Fortunately for their masters, the arriving slaves left a disease environment that included most of the illnesses that Europeans routinely faced and acquired immunities against. Unfortunately, however, they brought with them a few other maladies to which only they were resistant[27] – a matter that Philip Curtin discusses in his now classic look at 'Epidemiology and the Slave Trade' (Chapter 6).

Two of these diseases, *falciparum* malaria and yellow fever – which rank among the greatest tropical killers in human history – wrote an extraordinarily virulent chapter in the history of the Americas. The protozoa of *falciparum* malaria (the most lethal of all the malaria types) doubtless arrived in the blood of the first Africans to step ashore in the New World, and anopheline mosquitoes were on hand to greet the new arrivals and begin to spread the pathogens about. The virus of yellow fever, however, would have encountered far more difficulty in remaining alive during a transatlantic crossing, and most probably the favorite vector of yellow fever, the *Aedes aegypti* mosquito, was not native to the Americas and also had to be imported from Africa. Thus yellow fever's official debut in the Americas was delayed until 1647, although many suspect that it made some earlier appearances.[28]

These African diseases joined with those from Europe in further eradicating the Indians in low-lying areas to the point where, save for a handful, they completely disappeared from the Caribbean. A stark illustration of the virulence of these mosquito-borne plagues begins in the highlands of Mexico and the Andes where the mosquito vectors that transmitted them seldom reached. There, native populations, having only to face the pathogens carried by the Europeans, eventually developed immunities to defend against those germs, recovered from a downward demographic spiral and began to grow once again. The illustration is completed in those areas where populations faced waves of both European and African illnesses. In these instances there were no populations left alive to recover.[29]

Although much remains to be elucidated, the nature of black resistance to *falciparum* malaria and yellow fever is at least partially understood by modern medicine in immunological terms. In earlier times, however, it was thought of as 'racial' resistance, and as both diseases slaughtered whites but not blacks on

---

[27] Kiple, *Caribbean Slave*, pp. 3–4, 8–13.

[28] Kenneth F. Kiple and Virginia H. King, *Another Dimension to the Black Diaspora: Diet, Disease, and Racism* (Cambridge, 1981), pp. 23, 31–7, 48–51; Kiple, *Caribbean Slave*, pp. 19–20, 161–8.

[29] Cook and Borah, *Essays in Population History*, Vol. 1, *passim*; Dobyns, *Their Number Become Thinned, passim*; John Hemming, *Red Gold: The Conquest of the Brazilian Indians* (Cambridge, Mass., 1978), p. 4; Kiple, *Caribbean Slave*, pp. 4, 9–11.

plantations and in battle alike, the African ironically became ever more valuable in the eyes of the European.[30] Francisco Guerra treats this and other themes in his examination of 'The Influence of Disease on Race, Logistics and Colonization in the Antilles' (Chapter 7).

It was a bitter irony that although they had the blacks to do the hard work for them in hot places, whites nonetheless had to be present to ensure that the work got done. And such a presence left them exposed to fevers that were lethal for whites but not for blacks. When yellow fever struck Barbados in 1647–8 and then swept the Caribbean, thousands of whites – perhaps 6,000 in Barbados alone – went to yellow fever graves dug by slaves that the disease had seemingly left untouched. For whites to move inland, however, away from the yellow fever of coastal cities meant courting the 'ague' – frequently *falciparum* malaria – and the kind of nasty death that it could provoke.[31] No wonder that there developed a 'Fear of Hot Climates in the Anglo-American Colonial Experience' (Chapter 8), which is discussed by Karen Ordahl Kupperman.

As this title indicates, such a fear was not limited to the West Indies. Rather, the range of the African diseases was such that yellow fever struck New York in 1668, Philadelphia and Charleston in 1690, and Boston in 1691. In the eighteenth century the disease became a regular summer visitor to cities of the eastern seaboard, and in the nineteenth century a scourge of the Gulf coast as well.[32]

Meanwhile, in less dramatic fashion, *falciparum* malaria had also become a part of the North American disease environment. The milder *vivax* malaria, which had migrated in the blood of the colonists from Europe, was an old curse for Englishmen. But toward the end of the seventeenth century a new kind of malaria had set upon settlers in South Carolina that was so 'extraordinarie sicklie that sickness quickly seased many of our numbers'. Such a sudden 'seasing' of lives, coinciding with the arrival of colonists from the West Indies on the one hand and the beginning of the African slave trade to North America on the other hand, seems like a trumpet-call announcing the arrival of *falciparum* malaria.[33] These same circumstances probably account for the establishment of the disease in the

---

[30] Kenneth F. Kiple and Brian Higgins, 'Yellow Fever and the Africanization of the Caribbean', in eds. John W. Verano and Douglas H. Ubelaker, *Disease and Demography in the Americas* (Washington, 1992), *passim*; Kiple and King, *Another Dimension*, pp. 29–68.

[31] Kiple, *Caribbean Slave*, pp. 20, 163–5.

[32] K. David Patterson, 'Yellow Fever Epidemics and Mortality in the United States, 1693–1905', *Social Science and Medicine* XXXIV, no. 8 (1992), pp. 855–65; Donald B. Cooper and Kenneth F. Kiple, 'Yellow Fever', in ed. Kenneth F. Kiple, *Cambridge World History of Human Disease*, pp. 1100–1107.

[33] Wyndham Bolling Blanton, *Medicine in Virginia in the Eighteenth Century* (Richmond, 1931), pp. 54–5; John Duffy, *Epidemics in Colonial America* (Baton Rouge, 1953), p. 204; Peter H. Wood, *Black Majority: Negroes in Colonial South Carolina from 1670 through the Stono Rebellion* (New York, 1974), Chap. 3; Kiple and King, *Another Dimension*, p. 51.

Chesapeake Bay region at about the same time. Darrett B. Rutman and Anita H. Rutman probe the circumstances 'Of Agues and Fevers: Malaria in the Early Chesapeake' (Chapter 9), and compare the society, economy, and culture that developed there with that of nearby New England where the disaster was relatively rare.

But if African pathogens had moved north to loose themselves among the Europeans, so too had the diseases that, having previously conquered the Aztecs and the Incas, were now racing pell-mell through the bodies of the native North Americans. '[T]hey dye like rotten sheep ...' declared William Bradford, with no little satisfaction, whereas '... not one of the English was so much as sicke, or in the least measure tainted with this disease'.[34] This quotation was taken from John Duffy's survey of 'Smallpox and the Indians in the American Colonies' (Chapter 10), which, in tandem with Sherburne F. Cook's examination of 'The Significance of Disease in the Extinction of the New England Indians' (Chapter 11), speak volumes about the demise of the major Indian groups of North America beginning about a century after Cortez first set foot in Mexico.[35]

As in the Americas, European contact in the Pacific was spearheaded by the Spaniards. It began with Magellan's voyage, was extended by the Spanish trade route from Mexico to the Philippines, and expanded as Spanish explorers and missionaries fanned out among the islands. In the seventeenth century they were joined by Dutch traders, and in the eighteenth century by British explorers.[36] And as in the Americas, the end of isolation from the Eurasian civilizations, and thus from Eurasian pathogens, meant death and depopulation.

Yet because island communities were typically small, diseases were normally confined to an island or two with the result that, initially at least, there were no widespread epidemics of the spectacular sort that the New World had experienced.

---

[34] Duffy, p. 237 of this volume.

[35] For further discussion of early North American disease exchanges, see Crosby, *Ecological Imperialism*, pp. 200–3; Reff, 'Old World Diseases and Dynamics of Indian and Jesuit Relations', *passim*; Ewers, 'Influence of Epidemics on Indian Populations', *passim*; Phillip L. Walker, Patricia Lambert, and Michael J. DeNiro, 'The Effect of European Contact on the Health of Alta California Indians', in Thomas, *Columbian Consequences*, Vol. 1, p. 64; Clark Spencer Larsen et al., 'Beyond Demographic Collapse: Biological Adaptation and Change in Native Populations of La Florida', in Thomas, *Columbian Consequences*, Vol. 2, pp. 409–28; Timothy K. Perttula, 'European Contact and Its Effects on Aboriginal Caddoan Populations between AD 1520 and AD 1680', in Thomas, *Columbian Consequences*, Vol. 3, pp. 501–518; Dean R. Snow and Kim M. Lanphear, 'European Contact and Indian Depopulation in the Northeast: The Timing of the First Epidemics', *Ethnohistory* XXXV, no. 1 (1988), pp. 15–33; and Robert Fortuine, 'The Health of the Eskimos, as Portrayed in the Earliest Written Accounts', *Bulletin of the History of Medicine* :LXV, no. 2 (1971), pp. 97–114.

[36] J.H. Parry, *The Age of Reconnaissance* (Berkeley, 1963), pp. 159–161, 194–201; Crosby, *Ecological Imperialism*, pp. 122–30. See also J.C. Beaglehole, *The Exploration of the Pacific* (London, 1934).

Moreover, because populations were too small to maintain them, the new diseases had to be continually reintroduced. Thus although influenza probably pummeled the islanders from the beginning of contact with the Europeans, the first report we have of the disease is from Tahiti in 1772. Similarly, syphilis (and gonorrhea) may have reached the Pacific with early explorers and traders, but reports of it only came with the voyages of James Cook in the late 1760s and again in the late 1770s. In the case of smallpox, its first recorded epidemic took place close to a century earlier (1688) in Guam, which was right on the route of the Manila galleons sailing from Mexico.[37] But after this we hear little about the disease for another century until it exploded among the aborigines of Australia and began the grim work of nearly halving their numbers as is shown in Judy Campbell's discussion of 'Smallpox in Aboriginal Australia, 1829–1831' (Chapter 12).[38]

And finally in the Pacific, Hawaii, which can probably serve in microcosmic fashion as a model of the demographic tragedy which befell all of that vast region of the world, is the focus of David E. Stannard's examination of 'Disease and Infertility: A New Look at the Demographic Collapse of Native Populations in the Wake of Western Contact' (Chapter 13).[39]

We close this volume by noting that the ecological disruption of much of the globe occasioned by the expansion of Europe went far beyond uniting New World peoples with Old World pathogens. As Alfred Crosby has so brilliantly portrayed the process in his study of *Ecological Imperialism*, Old World plants, animals, and insects were as aggressive as micro-organisms in colonizing new areas, and just as spectacularly successful in working their own ecological mischief.[40]

---

[37] Leslie B. Marshall, 'Disease Ecologies of Australia and Oceania', in ed. Kenneth F. Kiple *Cambridge World History of Human Disease*, pp. 482–496.

[38] As Campbell suggests, however, it seems likely that at various times smallpox was introduced into Australia by Asians as well as by Europeans. For more on smallpox in Australia, see Campbell's later article, 'Smallpox in Aboriginal Australia, The Early 1830s', *Historical Studies* XXI, no. 84 (1985), pp. 336–358; N.G. Butlin, 'Macassans and Aboriginal Smallpox: The "1789" and "1829" Epidemics', *Historical Studies* XXI, no. 84 (1985), pp. 315–335; and Crosby's discussions of the initial Australian smallpox epidemic in *Ecological Imperialism*, pp. 205–207, 309–311.

[39] For more on Oceania's (and especially Hawaii's) experience with European diseases, see David E. Stannard, *Before the Horror: The Population of Hawai'i on the Eve of Western Contact* (Honolulu, 1989); Andrew F. Bushnell, '"The Horror" Reconsidered: An Evaluation of the Historical Evidence for Population Decline in Hawai'i, 1778–1803', *Pacific Studies* XVI, no. 3 (1993), pp. 115–161; James Watt, 'Medical Aspects and Consequences of Cook's Voyages', in ed. Robin Fisher and Hugh Johnston *Captain James Cook and His Times* (Seattle, 1979), pp. 129–157; William Shainline Middleton, 'Early Medical Experiences in Hawaii', *Bulletin of the History of Medicine* XLV, no. 5 (1971), pp. 444–460; and Robert C. Schmitt, 'The Okuu - Hawaii's Greatest Epidemic', *Hawaii Medical Journal* XXIX, no. 5 (1970), pp. 359–364.

[40] Crosby, *Ecological Imperialism*, pp. 145–194 and *passim*. On this point and what follows, see also Crosby's *Germs, Seeds, and Animals: Studies in Ecological History* (Armonk, N.Y., 1994).

E.L. Jones provides us with one example in his look at 'Creative Disruptions in American Agriculture, 1620–1820' (Chapter 14), with the disruptions in question brought on by the effort to transfer European agriculture to North America. Deforestation opened the way for Old World weeds, and fields and livestock attracted an astounding variety of pests and predators, all of which set about rearranging the continent and – although Jones does not mention it – likely making life quite literally as difficult for the Native Americans as the Eurasian pathogens that were ricocheting about.[41]

Yet if European plants did harm to the Americas, American plants proved marvelously useful for the Europeans. Maize and manioc sent to Africa triggered a population explosion that fueled the flow of slaves back to the homeland of the plants. And in Europe maize fed to livestock meant that more could be overwintered with more available protein the result, whereas the potato entered the human stomach directly.[42] Indeed, as William L. Langer points out, the potato may have been the root at the heart of 'Europe's Initial Population Explosion' (Chapter 15).

Clearly, in the exchange of plants and pathogens that characterized the expansion of Europe, the Europeans, at least in the relatively short run, were the only winners.

Bibliography and Suggested Readings

Ackerknecht, Erwin H., *History and Geography of the Most Important Diseases* (New York, 1965).

Ashburn, P.M., *The Ranks of Death: A Medical History of the Conquest of America* (New York, 1947).

Barua, Dhiman, and William Burrows, eds., *Cholera* (Philadelphia, 1974).

Beaglehole, J.C., *The Exploration of the Pacific* (London, 1934).

Blanton, Wyndham Bolling, *Medicine in Virginia in the Eighteenth Century* (Richmond, 1931).

Carpenter, Kenneth J., *The History of Scurvy and Vitamin C* (Cambridge, 1986).

---

[41] For other views on such ecological disturbance, and Indian reactions to it, see Robert S. Santley, Thomas Killion, and Mark Lycett, 'On the Maya Collapse', *Journal of Anthropological Research* XLII, no. 2 (1986), pp. 123–159; James H. Merrell, 'The Indians' New World: The Catawba Experience', *William and Mary Quarterly* (3rd series) XLI, no. 4 (1984), pp. 537–565; and Calvin Martin, 'The European Impact on the Culture of a Northeastern Algonquian Tribe: An Ecological Interpretation', *William and Mary Quarterly* (3rd series) XXXI, no. 1 (1974), pp. 3–26.

[42] Crosby, *Germs, Seeds, and Animals*, pp. 92, 149–156, 172–173; Kiple, *Caribbean Slave*, p. 25; Kiple and King, *Another Dimension*, pp. 8–9.

Cartwright, Frederick F., *Disease and History* (New York, 1972).

Cohen, Mark Nathan, *Health and the Rise of Civilization* (New Haven, 1989).

Cook, Sherburne F., *The Conflict between the California Indian and White Civilization* (Berkeley, 1943).

Cook, Sherburne, F., and Woodrow Borah, *Essays in Population History: Mexico and the Caribbean*, 3 vols. (Berkeley, 1971–9).

Cronon, William, *Changes in the Land: Indians, Colonists and the Ecology of New England* (New York, 1983).

Crosby, Alfred W., *The Columbian Exchange: Biological and Cultural Consequences of 1492* (Westport, Conn., 1972).

Crosby, Alfred W., *Ecological Imperialism: The Biological Expansion of Europe, 900–1900* (New York, 1986).

Crosby, Alfred W., *Germs, Seeds, and Animals: Studies in Ecological History* (Armonk, N.Y., 1994).

Curtin, Philip D., *Death by Migration* (New York, 1989).

Denevan, William M., *The Native Population of the Americas in 1492* (Madison, Wis., 1992).

Dennie, Charles Clayton, *The Gift of Columbus* (Kansas City, 1936).

Dobyns, Henry F., *Their Number Become Thinned* (Knoxville, 1983).

Duffy, John, *Epidemics in Colonial America* (Baton Rouge, 1953).

Fisher, Robin, and Hugh Johnston, eds., *Captain James Cook and His Times* (Seattle, 1979).

Harrison, G., *Mosquitoes, Malaria, and Man* (New York, 1978).

Hemming, John, *Red Gold: The Conquest of the Brazilian Indians* (Cambridge, Mass., 1978).

Hopkins, Donald, *Princess and Peasants: Smallpox in History* (Chicago, 1983).

Kiple, Kenneth F., ed., *The African Exchange: Toward a Biological History of Black People* (Durham, N.C., 1988).

Kiple, Kenneth F., ed., *The Cambridge World History of Human Disease* (New York, 1993).

Kiple, Kenneth F., *The Caribbean Slave: A Biological History* (Cambridge, 1984).

Kiple, Kenneth F., and Virginia H. King, *Another Dimension to the Black Diaspora: Diet, Disease, and Racism* (Cambridge, 1981).

Kunitz, Stephen J., *Disease and Social Diversity: The European Impact on the Health of Non-Europeans* (New York, 1994).

McNeill, William H., *Plagues and Peoples* (New York, 1977).

Parry, J.H., *The Age of Reconnaissance* (Berkeley, 1963).

Stannard, David E., *American Holocaust: The Conquest of the New World* (New York, 1992).

Stannard, David E., *Before the Horror: The Population of Hawai'i on the Eve of Western Contact* (Honolulu, 1989).

Thomas, David Hurst, ed., *Columbian Consequences*, 3 vols. (Washington, 1989–91).

Verano, John W., and Douglas H. Ubelaker, eds., *Disease and Demography in the Americas* (Washington, 1992).

Ziegler, Philip, *The Black Death* (New York, 1969).

Zinsser, Hans, *Rats, Lice, and History* (Boston, 1963).

This volume is dedicated to
Tascha, Tina, and Coneè

1

The Origin and Antiquity of Syphilis:
Paleopathological Diagnosis and Interpretation

Brenda J. Baker and George J. Armelagos

Despite Thomas Gann's 1901 publication of "Recent Discoveries in Central America Proving the Pre-Columbian Existence of Syphilis in the New World," the controversy concerning the origin and antiquity of syphilis remains. As the Columbian quincentenary draws near, it is appropriate to reassess the documentary and skeletal evidence regarding the origin of syphilis and its dispersion throughout the world in the light of paleopathological diagnosis and interpretation. A review of the literature strongly suggests a New World origin of the treponemal infections. Whereas the evidence for pre-Columbian treponematosis in the Old World is documentary and equivocal, there is a vast array of skeletal evidence indicating the presence of a nonvenereal form of treponemal infection in the Americas prior to Columbus's arrival.

Hypotheses on the Origin of Syphilis

Three hypotheses have been advanced to explain the origin and subsequent spread of venereal syphilis throughout the world.

The Columbian hypothesis, proposed by Crosby (1969), Dennie (1962), Goff (1967), Harrison (1959), and others, is that syphilis originated in the Americas and was carried to Europe by Columbus's crew in 1493. Subsequently, a syphilis epidemic occurred in Europe about 1500. The rapid spread of syphilis throughout Europe at

that time suggests the introduction of a virulent disease into a population that had not previously been exposed to it and had no immunity to it.

Proponents of the diametrically opposed pre-Columbian hypothesis (e.g., Hackett 1963, 1967; Holcomb 1934, 1935) assert that venereal syphilis was present in Europe prior to Columbus's voyage but was not distinguished from "leprosy." The alleged epidemic resulted from the recognition of syphilis as a separate disease in the 1490s. Cockburn (1961; 1963:153–59) provides an evolutionary framework for the pre-Columbian origin of syphilis in which geographical isolation led to speciation of *Treponema*. Throughout most of human history, treponemal infection (i.e., pinta, yaws, endemic syphilis, and venereal syphilis) was mild and chronic because populations were small. As population size increased, more acute infections were selected for and spread by direct skin-to-skin contact among children. By 1492, European living standards had improved to the point of differentially affecting the transmission of *Treponema* species. Those dependent upon skin contact were disadvantaged and replaced by a hardier strain that was sexually transmitted (Cockburn 1961:226). Thus in Cockburn's view the discovery of America and the appearance of venereal syphilis are not cause and effect; rather, both resulted from other social and economic events.

A third, unitarian hypothesis is that the agent of

704 | CURRENT ANTHROPOLOGY Volume 29, Number 5, December 1988

syphilis has evolved with human populations and was present in both the Old and the New World at the time of Columbus's discovery. Hudson (1963a, b, 1965a, b, 1968) maintains that pinta, yaws, endemic (nonvenereal) syphilis, and venereal syphilis are four syndromes of treponematosis, a single disease caused by *Treponema pallidum*, which evolved simultaneously with humans. The syndromes form a biological gradient in which various social and environmental factors produce different manifestations of treponematosis (Hudson 1965a). Although Hudson and Cockburn agree on the role of improved hygiene in the appearance of venereal syphilis, they disagree on several aspects of its etiology and epidemiology.

According to Hudson (1963a, 1965a), treponematosis originated during the Paleolithic period as a childhood disease (yaws) transmitted by skin-to-skin contact in the hot, humid climate of sub-Saharan Africa. The infection accompanied gatherer-hunters in their migrations throughout the world. As groups moved into drier zones bordering the tropics, the focus of treponemal activity retreated to the moist areas of the body (mouth, armpits, and crotch), as in endemic syphilis (Hudson 1965a:891). Treponematosis in the form of endemic syphilis was carried into the New World by the earliest migrants from the Old World. As the tropical zones of the Americas were populated, the climatic change caused the shift back to yaws (p. 893). The appearance of villages in the Neolithic period did not alter the nonvenereal nature of the infection; crowded, unsanitary conditions and increased frequency of child-to-child contact in village settings facilitated its spread (1963a:1042–43; 1965a:892–93).

Urbanization, beginning in Mesopotamia and Egypt by 4000 B.C., was accompanied by an improvement in personal and community hygiene (Hudson 1963a:1043). Although it seems counterintuitive for sanitation to have improved in cities, Hudson (1965a:895) points out that "hygienic barriers do not have to be very high to prevent the spread of touch-contact syphilis." Availability of water, washing and bathing with soap, separate sleeping quarters, and the like became adequate barriers to the proliferation of treponematosis by casual contact among children. As a result, individuals reached sexual maturity without prior exposure to it. Hence, "coitus . . . became the only personal contact of sufficient intimacy to permit transmission of treponemas," and adults disseminated the disease in a society in which there was "promiscuity and prostitution" (p. 895).

Hudson (1965b:738) indicates that both venereal and nonvenereal forms of treponematosis may be present within a narrow geographical area, for example, where a city characterized by venereal syphilis is surrounded by a rural area characterized by yaws. Despite identical climates, the higher hygienic level and different social customs in the city promote venereal transmission. Dissolution of urban life would result in a shift from venereal to nonvenereal forms of treponematosis (either endemic syphilis or yaws, depending upon the climate).

Syphilis and Leprosy

Because the pre-Columbian and unitarian hypotheses suggest that diseases such as yaws, endemic syphilis, venereal syphilis, and leprosy were confused from ancient times and grouped under the term "leprosy" (Holcomb 1935:277; 1940:177; Hudson 1965a:896), before examining the evidence it is necessary to discuss the differential diagnosis of these diseases.

Venereal syphilis has an incubation period of 10–90 days before the primary lesion appears in the anogenital region (Olansky 1981:299). Secondary lesions usually develop on the skin and mucous membranes. Prior to the advent of penicillin treatment, the prevalence of syphilis was about 5% in mostly urban adult populations (Steinbock 1976:110). Steinbock's survey of the clinical literature predating penicillin use indicates skeletal involvement in 10–20% of cases (cf. Hackett 1976:108, who cites a single study in which osseous lesions developed in only 1% of untreated patients). Since asymptomatic bone lesions often go undetected in early syphilis, skeletal involvement may be underestimated (Hansen et al. 1984; Steinbock 1976:109). Following Steinbock's (p. 110) arithmetic, however, one obtains a frequency of osseous involvement in 1 of every 100–200 individuals in a skeletal series representing an adult urban population (a prevalence of 0.5–1% in skeletal populations). Hackett (1976:108, 114) indicates that only 1 in 1,000 adults would develop syphilitic bone lesions.

Skeletal involvement in venereal syphilis most often affects the cranial vault, the nasal area, and the tibia. Together, these three locations comprise 70% of all tertiary syphilitic bone lesions (Ortner and Putschar 1985:182). The major diagnostic criterion of skeletal syphilis is the caries sicca sequence, described in detail by Hackett (1976:30–49), which results in the "worm-eaten" appearance of the outer table of the cranial vault, characterized by the formation of stellate scars. Caries sicca is usually accompanied by naso-palatine destruction. This destruction, more extensive and rapid than in leprosy, usually involves the nasal bones and is accompanied by healing and sclerosis (Hackett 1976:63–65; Ortner and Putschar 1985:192, 197; Steinbock 1976:145, 208). Where there is gross destruction of the naso-palatine region, there is often maxillary alveolar damage as well (Hackett 1976:65).

Postcranially, formation of subperiosteal bone begins in the metaphyses of the long bones, with the tibiae being most often involved. Inflammation of the entire periosteum initiates a subperiosteal response resulting in thickening and possible bone deformation (Steinbock 1976:115). Hackett (1976:79–90) proposes a sequence for nongummatous periostitis that ranges from finely striated nodes and expansions to grossly rugose expansions, which he tentatively considers diagnostic criteria of syphilis. Gummatous lesions—nodes/expansion with superficial cavitation—he regards as certainly diagnostic (pp. 93–97). Gumma formation may occur periosteally or in the medullary cavity, resulting in both proliferative and degenerative changes. Syphilis lacks the smooth cloacae and the sequestrum and involucrum formation of pyogenic osteomyelitis (Hackett 1976:95; Steinbock 1976:137). Generally, the affected bone appears roughened and irregular because of thickening and increased density. The medullary cavity, particularly in the tibia, is greatly narrowed by cortical thickening (Steinbock 1976:117, 123). Hands and feet are rarely affected.

Pinta, yaws, endemic (nonvenereal) syphilis, and venereal syphilis have been thought to be caused by different species of *Treponema* (respectively, *T. carateum, T. pertenue,* and two subspecies of *T. pallidum*). The causative organisms of each disease, however, cannot be distinguished from each other by any known test. In electron microscope studies, the "species" of *Treponema* are morphologically identical (Hovind-Hougen 1983:5). Their antigenic structures differ only quantitatively (Hudson 1965a:886). DNA sequence homology analysis indicates that *T. pertenue* and the subspecies of *T. pallidum* are identical and "might be regarded as a single species" (Fieldsteel 1983:50). Partial cross-immunity exists between the treponemal syndromes (Cannefax, Norins, and Gillespie 1967:473–74). Clinically, yaws and endemic and venereal syphilis closely resemble each other in the prolonged course of the disease, with early and late manifestations. Primary yaws is similar to primary syphilis; secondary yaws resembles secondary syphilis, although the skin lesions of the former are often larger and more exuberant; and lesions of tertiary yaws, characterized by gummatous lesions of the skin, soft tissue, bones, and naso-palatine area, are indistinguishable from those of tertiary syphilis (Musher and Knox 1983:114–15). Where (as in all forms except pinta) bone lesions result from the treponemal syndromes, they are also indistinguishable from each other (Hackett 1976:113). Except for the dental stigmata and osteochondritis found only in congenital syphilis, the bone lesions found in one disease are identical to those found in the others (Steinbock 1976:139, 143). Steinbock stresses that the differences in skeletal involvement are merely quantitative. For example, in endemic syphilis and yaws, the cranial vault is infrequently affected in comparison with venereal syphilis, whereas tibial lesions are much more common.

Skeletal series in areas in which either endemic syphilis or yaws occurs are expected to reveal bone lesions in approximately 1–5% of the entire series (Steinbock 1976:139, 143).

Leprosy (now known as Hansen's disease) is a chronic infectious disease caused by the bacillus *Mycobacterium leprae.* The incubation period averages at least three to five years (World Health Organization 1980:16). A prevalence of about 0.5% (4.6 per 1,000) is found in modern Africa, where leprosy is endemic (p. 10). In clinical studies, skeletal manifestations occur in 15–68% of leprosarium patients (Chamberlain, Wayson, and Garland 1931, Esguerra-Gómez and Acosta 1948, Faget and Mayoral 1944, Murdock and Hutter 1932, Paterson

1961). Although leprosy is best known as a skin disease, its effects on the nervous and skeletal systems are well known. Skin changes usually consist of rough, dry macules, in which hypopigmentation may occur (Drutz 1981, World Health Organization 1980).

Skeletal manifestations of leprosy have been described in detail by Møller-Christensen (1967), Møller-Christensen and Faber (1952), Møller-Christensen and Inkster (1965), and Paterson (1959). The most reliable diagnostic criterion of leprosy is the occurrence of facies leprosa in the skull. This condition is characterized by atrophy of the anterior nasal spine, atrophy of the maxillary alveolar margin, mainly in the incisor region, and inflammatory changes of the superior surface of the hard palate. Facies leprosa has been identified in 60–82% of modern leprosy patients (Steinbock 1976:201). Postcranial changes accompanying facies leprosa include atrophy and resorption of the phalanges in the hands, beginning distally, and at the metatarsophalangeal joints in the feet. At a medieval Danish leper cemetery (St. George's Hospital, Naestved), 71.3% of 185 adequately preserved skeletons exhibited both facies leprosa and changes in the hands and feet (Weiss and Møller-Christensen 1971:262–63). Changes affecting only the hands and feet occurred in 26.5% and changes in the skull alone in 2.2% (Weiss and Møller-Christensen 1971:262–63). Examination of the hands and feet is therefore important in differentiating other diseases, such as syphilis, from leprosy. Subperiosteal bone deposits occur occasionally in the tibia and fibula in leprosy, but other long bones remain uninvolved. In contrast to the situation in syphilis, where extensive bone destruction is always accompanied by reactive new bone formation (Møller-Christensen 1952:106–7), bone resorption is not accompanied by proliferation.

Documentary Evidence

In the absence of extensive skeletal evidence for syphilis, medical historians have turned to ancient and medieval documents in an effort to establish the antiquity of syphilis in the Old World (Baker 1985). Supporters of the pre-Columbian and unitarian hypotheses argue that syphilis was confused with leprosy in the ancient literature and have sought passages purported to delineate the venereal communication of the disease. Columbianists discount such descriptions and point to accounts of a new disease of foreign origin at the close of the 15th century.

BIBLICAL REFERENCES TO "LEPROSY"

The Old Testament (written between the 8th and 2d centuries B.C.) is the most frequently cited text in reference to leprosy. The Hebrew word *tsara'at,* which is translated into Greek as *lepra,* "scaly," denotes ritual uncleanliness and probably refers to a wide range of diseases with dermatological manifestations (Cochrane 1959:viii; Hulse 1975; Møller-Christensen 1967:304–5). Lepromatous leprosy, originally described by the Alexandrian medical school about 300 B.C., is referred to as elephantiasis because of the thickening and corrugation of the skin (Dols 1979:315). As a result of inexact translation, the biblical term "leprosy" could, therefore, refer to syphilis.

Biblical passages suggesting syphilis have been reviewed at length by Willcox (1949; see also Hudson 1961:552–54 and Rosebury 1971:98–104). Moses describes punishment for disobedience as manifesting "emerods," scabs, itches that cannot be healed, madness, and blindness (Deuteronomy 28:27–28). Job (Job 16, 19, 30) suffered from a genital lesion, and boils covered his body; iritis is suspected from his failing sight and mucous patches from his corrupt breath. David's illness (Psalms 38:1–11) is also cited as a case of pre-Columbian syphilis masquerading as "leprosy." David suffered from shooting pains and odoriferous lesions, and his "loins are filled with a loathsome disease." Like Job, he had failing vision and recovered from his illness. David believed his condition to have resulted from sleeping with Bathsheba, who was "unclean" at the time (2 Samuel 2–5).

Leviticus 13 and 22:4 and Numbers 5:2 are among passages discussing the skin lesions of "leprosy" and the restrictions placed upon the "unclean" in great detail (see Brody 1974:108–14 for further explication of biblical references to leprosy). Depigmentation and discoloration characterize the lesions reported. The lengthy description in Leviticus is actually a list used by priests to differentiate among diseases that may or may not result in ritual impurity (Hulse 1975; Sussman 1967:211).

If the foregoing passages are references to venereal syphilis, one would also expect biblical descriptions of congenital syphilis. In Jeremiah 31:29, where "the fathers have eaten sour grapes and the children's teeth are set on edge," the dental condition is suggestive of Hutchinson's teeth, a sign of congenital syphilis (Willcox 1949:32). Willcox also points to Exodus 20:5, where "the iniquity of the fathers" is visited "upon the children to the third and fourth generation." Although syphilis can be inherited only by the second generation, Brown et al. (1970:2) find this passage significant because "syphilis is one of the few known communicable diseases that can be passed from one generation to another."

Miriam's "leprosy" is described in Numbers (12:9–15). A possible macerated syphilitic fetus is suggested by Aaron's statement, "Let her not be as one dead, of whom the flesh is half consumed when he cometh out of his mother's womb." Leviticus (21:16–20) states that "he who hath a flat nose," perhaps indicative of congenital saddle nose, was ostracized. Similarly, in 2 Samuel 12 it is said that the child conceived from the adulterous and unclean union of David and Bathsheba died seven days after birth. If David's subsequent disease was syphilis, the baby may also have been afflicted.

OTHER ANCIENT REFERENCES
SUGGESTIVE OF SYPHILIS

Several Greek and Roman physicians and historians including Hippocrates, Martial, Pliny, and Celsus described genital lesions following sexual activity (Brown et al. 1970:3; Hudson 1961; 1963b:646; Kampmeier 1984:22–23; Rosebury 1971:105–7). During the 1st century A.D., Celsus described hard and soft genital sores, reporting that the latter exuded a malodorous discharge (Hudson 1961:555). Galen (born in A.D. 131) differentiated dry ulcers from moist ulcerating tubercles, analogous to mucous patches (Kampmeier 1984:22). Such lesions were described by both Greeks and Romans as resembling mulberries or figs, which Hudson (1961) and others (see Kampmeier 1984:22) interpret as genital condylomata diagnostic of syphilis. Martial and Pliny (1st century A.D.) refer to mentagra, a term derived from the Latin mentum, "chin," from which mentula, "little chin," also originated. Hudson (1961:554–55; 1963b:646) points out that the latter term was euphemistic for the pubic area and concludes that the lesions and contagious nature of mentagra were venereal. Byzantine physicians of the 3d through 7th centuries documented several types of genital lesions that have been attributed to gonorrhea and syphilis (Kampmeier 1984:23). Finally, Hudson (1961:551), in his thorough etymological treatise, links the term bubas to Greek and Latin terms denoting "serpent." Diaz de Isla employed this term to describe syphilis in 1539, noting that it was previously used in Spain to describe "leprosy" and the Romans' mentagra.

The ancient literatures of India and China have also been cited as containing "unmistakable proofs" that genital lesions were associated with sexual activity (Hyde 1891:117). Kampmeier (1984:22) indicates that the Sanskrit Veda contains several references to genital disease, which some have interpreted as syphilis. Lu and Needham (1967) mention no disease resembling syphilis in ancient China, and Crosby (1969:219) quotes Wong and Wu (1936:218) as saying that no Chinese writer "has ever described syphilis as being mentioned in ancient literature." Wong and Wu, however, assert in the following sentence that these writers "did not know the connection between chancres and syphilides, for the former were mentioned as early as the 7th century A.D." As to whether these chancres are syphilitic, they indicate (p. 219) that "the original texts are too brief to enable us to form any definite conclusion." Clinical descriptions of leprosy in China and India from as early as 600 B.C. are, in contrast, quite clear (Browne 1970:641; Lu and Needham 1967:226, 236–37; Steinbock 1976:192).

MEDIEVAL "LEPROSY"

Medieval texts have also been studied for evidence that syphilis was included with other diseases under the term "leprosy." True leprosy was apparently unknown in the Mediterranean region prior to 300 B.C. Andersen

BAKER AND ARMELAGOS The Origin and Antiquity of Syphilis | 707

(1969:123) has proposed an introduction from India after Alexander the Great's campaign in 327–326 B.C. Celsus, Pliny the Elder, Galen, and Aretaeus were the first to describe the disease, which they called elephantiasis, in the first two centuries A.D. (Dols 1979:315; see also Patrick 1967:245). The generic term *lepra* was not applied to true leprosy until the 8th century A.D. (Steinbock 1976:192–93) in the translation of Arab medical texts into Latin (Richards 1977:9). Thus, a previously distinct and well-defined disease of no religious significance was blended with the biblical concept of impurity and acquired the stigma still attached to the word "leper" (Richards 1977:9–10). As a result, the medieval diagnosis of leprosy may have incorporated several afflictions, including true leprosy and syphilis.

The mode of transmission of medieval leprosy is confused. Bartholomeus Anglicus (ca. 1230–50) wrote that leprosy was caused by "intercourse with a woman after she had been with a leprous man, heredity, and feeding a child with the milk of a leprous nurse" (Rubin 1974:153; see also Gordon 1959:493–94). Theodoric of Cervia (1205–98) provides one of the more detailed descriptions of the disease within the prevailing humoral theory (7 of his 12 common signs of leprosy correspond to those found by modern diagnosticians), but he also insists that those "lying with a woman with whom a leper has lain" will be infected (Brody 1974:34–41). Numerous medieval scholars refer to "venereal leprosy," "hereditary leprosy," and "leper whore" and describe genital lesions (Brody 1974:54–56: Holcomb 1935:297–303; Hudson 1961:548; 1972:150–51; Kampmeier 1984:23–24). Leprosy is neither hereditary nor sexually transmitted. It does show a strong family incidence (4.4–12% of household contacts of lepromatous leprosy patients show signs of the disease within five years [World Health Organization 1980]), but both husband and wife are affected in less than 5% of couples (Richards 1977:xvi).

Leper hospitals were established throughout Europe prior to the Crusades (A.D. 1096–1221) in an effort to separate lepers from society. "Leprosy" reached its peak prevalence in Europe in the 11th through 13th centuries (Rubin 1974:151), coinciding with the Crusades. Hudson (1963b) has outlined the importance of concurrent pilgrimage to the Middle East in disseminating disease, which he contends included treponemal infection disguised as "leprosy." As supporting evidence he cites the use of "Saracen ointment," which contained mercury, by the returning lepers (1961:548; 1963b:648; see also Hackett 1967:163–64). Mercury has no effect on true leprosy but was the mainstay in treating syphilis until the early 20th century (Steinbock 1976:88).

Perhaps the most explicit description of medieval "leprosy" is found in Robert Henryson's poem "The Testament of Cresseid." Written in Scotland prior to 1492, the poem has been variously claimed as a delineation of venereal syphilis (Hudson 1972) and as a sensitive portrayal of an individual afflicted with leprosy (Richards 1977:6–8). The poem, a contemporary version of the myth of the Trojan lovers, Troilus and Cressida, depicts a fallen woman who acquired an "incurable disease" and died "a leper" (Hudson 1972:146). Cresseid's face became "o'erspread with black boils," her "clear voice" became "hoarse," "rough and raucous" (quoted in Richards 1977:6–7). Cresseid's condition resulted from her lustful life. She was confined to a leper house to prevent the spread of her infection to others. Her life as a leper is detailed, including the last will and testament required for entrance into the leper hospital, her wandering with cup and clapper, and her diet of "mouldy bread, perry, and cider sour" (quoted in Richards 1977:6–8). Henryson called Cresseid's disease leprosy, but Hudson (1972:149) suggests that because it is associated with immorality and sex it is venereal syphilis. Richards (1977:6) finds Henryson so compassionate in his portrayal of the "leper" that he must have had firsthand knowledge of leprosy and "of lives broken by it."

THE EPIDEMIC OF 1500

By 1500, a "new" disease, which we know as syphilis, was being described in Europe (see Crosby 1969, Dennie 1962, Holcomb 1934, Williams, Rice, and Renato Lacayo 1927). As syphilis became widely recognized and described, "leprosy" became less common. Historical events unrelated to the return of Columbus may explain this trend. For example, the invention of the printing press in the mid-15th century led to rapid diffusion of information. By 1566, 58 books had been published on the subject of syphilis. Kampmeier (1984:24) argues that the proliferation of such publications led to the widespread recognition of the disease at this time, making it appear as if it were a new disease of epidemic proportions. This dissemination of knowledge was accompanied by historical events that caused the displacement of people throughout Europe.

Papal proclamations in 1490 and 1505 abolished all leper houses (Holcomb 1935:282), allowing the dispersal of thousands with "leprosy." Holcomb notes (p. 278) that Matthew Paris, an English monk who died in 1259, records "in somewhat ambiguous terms" the existence of 19,000 leper houses in Europe. While this figure may be exaggerated, Gordon (1959:493) indicates that "France and Germany alone had nearly 10,000 leprosaria" in 1400, and Richards (1977:11) notes approximately 200 leper hospitals "in their thirteenth- and fourteenth-century heyday" in Britain. It should be cautioned, however, that most leper hospitals were ecclesiastical foundations that accommodated only about ten lepers and at least as many chaplains and sisters (Richards 1977:11). Richards (see also Creighton 1965 [1894]:86–100) concludes that the number of hospitals is not a reliable estimate of the number of lepers because of the propensity of the church to establish the institutions to garner perpetual charity. Whatever the motive for establishing the hospitals, they did house thousands throughout Europe. If the diseases were confused, it is possible that some of the inhabitants were syphilitic and therefore that when the hospitals were closed syphilis was dispersed.

Hudson (1964; 1968:11) claims that treponemal infection existed in venereal and nonvenereal forms in pre-Columbian Spain and Portugal because of the Moorish occupation and the importation of slaves from sub-Saharan Africa. When an estimated 160,000 to 400,000 Jews were expelled from Spain in 1492, they allegedly carried syphilis throughout Europe (Holcomb 1935:284). The expulsion of Jews and lepers coincided with the discovery of America and the apparent epidemic of syphilis.

In late 1494, Charles VIII of France conducted a campaign against Naples. The city fell in February of 1495 as a plague broke out among the mercenary troops. They subsequently disbanded, carrying their disease throughout Europe (Brown et al. 1970:5; Williams, Rice, and Renato Lacayo 1927:683). It is generally agreed that this disease was syphilis; the controversy concerns the time of arrival of Spanish troops purported to have contracted the disease from Columbian contacts and the issue of several edicts regarding the disease elsewhere in Europe. Holcomb (1934:419; see also Hudson 1968:5–6; 1972:152) claims that Charles's army left Naples on May 20, 1495, and the Spaniards did not arrive until June. Although Charles did not reach France until October 27, 1495, an edict had been issued by the Diet of Worms more than two months earlier (August 7, 1495), indicating that syphilis was already widespread in Germany (Gordon 1959:536; Holcomb 1935:289, 427; see also Harrison 1959:4). While this would seem to vindicate Charles VIII, Waugh (1982:92) has pointed to problems in dating events of the time due to the variety of calendars in use (e.g., Gregorian vs. French).

Further confusion in the dates of early edicts on syphilis has resulted from modern errors. Holcomb (1935:293) laments the penchant of some writers (Columbianists) for accepting ideas "without first assuring themselves of the correctness of the historical data that they introduce." Reliance upon Sudhoff's archival work, however, has led to wide acceptance of the 1495 date of the aforementioned edict of the Diet of Worms. Sudhoff later amended the date to August 8, 1496, and subsequent research by Haustein revealed that the text was actually drafted by the Diet of Lindau on January 12, 1497 (cited in Temkin 1966:32–33). Thus, it is possible that the passage regarding syphilis was a response to its dissemination by soldiers returning from Italy.

Holcomb's pre-Columbian thesis hinges largely upon an edict issued in Paris that bars those with grosse verole (syphilis) from the city. Holcomb (1934:416, 421; 1935:293) dates this edict to March 25, 1493, or ten days after Columbus returned to Spain from his first voyage. This would render it impossible for the disease to have been imported from America. In an attempt to verify this date, Harrison (1959:4–6) followed a series of errors in later compilations of ancient French laws (one of which was cited by Holcomb) and discovered that the ordinance with the text in question was actually issued on June 25, 1498 (verified by Haustein's research, cited

in Temkin 1966:33). A thorough search of the French archives revealed that the earliest Parisian reference to the disease was contained in an edict promulgated by the Paris parliament on March 6, 1497 (Harrison 1959:4–6; see also Creighton 1965:[1894]:436), nearly four years after Columbus's crew returned from the first voyage. Holcomb (1934:428) misdates this edict as well, stating that it was issued on March 16, 1496.

Several edicts ostracizing people infected with syphilis were issued elsewhere in Europe beginning in 1496. In that year, 12 such ordinances were passed at Nuremberg, and syphilitics were barred from the baths of Zurich and other municipalities throughout Switzerland and Germany (Holcomb 1934:428; Kampmeier 1984:24–25). Ten persons with "the Neapolitan disease" were expelled from Besançon, France, in April of 1496, while an edict at Lyon, dated August 12, 1497, required those with the disease to report within ten days or be apprehended (Harrison 1959:4, 6). Early reference to syphilis in Britain is from an ordinance of Aberdeen dated April 21, 1497, in which it is stated that "the infirmity came out of France" (Creighton 1965 [1894]:417). A proclamation issued in Edinburgh by James IV on September 22, 1497, requires those with "Grandgor" (syphilis) to go to the island of Inch Keith in the Firth of Forth, "there to remain until God provide for their health" (Creighton 1965 [1894]:417–18). Hospitals for the syphilitic such as St. Jobsgasthuis, founded in Utrecht in 1504 (Fuldauer, Bracht, and Perizonius 1984), were established throughout Europe by the beginning of the 16th century.

It would appear from the dates of European edicts that a new disease swept the continent within three or four years of the return of the first Columbian voyagers. The concurrence of these events has been challenged, however, by those who point out that edicts after 1493 closely resemble those previously issued to isolate lepers. For example, a Parisian edict of 1488 is directed against les lepreux, while those following the papal proclamation of 1490 refer to syphilis (Creighton 1965 [1894]:73; Holcomb 1934:416: 1935:282). Creighton questions the sudden reappearance of leprosy in the late 15th century, especially since the Paris edict is so close in date to those concerning syphilis. Thus, one is left to wonder whether these ordinances were issued as a consequence of the importation of syphilis or if the discovery of America was merely coincidental with the recognition and renaming of the disease as it was differentiated from "leprosy."

LATE 15TH- AND EARLY 16TH-CENTURY TREATISES ON SYPHILIS

Treatises on syphilis proliferated in the late 1490s and early 1500s (for reviews see, e.g., Crosby 1969, Dennie 1962, Holcomb 1934, Hudson 1961). Williams, Rice, and Renato Lacayo (1927) provide translations of large portions of early Spanish works, the most important of which is Ruy Diaz de Isla's "Treatise on the Serpentine

Malady, Which in Spain is Commonly Called Bubas, which was drawn up in the Hospital of All Saints in Lisbon," first printed in ⊧539. In it, he claims that the serpentine disease (syphilis) appeared in Barcelona in 1493, originated on the island of Española (Haiti), and was brought to Europe by Columbus's crew (p. 693). He goes on to say that in the following year Charles VIII entered Italy with "many Spaniards infected with this disease." Not knowing what it was, "the French called it the disease of Naples," and the Italians, "as they had never had acquaintance with a like disease, called it the French disease." This portion of Diaz de Isla's account is confirmed by Gonzalo Fernández Oviedo y Valdés (1478–1557): "Many times in Italy I did laugh, hearing the Italians say the French disease and the French calling it the disease of Naples; and in truth both would have hit on the right name if they had called it the disease from the Indies." Oviedo also verifies that among Charles VIII's army were Spaniards "touched with this disease," but he indicates that they did not join the French until 1496 (see Williams et al. 1927:687–89 and Crosby 1969:222). Much has been made of this discrepancy in dates (e.g., Holcomb [1935:292] uses it to dismiss Oviedo's entire account); Waugh's (1982:92) caution regarding the difficulty in dating such events must be borne in mind.

Critics of the 16th-century treatises, such as Holcomb (1934, 1935), point out that no mention is made of an American origin of syphilis for more than 30 years after the discovery of the New World. Earlier texts attribute the disease to divine wrath visited upon a sinful populace, astrologic convergences, and the weather; Oviedo's work is among the first to mention an American origin. His "Summaria of the Natural History of the Indies" was published in 1526 and is purported to have been written from memory. His larger work, "General and Natural History of the Indies," was first printed in 1535 (Holcomb 1934:406–7; Williams et al. 1927:687). In it he says that, while he is writing from memory, he is referring to "notes which were written at the time when the things described in them happened." Holcomb (1934:407) points out that taking such notes is not the usual activity of a teenager (Oviedo was only 15 when Columbus returned from his first voyage). Crosby (1969:222) maintains that Oviedo was quite friendly with the explorer's sons and cites a passage in which Oviedo asked several of his friends sailing with Columbus in 1493 (second voyage) to provide him with detailed reports (his affiliation with several crew members is also recorded in the translation by Williams et al. 1927:688).

The original manuscript of Diaz de Isla's account is dedicated to King Manuel of Portugal, who died in 1521 (Williams et al. 1927:695). In a paragraph omitted from the printed versions, he writes of an island "discovered and found by the Admiral Dom Cristoual Colon at present holding intercourse and communication with the Indies" (Williams et al. 1927:695). Since Columbus's last voyage culminated in his death in the New World in 1506, it seems that the manuscript must have been written prior to that event. Furthermore, Diaz de Isla states that "in the year 1504 there were given me in writing all the remedies that the Indians used for this disease," indicating that his belief in its American origin dated to within 11 years of its alleged importation. Thus, the manuscript, usually ascribed to the period 1510–20, would appear more likely to have been written in 1505 or 1506. Holcomb (1934:412–13), however, asserts that Diaz de Isla "frequently states he had 40 years' experience in the treatment of the disease" and therefore acceptance of such dates would place his treatment well before the discovery of America. Holcomb's observation is not apparent in the translation provided by Williams et al. (1927:694), in which Diaz de Isla writes only that he has had "long experience." It seems that a decade or more would qualify as such.

Several 16th-century tracts written by European scholars in the New World document the lifeways, languages, and mythologies of various native groups and refer to a disease much like syphilis among them. These documents have been employed to support the Columbian hypothesis in publications of the past century (e.g., Brühl 1890, Crosby 1969, Williams et al. 1927), while others (e.g., Holcomb 1934:417–18) attribute such references to the introduction of the disease by Europeans. The biography of Christopher Columbus, by his son Ferdinand, includes a 1495 manuscript by Fray Roman Pane recording an Arawak myth in which the hero, Guagagiona, "saw a woman . . . from whom he had great pleasure, and immediately he sought many lotions to cleanse himself, on account of being plagued with the disease that we call French," and afterwards went to a secluded place "where he recovered from his ulcers" (Williams et al. 1927:687; see also Brühl 1890:276 and Crosby 1969:221–22). Crosby, reminding the reader that folklore is very slow to change, finds it unlikely that the Arawaks would have altered their legend to give the hero a new disease, thus implying that the malady was extant among the natives long before the Europeans arrived. This is corroborated by Bartolomé de las Casas, who questioned the natives as to the origin of the disease and was told they had had it from time immemorial (Crosby 1969:222; Williams et al. 1927:690). Further examples of "syphilis" in native mythology, as well as differential burial treatment of those afflicted, were documented by Bernardino de Sahagún, who lived in Mexico from 1529 to 1590 (Brühl 1890:275–76; Williams et al. 1927:690–91).

Linguistic evidence compiled by Montejo y Robledo from 16th- and 17th-century dictionaries of native Mexican and Central and South American languages reveals indigenous terms for *bubas* and related European expressions (Williams et al. 1927:685–86). Brühl (1890:278–80) counters the view that these terms were invented after the arrival of Europeans by reviewing the ways in which names were assigned to previously unknown things—adopting the European word with little or no change or deriving the name from a conspicuous feature of the object. While the terms for previously unknown diseases described a prominent symptom, the words synonymous with European appellations for syphilis were "formed at the development of the respective languages" and, in many cases, associated with chieftains and gods (Brühl 1890:279).

Skeletal Evidence

The preceding review of ancient and medieval documentary sources reveals many ambiguities in disease description and the dating of events. The ensuing interpretations of these passages remain controversial. Skeletal evidence of pre-Columbian syphilis is subject to similar disagreement. As Williams (1932:780) states, "one must have proof that a bone is ancient and that it is syphilitic. It is owing to a difference of opinion as to what constitutes proof that the controversy continues." Unfortunately, many of the remains thought to be syphilitic (primarily those recovered prior to Williams's review) lack archaeological provenience and cannot, therefore, be assumed pre-Columbian. Further difficulties arise in interpreting many late 19th- and early 20th-century descriptions of syphilitic specimens. These reports often present descriptions of an isolated skeletal element. Since skeletal lesions resulting from yaws, endemic syphilis, and venereal syphilis are identical, speculation regarding the mode of transmission of the treponeme in a single individual is impossible (i.e., an isolated case of treponematosis cannot be assumed to have resulted from venereal transmission). Reliable conclusions regarding the prehistoric distribution of treponemal disease may, however, be drawn from skeletal evidence. The pattern of treponemal infection discerned in entire skeletal series, viewed in conjunction with social and climatological factors, may permit epidemiological inferences.

OLD WORLD REMAINS

Although numerous cases of alleged pre-Columbian Old World syphilis have been described in the literature of the past century, few have withstood reexamination. Once Parrot (1879) had aroused European interest in the paleopathological identification of syphilis, nearly every French anthropologist discovered syphilitic specimens (Sigerist 1951:56). Parrot, however, confused the manifestations of congenital syphilis and rickets, delineating a "rachitic period" of congenital syphilis for which "swelling . . . of the articular ends of the bones" and "cranial osteophytes" resulting in "the form of a cross" on the skull vault were diagnostic (1879:697–98). Thus he reported syphilis in prehistoric Ecuador, Peru, and France solely on the basis of cranial vaults exhibiting circumscribed areas of bone deposition (i.e., cranial bossing) that were more likely due to rickets, iron deficiency anemia, or congenital anemia (Steinbock 1976:101). Reliance on Parrot's diagnostic criteria underlies Wright's (1971) contention that syphilis is evident in Neanderthal remains in the form of cranial bossing, thinning and pit-

ting of the occipital and parietals, and "the relative depression of the bridge of the nose" in both children and adults. Worn taurodont molars are suggested to resemble the mulberry molars of congenital syphilis. Bowing of the femur is attributed to syphilitic osteitis, also hypothesized to "account for Neanderthal long bones being so short and stout." Many of the lesions Wright describes are diagnostic of rickets, while the general skeletal variations he attributes to syphilis are the consequence of genetic and biomechanical differences between Neanderthal and modern populations.

The alleged skeletal evidence of pre-Columbian syphilis was thoroughly reviewed by Williams in 1932. Prior to investigating archaeological specimens, he examined the bones of over 500 modern individuals known to be syphilitic in order to establish diagnostic criteria. Various specimens described in the early literature as syphilitic had apparently been lost by the time of his research, and others were too incomplete for diagnosis to be attempted. In many of the remaining cases, the supposedly syphilitic lesions could be attributed to other causes. For example, several Egyptian cases had actually suffered postmortem damage by rodents or insects (pp. 802–3), and the lesions on Parrot's (1879:698) Peruvian crania were attributable to porotic hyperostosis (Williams 1929:852; 1932:971). Williams considered five cases of reputed Old World syphilis "suspicious." In the case of a tibia and fibula from Japanese shell middens, said to be more than 2,500 years old, he thought trauma or healed osteomyelitis the cause of the lesions described (p. 802) and judged the antiquity of the remains questionable in any event (p. 974). For a Nubian femur and tibia dated to 1000 B.C., insofar as his examination of the published illustrations permitted, he found the diagnosis of syphilis plausible, although "other causes of periostitis would be equally probable" (pp. 803, 975). For the remaining "suspicious" instances, all from France—a tibia from Solutré, a humerus and ulna from the Marne Valley, and an ulna, femur, and femur fragment from the museum at Saint-Germain (pp. 805–9, 975)—he found the diagnosis of syphilis equivocal. The few possible instances of pre-Columbian syphilis consist of isolated long bones with inadequate archaeological provenience (Sigerist 1951:56; Williams 1932:974). Jeanselme, Pales, and others concur that the Old World evidence presented prior to 1930 is inconclusive or negative (Williams 1932:975–76; see also Sigerist 1951:56 and Steinbock 1976:97).

Possible skeletal evidence accumulated since 1930 is sparse. Steinbock (1976:97) regards Siberian material consisting of several tibiae, a radius, and an ulna dated 1000–800 B.C. as the earliest indication of possible Old World syphilis. In addition, two tibiae dated 500–200 B.C. and three crania dated A.D. 100–700 are reported to show syphilitic lesions (cf. Hackett 1976:18, who indicates that the dates may be unacceptable). Evidence of pre-Columbian syphilis reported since 1930 in Europe is tantalizing but inconclusive. The skull of an adult female from Spitalfields Market in London presents the diagnostic stellate scars of caries sicca (Brothwell

1961:324–25; Morant and Hoadley 1931:222, pl. 3; Steinbock 1976:97). Historical records indicate that the site was part of the cemetery at the church of St. Mary Spittle, used A.D. 1197–1537 (Morant and Hoadley 1931:202). Brothwell (1961:324–25) finds it a "remarkable coincidence" that the woman succumbed to syphilis within 35 years of its supposed appearance in London, but the possibility cannot be dismissed. Similarly, excavations at the Helgeandsholmen cemetery in Stockholm, used from A.D. 1300 to 1531, have yielded syphilitic remains (Madrid 1986).

Hudson (1961:547–48) contends that "syphilitic skulls and other bones have been found in 'leper cemeteries' and doubtless many a European 'leper' lost his nose and his voice, or was covered with purulent crusts, as a result of treponemal infection." If he is correct, then excavations of cemeteries associated with medieval leprosaria should reveal skeletons of syphilitics in addition to lepers (his citations are to publications of 1868 and 1891, prior to the establishment of diagnostic criteria for syphilis and leprosy). Excavations at Danish leper hospitals and medieval churchyards and extensive examination of European skeletal collections reveal no evidence of pre-Columbian treponemal disease (e.g., Møller-Christensen 1952, 1967; Møller-Christensen and Faber 1952; Weiss and Møller-Christensen 1971).

Yaws and/or endemic syphilis have occasionally been reported in skeletal material from the Old World. An isolated skull from Iraq, dated prior to A.D. 500, exhibits a large crater-like depression on the mid-frontal and a smaller, slightly depressed area on the right side of the frontal bone that have been attributed to treponematosis (Guthe and Willcox 1954:fig. 2; Steinbock 1976:141). An elliptical area of porosity on the occipital of an eight-year-old child (INM 196) from the Chalcolithic site of Inamgaon in western India (dated 1000–700 B.C.) is interpreted as evidence of yaws (Lukacs and Walimbe 1984:123–24, fig. 7). This attribution is tenuous, however, since there is no other skeletal involvement and treponemal lesions are infrequent on the occipital.

Australia and the Pacific islands have yielded many examples of treponematosis in skeletal remains. Hackett (1976:109, 114) found treponemal changes in 1% of the 4,500 Australian Aboriginal crania he examined and argues that treponemal infection has probably existed in Australia "for some thousands of years." Unfortunately, no information regarding the antiquity of these remains is furnished, and it is uncertain if they predate European contact (see Steinbock 1976:141, 158). Two subadults from Tinian, in the Mariana Islands, display treponemal lesions thought to result from yaws (Stewart and Spoehr 1967(1952)). Pathological changes consist of a crater-like depression surrounded by an irregular zone of porosity on the frontal bone of one individual and similar lesions on the parietals. Parts of a femur, humerus, and radius from the same individual exhibit periostitis with cavitation. The incomplete tibia from the second subadult shows prominent thickening of the cortex along the anterior aspect (saber shin) accompanied by pitting and

cavitation (Stewart and Spoehr 1967(1952):311–17; see also Steinbock 1976:153, 158). The site is radiocarbon-dated to A.D. 854 ± 145, thus predating European contact by a considerable margin (Stewart and Spoehr 1967(1952):311). Yaws has also been described in a precontact skeletal series from Tonga (Steinbock 1976:159).

NEW WORLD REMAINS

Interest in prehistoric skeletal evidence of syphilis developed in America at about the same time as in Europe. The earliest discussion is usually attributed to Jones (1876), although Williams (1932:931) cites an 1875 account, by R. J. Farquharson, of syphilitic lesions in skeletal remains from mounds near Davenport, Iowa. Jones's (1876:49, 65–67, 71–72, 85) detailed descriptions of skeletal lesions in ancient inhabitants of Tennessee and Kentucky support his conclusion that syphilis (i.e., a treponemal infection) was the cause of pathology observed in several individuals. Jones remarks (p. 66) that the tibiae are, in many cases, "thoroughly diseased, enlarged, and thickened, with the medullary cavity completely obliterated by the effects of inflammatory action, and with the surface eroded in many places." Skeletal involvement was not confined to the tibial shafts but included the cranium, clavicle, sternum, and other long bones. Significantly, Jones notes the symmetrical distribution of the skeletal lesions. The crania are described (p. 66) as exhibiting lesions "in which a network of periosteal deposit had been formed, and which had been perforated by ulcers, subsequently forming and assuming the annular type." Williams (1932:966) examined some of the skulls in the Jones collection and verified the presence of stellate scars in one specimen that he also attributed to syphilis. Soon after Jones's disclosure, claims of pre-Columbian syphilis in the Americas proliferated (e.g., Gann 1901, Lamb 1898, Langdon 1881, Orton 1905, Parrot 1879), although much of the purported evidence was deemed inconclusive by others (e.g., Hyde 1891; Putnam 1878:305; Whitney 1883). As with the European material, difficulty in differentiating disease processes, incomplete skeletons, and absence of archaeological context precluded reliable diagnoses in most cases. Even the most conservative, however, described skeletal lesions in ancient American remains that they admitted might have been due to syphilis (e.g., Hyde 1891:128; Whitney 1883:366). Williams (1932:976–77) considered reported cases of syphilis from several areas in North and South America "as nearly free from suspicion as any that can be found."

In the Southeastern United States, reported evidence of pre-Columbian treponematosis abounds. Following Jones's (1876) report, Lamb (1898) described syphilitic lesions in a skeleton excavated by Clarence B. Moore at Lighthouse Mound, in northeastern Florida. Moore (quoted in Bullen 1972:157) found the percentage of pathological specimens and degree of skeletal involvement in the 74 individuals recovered remarkable and indicated that "cranial nodes" were apparent. The skeleton examined by Lamb (1898:63–64) was not accompanied by the skull but exhibited "lesions of osteoperiostitis, both hyperostotic and ulcerative," on the shafts of the long bones. Williams (1932:968) also examined this individual and agreed that the lesions "were in all probability syphilitic."

Bullen's (1972) survey of prehistoric skeletal material from Florida reveals considerable evidence suggestive of treponematosis. Enlarged long bones exhibiting encroachment upon the medullary cavity have been recovered from the Tick Island Archaic site, radiocarbon-dated to 3300 B.C. (p. 166). Burial 352 from Palmer Mound (FSM 97527) presents the most convincing case of pre-Columbian treponemal infection in Florida (pp. 138–50). The site belongs to the Weeden Island period and dates to A.D. 850. The nearlry complete skeleton of an adult female displays cranial caries sicca (see also Hackett 1976:110) and lesions on several long bones. The right humerus shows focal areas of destruction surrounded by diffuse osteitis and dense reparative bone, the radii and left fibula are slightly thickened with some periosteal new bone formation, and the left tibia is expanded and irregular. A radiograph of the left tibia reveals multiple lytic areas surrounded by sclerotic bone that Hackett (1976:110) has identified as superficial cavitation of nodes—diagnostic of syphilis. Additional remains from Palmer and several other prehistoric sites (mostly Weeden Island, A.D. 850–1350) exhibit treponemal lesions (Brothwell and Burleigh 1975:394; Bullen 1972:150–62; Iscan and Miller-Shaivitz 1985), indicating that the Palmer burial is by no means an isolated case.

Treponematosis has also been identified in a prehistoric skeletal series from Georgia. The remains of 265 individuals from Irene Mound (A.D. 1200–1450), near Savannah, reveal widespread inflammatory response with marked diaphyseal expansion in the lower legs and arms (Powell 1988c). Few cranial and naso-palatine lesions are noted, but in some cases focal lytic lesions of the skull vault are apparent. The demographic and anatomical patterning of skeletal lesions suggests endemicity rather than venereal transmission.

Syphilis is proposed as the cause of bone pathology in several specimens from northern Alabama, including a cranium in which the palate has been almost completely eroded and only the remodeled edges remain (Rabkin 1942:220–21, fig. 6). No specific provenience is provided for the syphilitic remains, but the sample includes material from as late as A.D. 1400–1600 (p. 218). Prehistoric pathological remains suggestive of syphilis at Moundville, Alabama, were first noted by Moore (1907:339–40). One skull that has received considerable attention in the literature (e.g., Bullen 1972:163–64; Hackett 1976:109–10; Haltom and Shands 1938; Williams 1936:785–86) displays extensive erosion and new bone formation on the frontal, resulting in the stellate scars characteristic of caries sicca. Hackett (1976:110) indicates that although the changes in this skull are not typical caries sicca, "in which the nodules are smaller and of more regular size," the diagnosis of treponematosis is "fully supported by the presence of similar changes in [crania found in] European medical museums

and in Australian anthropological collections." Two tibiae from another individual present thickening due to osteoperiostitis, probably a result of treponemal infection (Williams 1936:786).

In an examination of over 500 individuals at Moundville, Powell (1988a) observed a "high prevalence of subperiosteal apposition on lower limb long bone shafts and moderate prevalence of cranial stellate lesions." Periostitis of major long bones is reported in 207 cases, of which 72% appear minor in extent and well-healed at death (Powell 1988b). The absence of the dental stigmata associated with congenital syphilis and the frequency of healed tibial lesions have led Powell (1988a,b) to attribute the observed pathology to a nonvenereal treponemal syndrome (yaws or endemic syphilis).

A possible case of treponematosis from the Late Woodland Hardin site in the North Carolina piedmont has been described by Reichs (1987). The skeleton exhibits destructive and proliferative changes resulting in node formation, expansion and cortical thickening of long bone shafts, medullary encroachment, and pathological fracture, with both cranial and postcranial involvement. Although the lesions are suggestive of treponematosis, Reichs recognizes that the overall pattern of pathology in this individual may be due to the synergistic effects of multiple diseases.

An apparent case of congenital syphilis in a six-to-seven-year-old child (U.S. National Museum of Natural History, Smithsonian Institution collection [hereafter NMNH], No. 379177) from Virginia dates prior to A.D. 1400 (Ortner and Putschar 1985:207–10). Abnormal reactive bone is evident in a frontal lesion, and the surface of the nasal aperture displays thickened, porous, periosteal bone. The extant deciduous incisors have hypoplastic defects so severe that, in three, the superior portion of the crown had broken off before death. The deciduous and first permanent molars are unaffected, as is an observable unerupted permanent incisor. Postcranial skeletal involvement is extensive. The shafts of both tibiae are thickened, with periosteal expansion occurring primarily on the anterior aspect. The other long bones also exhibit periosteal apposition and diaphyseal expansion, although to a lesser degree. A similar process is apparent in several metacarpals and metatarsals. Dactylitis is more common in yaws than in syphilis (Steinbock 1976:143); however, a congenital disease is indicated by the development of hypoplastic dental defects at about the seventh fetal month (Ortner and Putschar 1985:210). Thus, a pattern in which the bones with minimal overlying tissue are most severely affected, as is commonly observed in treponematosis, accompanied by congenital dental defects suggestive of Hutchinson's teeth is strong evidence of congenital syphilis. Although such dental stigmata are not pathognomonic of congenital syphilis, they are associated with characteristic bone lesions in about 50% of all cases, and the diagnosis in such instances is "very reliable" (Steinbock 1976:106).

The skeleton of a 25–35-year-old male (NMNH 385788) from a site radiocarbon-dated to A.D. 925 provides additional evidence of treponematosis in prehistoric Virginia (Ortner 1986). Remains from tidewater and piedmont sites in Delaware, Maryland, and Virginia that exhibit inflammatory lesions on the frontal and associated long bones are in some cases suggestive of syphilis (Stewart and Quade 1969). Hackett (1976:110) indicates that the skull from Accokeek, Maryland (NMNH 378196 [Stewart and Quade 1969:pl. 1-C]), exhibits serpiginous cavitation (diagnostic of treponematosis). Although the piedmont sites are late prehistoric, the tidewater sites discussed by Stewart and Quade (1969:92–93), including Accokeek, date from A.D. 1200–1600; it is therefore uncertain if the remains are pre-Columbian.

A possible case of pre-Columbian treponematosis from the Veddar site (Cnj 43-2, also known as the Palatine Bridge site) in the Mohawk Valley of New York is the only evidence reported in northeastern North America (Elting and Starna 1984). The remains in question are thought to date to the Early Woodland component of the site (500 B.C.) and are undoubtedly pre-Columbian. The tibiae and fibulae of one individual exhibit diffuse periosteal inflammation and new bone formation with narrowing of the medullary canals. Coarse striations and nodes with superficial cavitation are described, and the latter is noted to be one of Hackett's (1976) diagnostic criteria. The changes evident from the photographs (Elting and Starna 1984:270–71, figs. 2 and 3) may more closely correspond to Hackett's (1976:82–83) coarsely striated and pitted expansions, only tentatively considered diagnostic. The absence of sequestrum and cloaca formation, however, rules out osteomyelitis, and the changes apparent in the medullary canals indicate that "a diagnosis of treponematosis is reasonably secure" (Elting and Starna 1984:272).

Syphilis was reported in remains from the Ohio Valley as early as 1881 (Landgon 1881:254–56). William C. Mills's excavations at several Ohio sites in the early 1900s revealed a large number of burials, many of which were pathological. For example, of 127 individuals from the Baum site (A.D. 950–1250), 21 were diseased, and at least 12 were deemed syphilitic by Orton (Mills 1906:126–35; Orton 1905). Williams (1932:954–62) examined much of the prehistoric skeletal material from the Ohio State Museum and found long bones with possible syphilitic lesions in 15 individuals (at least one of which had been previously described by Means [1925]). In 9 cases, three different roentgenologists agreed that the proliferative bone changes resulted from syphilis. Six tibiae from 4 different individuals are depicted and described in detail. In general, they display thickening of the anterior aspect, with a slightly nodular surface perforated by small openings. Where both tibiae are presented, the involvement is bilateral. Hackett (1976:109) indicates that these specimens do not exhibit diagnostic criteria of treponematosis. Williams (1932:955), however, states that the bones he described were "only a portion of the ancient diseased, probably syphilitic, bones that have been disclosed by the investigations of the Ohio State Museum."

Nine individuals from May's Lick, Kentucky, radiocarbon-dated to A.D. 1325 (580 ± 108 B.P.), show cranial vault changes suggestive of treponematosis (Brothwell and Burleigh 1975:394). At least two skeletons from Indian Knoll, Kentucky (radiocarbon-dated ca. 3350 B.C.), exhibit such lesions (Brothwell and Burleigh 1975:393; Steinbock 1976:96), thus extending the evidence in the Ohio Valley region to the Archaic period. Cassidy (1980:136–38; 1984:325, 330–32) has identified a "syndrome of disseminated periosteal reactions," distinct from localized inflammatory lesions, in skeletal series from Indian Knoll and the late Fort Ancient–period Hardin Village (ca. A.D. 1525–1675). This syndrome is characterized by thickening of the long bones, particularly those of the legs; development of "stripes of smooth billowed material or patches of rough porous material on the surfaces; and some diminution of the medullary canals in severe cases" (Cassidy 1980:136–37). Such lesions are indicative of a nonvenereal treponematosis that affected 2.4% of the Indian Knoll population and 31.4% of the Hardin Village series, where eight individuals display severe manifestations (Cassidy 1984:325, 330). The increase in incidence of this syndrome in the post-Columbian group is postulated to be a result of increased population size and sedentism (Cassidy 1980:137).

A considerable amount of purported treponematosis has been discovered in Woodland and Mississippian remains in Illinois. The material is from the lower Illinois River valley, in the west-central portion of the state. A high incidence of cranial lesions (attributed to various causes) in a skeletal series from the Jersey County Bluff mounds (A.D. 400–1400) is noted by Stewart and Quade (1969:95–96). Of 122 relatively complete skeletons, 4 (3.3%) exhibit both frontal and long bone lesions. Hackett (1976:110) indicates that one skull (NMNH 380044 [Stewart and Quade 1969:pl. 1-A]) from this series exhibits serpiginous cavitation and another (NMNH 379875 [Stewart and Quade 1969:pl. 2-C]) "a rather atypical caries sicca." The cranium and left tibia of an individual from the Middle Woodland (ca. 100 B.C.–A.D. 400) component of the Carter Mound Group (Burial 7, Mound 1) in adjacent Greene County illustrates the pathology usually reported in the literature as "syphilis" (Buikstra 1979:233). A 40-year-old Middle Woodland male from the Klunk site (C40, Burial 21) in Calhoun County also exhibits cranial and long bone lesions suggestive of treponematosis (Morse 1978:136–37, pl. 15 A–C).

Additional cases have been reported somewhat farther up the Illinois River in Schuyler and Fulton Counties. The skeleton of a 30–40-year-old male from the Rose Mound Group (Middle Mississippian, A.D. 1200–1400) in Schuyler County displays cranial and postcranial pathology suggestive of treponematosis (Morse 1967:48–52; 1978:53–55, 166–69, pls. 30 A and B, 31 A–E). The naso-palatine destruction is extensive, including the alveolar area, intranasal structures, and nasal bones. The maxillary incisors have been lost antemortem. Some healing is evident along the perimeter of the nasal cavity. There is slight involvement of the frontal bone. The anterior portions of both tibiae show periostitis and osteitis with cavitation, as do the distal portions of the humeri, the upper third of the right ulna, and the left

714 | CURRENT ANTHROPOLOGY Volume 29, Number 5, December 1988

clavicle. Hackett (1976:97) categorizes the long bone lesions as nodes/expansions with superficial cavitation and therefore diagnostic of treponematosis. A case described by Morse (1967:52–58; 1978:55–57, 166–69, pls. 30 C–E, 31 W–Z) in Fulton County consists of the fairly complete skeleton (T-6) of a 35-year-old male. The remains are from the Thompson site and date to the Early Mississippian period, approximately A.D. 1000. The anterior portion of the frontal displays subperiosteal thickening with cavitation of the outer table surrounded by slight erosion. Postcranial lesions are evident on the right tibia, radius, ulna, and humerus, both femora, and the right clavicle. Generally, they exhibit cortical thickening and sclerosis, with some focal destruction (pitting and sinus formation) and encroachment on the medullary cavity. Lesions on the sacrum and greater trochanter of the right femur are of a different nature and are attributed to bed sores. The skeleton of a Middle Woodland resident of Fulton County (originally described by Denninger) exhibits osteoperiostitis that Williams (1936:787) diagnoses as syphilis. Both tibiae and fibulae present bone proliferation of periosteal origin with some narrowing of the medullary cavity. Hackett (1976:97) notes the similarity of the "pronounced periostitis" on the anterior surfaces of the femora, tibiae, and fibulae in a Late Archaic Red Ocher burial (1500–1000 B.C.) from Fulton County to that in yaws patients in Uganda and in Australian Aboriginal bones. The skeleton of this 22-year-old female from the Morse site (F772, Burial 12) is described and illustrated by Morse (1978:17, 132–33, pl. 13 A and B). According to Hackett (1976:97), the long bones depicted exemplify the diagnostic nodes/expansions with superficial cavitation.

In an epidemiological study of Illinois Woodland populations, Cook (1976, 1984) observes a pattern of osteitis and periostitis suggestive of treponematosis. In the Late Archaic Klunk skeletal series, 31 of 123 individuals (25%) exhibit treponemal lesions, whereas Middle and Late Woodland populations show an overall prevalence of approximately 50% (Cook 1984:259). The Mississippian Schild site reveals a prevalence similar to that of the Woodland groups. The prevalence of the treponemal disease and absence of indicators of congenital infection, while atypical of venereal syphilis, are characteristic of nonvenereal treponematosis (Cook 1976, 1984). Thus, yaws or endemic syphilis seems to have existed in Illinois for nearly 3,000 years.

In Arkansas, the incomplete skeleton of an adult female (NMNH 258778) discovered during Moore's excavations on the St. Francis, White, and Black Rivers in the early part of the century includes several pathological bones (Ortner and Putschar 1985:210–14, figs. 329–32). The external table of the skull vault exhibits an "irregular lumpy appearance" with "typical gummatous lesions characterized by a mixture of bone formation and destruction" (Ortner and Putschar 1985:212). There is some involvement of the inner table. The proximal metaphysis of the left ulna and the proximal shaft of the left femur show expansion of the cortex. The entire shaft of the right femur and the left proximal tibia exhibit cortical enlargement with porosity. The anterior surfaces consist of raised plaques and spicules. The remains are thought to be pre-Columbian.

Remains from the Late Mississippian Nodena culture (ca. A.D. 1400–1700 [D. F. Morse 1973:83]) are reported to display evidence of treponematosis. Typical lesions are described in six skeletons 'and additional isolated bones from the "vicinity" of the mounds in Crittenden and Mississippi Counties in northeastern Arkansas (Wakefield, Dellinger, and Camp 1937). The tibial shaft is most often affected, and in some cases "the sharp anterior crest was replaced by a rounded surface and this thickening gave the shaft the appearance of having been bowed anteriorly" (p. 491, fig. 4). Fibulae, radii, ulnae, and clavicles show a similar "deforming osteitis." Erosion of the palate and nasal bones is evident in one skull. Extensive cranial and postcranial involvement in one skeleton (pp. 491–92, fig. 3) provides a convincing case. The cranial vault of this individual (No. 6) has a nodular surface typical of caries sicca, and the long bone X-rays reveal cortical thickening with encroachment upon the medullary canals. Although no European trade items were found with these burials, their apparent Nodena affiliation indicates that they may postdate 1492.

Morse (1973:50–52, 54–55) has also described Nodena material from Mississippi County with lesions suggestive of treponematosis. HM 916, an isolated skull of a 26-year-old female, displays "an area of sclerotic periosteal reaction with pitting over almost the entire left half of the frontal bone," substantial involvement occurring above the left orbit (fig. 27a). Steinbock (1976:96) agrees that this "closely resembles syphilis." An X-ray (Morse 1973: fig. 27b), however, reveals the presence of a mud-dauber nest inside the skull. In our opinion, the lesions are not diagnostic of treponematosis and are far more likely to have resulted from destruction by the wasps. HM 900 consists of the skull of a female aged 22 and exhibits cicatrization of the nasal aperture, with loss of the anterior nasal spine and nasal septum and involvement of the nasal bones. The entire palate is eroded, with healed sclerotic borders remaining. The maxillary sinuses have large eroded openings, and the involvement extends to the ethmoid and orbits. Morse (1973:54) attributes the observed pathology to a malignant tumor but does not rule out the possibility of treponematosis or leprosy. The lack of alveolar involvement would eliminate leprosy, and healing is not found in neoplasm (Hackett 1976:65). The absence of frontal pathology does not preclude the possibility of a treponemal lesion similar to the gangosa of yaws. Hackett (1976:63; see also Ortner and Putschar 1985:192, figs. 274–79, and Steinbock 1976:145, 151) indicates that such naso-palatine destruction is characterized by "an empty nasal cavity . . . presenting a smooth, 'bored out' tunnel-like passageway" and may be accompanied by opening of the ethmoid sinuses and partial or complete destruction of the palate and maxillary alveolus. Thus, "when extensive and healed," this type of naso-palatine destruction "is a *diagnostic criterion of syphilis*" (p. 65).

Despite excavation of nearly 2,000 Nodena burials,

few complete skeletons are extant. Early excavators did not consistently save skeletal material, and the majority of the collection consists of crania and pathological specimens. Thus, of 43 relatively complete individuals from the Upper Nodena site, 37 (86%) display inflammatory lesions, as do 9 of 16 such individuals (56.3%) from the Middle Nodena site (Powell 1988d). Powell reports that the lower long bones show "localized patches of mild to moderate periostitis, well-healed at death, most typically affecting the anterior crests and lateral aspects of . . . tibia shafts." Several tibiae are noted to display "saber shin." Five of the individuals with mild to moderate tibial periostitis exhibit remodeled cranial lesions. Six isolated crania (one identified as HM 900) also present focal lytic lesions, in one case described as "lesions of the distinctive 'stellate' configuration associated with the gummateous skin ulcers of treponemal infection" (Alabama Museum of Natural History, Nod 432 [Powell 1988d:pl. 1]). The lesions evident in the photograph correspond to Hackett's (1976:36) confluent clustered pits, diagnostic of treponematosis when accompanied by healing. From this evidence Powell concludes that an endemic treponematosis was present in the Nodena population. A high frequency of generalized periostitis, noted by several investigators (see Rose et al. 1984:414–15), is evident in skeletal series from Baytown (A.D. 300–700), Coles Creek (A.D. 700–1200), and Mississippian (A.D. 1200–1680) sites in eastern Arkansas and Louisiana, providing support for the long-standing occurrence of treponematosis in the lower Mississippi Valley.

Stewart and Quade (1969:91) describe frontal lesions in a Hopewellian skull (NMNH 379109) found near Kansas City, Missouri, as possibly due to treponematosis. The skull has three depressed scars on the middle of the frontal and similar scars around each parietal boss. At the precontact Morris site in southeastern Oklahoma, over a third of the adults exhibit "osteitis with tremendous swelling," primarily in the tibiae (Brues 1966:108–9). Brues describes a sequence of long bone lesions very similar to Hackett's (1976), culminating in the formation of pits. Cranial lesions similar to those illustrating syphilis are also noted. Two precontact skulls with "gnarled and pitted" surfaces are described by Goldstein (1957:302, pl. 1 b–d) as suggestive of syphilis. One skull (Cat. No. 411, Sanders Site, Lamar County) is accompanied by pathological tibiae, fibulae, and a femur (Goldstein 1957:pl. 1 c and d). The other (Cat. No. 660B, Willison Farm, Bell County) does not appear to be accompanied by postcranial remains. In South Dakota, several bones from the 14th-century Crow Creek site (39BF11) display varying degrees of periostitis, with considerable new bone formation and narrowing of the medullary cavity in some tibiae, resulting in a saber-shin appearance (Gregg, Allison, and Zimmerman 1981).

Osseous lesions from a possible syphilitic aortic aneurysm provide the only evidence of treponemal disease in a gatherer-hunter group from the northern Plains. The remains are from one of five individuals interred in the Bracken Cairn (DhOb-3) in southwestern Saskatchewan

(Walker 1983:499). The site, radiocarbon-dated to 515 B.C., is affiliated with the Pelican Lake phase of the Late Archaic period. Resorptive lesions appear on the right margin of the manubrium, the sternal end of the right clavicle, and the left side of the centra of the second and third thoracic vertebrae of a 36–46-year-old male. Walker suggests (pp. 501–2) that the erosion is due to pulsation of an aneurysm. Clinical descriptions indicate that syphilitic aneurysms typically occur on the ascending aorta and cause pulsation of the right sternoclavicular joint. In contrast, aneurysms due to atherosclerosis are very rare in the aortic arch and in the age-group of this individual.

Evidence of pre-Columbian treponematosis is lacking in northwestern North America. Syphilitic skeletal material abounds, however, in 18th- and 19th-century Alaskan material (see Cook 1985; Holcomb 1940; Meer 1985; Ortner and Putschar 1985:214–18, figs. 333–40), where venereal syphilis was apparently introduced after Russian contact. In California, nine individuals exhibiting periostitis suggestive of treponematosis were recovered from a Middle Horizon (500–200 B.C.) site in Sonoma County (Son 299; Roney 1966:101–2). A Late Horizon specimen (Scr.I.83.4434) has been radiocarbon-dated to A.D. 1105 (Brothwell and Burleigh 1975:394). Tenney's (1986) survey of osteological material in the Lowie Museum of Anthropology disclosed many individuals with generalized skeletal lesions like those expected in treponematosis. Nasal destruction, palatal perforation, cranial sclerotic new bone formation, and fusiform tibial lesions without cloacae are noted.

In the Southwestern United States, additional evidence of pre-Columbian treponematosis has accumulated. Hyde (1891:119–20, 124–28, fig. 6) reported two pathological tibiae from a prehistoric (Basketmaker?) burial found near the Animas River, about 45 miles from Durango, Colorado. The tibiae are enlarged, and the surfaces of both shafts are roughened and porous, with apparent striations and "superficial erosions" resulting from a "chronic inflammatory process." The left tibia appears bowed. While syphilis is not ruled out as the cause of this "chronic rarefying and formative osteitis, with osteomyelitis and chronic formative periostitis," it is indicated that such a diagnosis may not be justified (pp. 127–28). At Mesa Verde National Park, the remains of a 24-year-old male from the Pueblo III (A.D. 1100–1300) Mug House exhibits bilateral symmetrical enlargement and bowing of the tibiae in the anterior-posterior plane (Miles 1966:96; 1975:28, fig. 33). Although treponematosis is possible, the smooth periosteal surface does not support such a diagnosis (Miles 1975:28).

The skull and right femur of an adult female (Case 60455) from Pecos Pueblo, New Mexico, excavated by Kidder and originally described by Hooton (1930), show caries sicca on the frontal and parietals, partial destruction of the nasal bones, with subsequent healing, and dense periosteal bone apposition on the femur (Williams 1932:932–34). Hackett (1976:109) concurs with Williams's diagnosis of syphilis in this individual. Two

716 | CURRENT ANTHROPOLOGY Volume 29, Number 5, December 1988

other crania from Pecos Pueblo (Cases 59864 and 59814) exhibit cicatrization of the nasal and palatal areas (Williams 1932:934–37) similar to that described in the Arkansas HM 900 skull. Ceramics associated with these remains indicate that they date to the Pueblo IV period (A.D. 1300–1540). Case 59814 dates to the latter portion of this period and may not be pre-Columbian. Elsewhere in New Mexico, an isolated tibia (SM 56A) recovered from Smokey Bear Ruin exhibits periostitis and deformation due to considerable subperiosteal bone apposition (El-Najjar 1979:604, fig. 3b and c). Sequestra and cloacae are absent. Ceramics indicate that the site was used around A.D. 1250–1350.

Scattered sites in Arizona have yielded further evidence of treponematosis. Williams (1936:786–87) reports that a skeleton from the Basketmaker period (ca. 200 B.C.–A.D. 700) exhibits lesions in four long bones accompanied by a stellate scar on the skull, which he attributes to syphilis. Of some 400 burials from Tuzigoot Ruin, near Clarkdale (south of Flagstaff), one skull shows extensive destruction of the frontal and nasal bones and perforation of the palate (Denninger 1938). Tuzigoot was inhabited from about A.D. 1000–1350. A 20–25-year-old female (CdC No. 2) from a Pueblo II (A.D. 900–1100) site at Canyon de Chelly displays gummatous destruction and bone necrosis producing a "worm-eaten" appearance of the cranial vault (El-Najjar 1979:604–5, fig. 4 a and b). The photographs are illustrative of Hackett's (1976:43–45) diagnostic criteria of serpiginous and nodular cavitation. South of Canyon de Chelly, near Fort Apache, 2 of 57 individuals excavated at Kinishba and Vandal Cave are suspected of suffering from treponematosis. Tree-ring dates at Kinishba range from A.D. 1233 to 1306, while the Basketmaker II and Pueblo III occupations at Vandal Cave date from A.D. 608 to 683 and prior to A.D. 1300 respectively (Cole et al. 1955:231). Pronounced fusiform expansion and focal pitting of the cortex of the right tibia shaft accompany periosteal bone proliferation in the skull of A-17-0-17 from Kinishba (pp. 232–35, figs. 1–3). An isolated right tibia from Vandal Cave (VI-B-5) has a saber-shin appearance caused by deposition of new periosteal bone on the anterior aspect of the shaft (pp. 235–36, fig. 4). In the Salt River Valley, near Phoenix, excavations conducted at Los Muertos in the late 1890s revealed several skeletons that suggest the possibility of treponematosis. Matthews, Wortman, and Billings (1893:172) describe one individual with "irregular nodular hypertrophy" of the shafts of both tibiae, both ulnae, and the distal right fibula and other individuals with involvement of the tibial shafts alone. Los Muertos is a Classic Hohokam site, dating between A.D. 1100 and 1450 (Gumerman and Haury 1979).

Mexican remains also provide evidence of pre-Columbian treponematosis. Goff (1963; 1967:289–91, figs. 2–6, 9–11) attributes pathological changes in 20 skulls and several long bones from Cueva de la Candelaria, Coahuila, northeastern Mexico, to treponemal infection. The skulls exhibit osteitis and periostitis resulting in a nodular appearance. In one case (1967: fig. 3),

an active lesion surrounded by serpiginous and nodular cavitation is apparent. The long bones illustrated (figs. 9–11) present fusiform expansion of the shafts. Dating of the site does not seem well established and ranges from the 6th to the 16th century (p. 289). Williams (1936:784–85, fig. 1) reports that a pre-Hispanic Aztec skull from Santiago Tlaltelolco (near Mexico City) exhibits two lesions, one of which has destroyed nearly half of the frontal. This defect is accompanied by reactive bone formation at the perimeter, resulting in "the characteristic worm-eaten appearance seen on some syphilitic skulls," and resembles the active lesion described in the Candelaria skull. The skull of an adult male, dated to 300 B.C., from the Tehuacán Valley in Puebla exhibits similar destruction of the cranial vault (Anderson 1965).

Mayan remains from Central America also include individuals with apparent treponemal disease. Goff (1967: 288–89, fig. 7) refers to two crania from Zaculeu, Guatemala (A.D. 900–1000), as syphilitic. One shows apparent caries sicca on the frontal, while the other displays a large parietal defect with no evident healing and periostitis on the frontal. Inflammatory lesions in ten individuals (15.9% of adults) buried at Altar de Sacrificios, Guatemala, before A.D. 950 exhibit osteitis suggestive of treponematosis (Saul 1972). Cranial lesions alone are evident in two individuals (table 8). Burial No. 96 (fig. 10) exhibits periostitis, which is not diagnostic. Cranial lesions of Burial No. 129 (p. 42, fig. 7) may actually be due to postmortem insect damage. Six individuals show only postcranial involvement, while two have both cranial and postcranial lesions (table 8). Postcranial lesions consist of cortical thickening and enlargement of the long bone shafts, resulting in the saber-shin tibia evident in Burial No. 112 (figs. 22–24). In Belize, a Mayan tomb revealed the remains of an adult male with enlarged tibiae presenting a surface "covered with a number of small nodular outgrowths, between which were small pits or depressions" (Gann 1901:969). With this skeleton were three clay figures of men performing an operation with a pointed implement on the head of the disproportionately large penis and "a natural-sized model of the human penis in a state of semi-erection" on which "three longitudinal incisions" were made on the glans (p. 969). Gann takes this as evidence that the buried individual suffered from a venereal disease and that this disease, as indicated by osseous involvement of the tibiae, was syphilis.

South American evidence of pre-Columbian treponematosis comes primarily from Peru. At Paracas, two individuals from tombs excavated by Julio Tello in 1929 are considered by Williams (1932:937–46) to be syphilitic. The remains are affiliated with the early Nazca culture, approximately 200 B.C. (Lanning 1967:25–27, 122; Williams 1932:938). The first individual displays stellate scars (caries sicca) over much of the cranium. The accompanying long bones (both femurs and the left tibia, humerus, and ulna) show marked periosteal bone apposition with some encroachment upon the medullary canal and present nodular surfaces with small openings. The second, mummified individual suffered from a large ulcer on the roof of the mouth that had perforated the hard palate. The lower portion of the body was poorly preserved. Hackett (1976:109), referring to the photographs of the Paracas crania, indicates that the diagnosis of syphilis in both cases "may not be acceptable." Although his caution is justified, the photographs and description do lend credence to a diagnosis of treponemal infection in the first case.

A burial excavated by Kroeber in the Cañete Valley, Peru, dated about A.D. 500, is also described as syphilitic (Williams 1932:948–54). Although the skull is normal, a chronic inflammatory osteoperiostitis produced "dense, ivory-like bone" over the entire shaft of the left femur and both tibiae, with some encroachment upon the medullary canal. The left fibula is involved to a lesser extent. The lateral view of the right tibia indicates considerable bone apposition on the anterior aspect. Hackett (1976:109) states that these long bones do not exhibit lesions diagnostic of treponemal disease, but according to Williams (1932:948) "the absence of sequestrums and of deep sinuses tends to exclude nonsyphilitic periostitis and osteomyelitis."

An eight-year-old child from Machu Picchu (Peabody Museum, New Haven, No. 51–9210) dated ca. A.D. 1100–1200 allegedly exhibits congenital syphilis (Goff 1967:293, fig. 12; Williams 1932:972) Lesions are evident on the frontal and are accompanied by saber-shin tibiae. No reference is made to the dentition. Other tibiae in this series exhibit similar enlargement (Williams 1932:972). MacCurdy (1932:264, pls. 38, 41) reports three cases of possible syphilis at sites in the Urubamba Valley near Cuzco. The cranium of a six-year-old from Paucarcancha (Cat. No. 51) exhibits considerable necrosis of the left parietal and frontal. At Patallacta, the left parietal of an eight-year-old child (Cat. No. 938) has a circular area of necrosis 4.2 cm in diameter, and the cranium of a 26-year-old male (Cat. No. 635) displays an area of necrosis nearly 5 cm in diameter that has a large perforation at its center. In none of these cases is reactive new bone formation apparent; therefore treponematosis is probably not the cause. Williams (1932:972) agrees with this assessment in the first two cases but considers the adult male a possible example of syphilis. The apparent Inca affiliation of these sites indicates that they may be post-Columbian.

At Aguazuque, a preceramic site in central Colombia, 13 of 40 individuals (32.5%) demonstrate lesions associated with treponematosis, particularly in the tibia, in some resulting in a saber-shin deformity (Correal Urrego 1987). Three of these individuals also display caries sicca. A skeleton with both cranial and postcranial lesions is radiocarbon-dated to 2080 B.C. (4030 ± 80 B.P.). Correal Urrego suggests that since yaws is rare in this part of modern Colombia the pathology stems from venereal syphilis.

In Argentina, a pre-Columbian skull from Río Negro is regarded as above suspicion by Williams (1932:946–48, 976) although he did not personally examine it. It had previously been described as exhibiting "little elevations and depressions that were like scars" and pronounced syphilitic by Broca and other European authorities. From the Chubut River valley, a probably pre-Columbian skull shows gummatous lesions (p. 973). Another skull, from Calchaqui, exhibits a mass of smooth-edged scars, with thickening of adjacent areas and nasal destruction accompanied by healing (pp. 973–74).

Discussion

Review of the documentary and skeletal evidence for pre-Columbian syphilis reveals many ambiguities in dates and differential diagnosis. What, then, can be determined from this evidence?

Is it possible that syphilis and leprosy were confused before the 1490s? Ancient and medieval texts portray leprosy as a highly contagious disease with a short incubation period, associated with immorality, sexually and congenitally transmitted, and responding to mercury treatment (Holcomb 1935:297–303; Hudson 1972:149). Leprosy has none of these characteristics. Syphilis, however, is not the only disease that manifests such features. It is just as likely that such descriptions refer to other venereal or skin diseases. Drawing diagnostic conclusions from these accounts is "unconscionable," as one is "faced with a spectrum of dermatologic diseases, exanthems, leprosy, tuberculosis, and epidemics in the Middle Ages of louse-borne typhus, bubonic plague, and widespread ergotism" (Kampmeier 1984:28).

Many authorities (e.g., Brown et al. 1970:82; Harrison 1986:51; Kampmeier 1984:19, 21, 28; Sussman 1967:214; see also Rosebury 1971:20–21) attribute biblical and other ancient disease descriptions such as those previously summarized to gonorrhea rather than syphilis. Galen, in the 2d century A.D., invented the term "gonorrhea" (seed flow) to describe the discharge associated with the disease (Brown et al. 1970:82; Kampmeier 1984:28). The hard and soft genital sores described by Galen and Celsus may have been not syphilitic condylomata but evidence of chancroid, genital herpes, venereal warts, granuloma inguinale of leishmaniasis, or other nonvenereal skin diseases (Kampmeier 1984:26–27). Along with cutaneous lesions and granuloma inguinale, leishmaniasis may also cause destruction of the nasopharynx (Steinbock 1976:151). In addition to syphilis, several other diseases causing skin lesions can cross the placenta to infect the fetus. Among these are rubella (German measles), measles, smallpox (variola), chickenpox and shingles (varicella-zoster virus), genital herpes, and gonorrhea (Rosebury 1971:55–56). All of these are highly contagious diseases with short incubation periods, and the latter two are acquired through sexual intercourse.

Mercury treatment has been cited by proponents of the pre-Columbian hypothesis as proof that ancient "leprosy" was syphilis. Mercury, however, was commonly prescribed for many disorders. In his medical treatise of 1546, Fracastor advocates rubbing mercurial ointment on the inner arms to cure a severe headache (Rosebury 1971:47). Although application of mercury is

718 | CURRENT ANTHROPOLOGY Volume 29, Number 5, December 1988

known to have an effect on syphilis, it also results in a rapid reduction in gonorrheal discharge and probably relieved symptoms of several other diseases (Harrison 1959:6–7; cf. Hudson 1961:548–49).

Did an epidemic of syphilis begin in the late 1490s? The documentary evidence regarding the appearance of a new disease is ambiguous in terms of symptoms described, but the numerous ordinances passed throughout Europe in the late 1490s in an effort to control the disease and the proliferation of publications regarding it indicate that a highly contagious infection that caused genital and cutaneous lesions was raging at that time.

Was this epidemic the result of differentiation of syphilis and its widespread recognition as a disease distinct from "leprosy"? In support of the pre-Columbian hypothesis, it has been noted that leprosy declined at this time and that edicts regarding the new disease were quite similar to those previously issued to isolate lepers. The characteristic hard chancre of syphilis was first described in 1514 by de Vigo, and syphilitic and non-syphilitic condylomata were differentiated in 1563 (Brown et al. 1970:82; Kampmeier 1984:26–27). It is possible, however, that these lesions were not described prior to 1500 because they did not previously exist in the Old World. Holcomb (1934, 1935) has explained the decline in "leprosy" as a transference of the symptoms associated with that disease to syphilis. If the two diseases were differentiated by the late 1490s, why do 16th-century descriptions continue to apply the term "leprosy" to syphilis? Paracelsus (1493–1541), for example, thought that "leprosy and venereal bubas" (quoted by Brody [1974:56–57]) were the first stage of syphilis. His description is usually explained as confusion of syphilis with gonorrhea (Brown et al. 1970:82; Kampmeier 1984:26). Similar diagnostic difficulties plagued scholars of the 16th through 19th centuries until syphilis and gonorrhea were finally differentiated (Brown et al. 1970:82–83; Hackett 1963:29; Kampmeier 1984:26–28; Rosebury 1971:181). By the end of the 15th century, "leprosy" had become identified with syphilis to the extent that Job, once the patron saint of lepers, became the patron saint of syphilitics (Brody 1974:56–58, 191–92; Creighton 1965 [1894]:102). Although the symptoms were being transferred from one disease to another, it appears that syphilis was being grouped with ailments having similar symptoms rather than being differentiated from them. This would seem to indicate that syphilis was a new disease.

Was the epidemic of venereal syphilis due to increasing urbanization and improved hygiene in late 15th-century Europe? The decline in the incidence of leprosy actually began in the 14th century and has been attributed to improved living conditions (Clay 1966 [1909]:41–43; Rubin 1974:151–53). The incidence of nonvenereal treponematosis, if it had been present in Europe, would also have decreased with such improvements. Hudson (1961:548; 1965a:897) postulates that endemic syphilis was present in Europe from Roman times and retreated to rural areas in the Balkans, Russia, and Scandinavia as standards of living rose during the Middle Ages. In the meantime, the treponeme was in-

creasingly being transmitted sexually in the more advanced areas, culminating in the identification of syphilis at the end of the 15th century. Endemic syphilis, associated with poor hygiene and primitive living conditions, did exist in Europe until the mid-1800s—as sibbens in Scotland, button scurvy in Ireland, radesyge in Norway, saltfluss in Sweden, and spirocolon in Greece and Russia—but was not recognized until the middle of the 17th century (Morton 1967:374; Steinbock 1976:138). In Scotland, the introduction of endemic syphilis was blamed on Cromwell's army in 1650 (Morton 1967:374–75). In contrast, edicts concerning venereal syphilis were issued in Aberdeen and Edinburgh in 1497. Thus, while the cities and towns were ravaged by a venereal disease, treponemal infection seems to have spread slowly to the countryside, where social conditions allowed nonvenereal transmission to prevail. The epidemiological aspects of the unitarian hypothesis are supported. However, if syphilis was recognized as a distinct disease at the end of 15th century, documentary evidence indicates that the venereal form of treponematosis was the first to appear, followed by reversion to an endemic form in rural areas. Again, rather than supporting the pre-Columbian existence of treponematosis, a case can be made for the appearance of a new disease which was subsequently included in a category of maladies manifesting similar lesions.

As Hudson (1968:6) indicates, "by selecting the 'right' witnesses and dates and discarding the rest, it is possible to build a case for either view, depending on the credibility of the witnesses and the credulity of the reader." On the basis of the documentary evidence prior to 1492, syphilis cannot be excluded from the list of diseases that may have been grouped under the term "leprosy." The lack of syphilitic skeletal material in European leper cemeteries, combined with the dearth of Old World remains that have even been suggested to exhibit treponemal lesions, however, precludes this possibility. If treponematosis evolved with Homo, as postulated in the unitarian hypothesis, and was among the diseases described in biblical, Greek, Roman, and medieval texts, then skeletal evidence suggestive of treponematosis should be abundant in the materials recovered from Old World sites. The case for pre-Columbian syphilis in the Old World rests solely on vague and ambiguous disease descriptions and must, therefore, be rejected.

Was syphilis present in the New World before 1492? A substantial amount of documentary evidence from the early 16th century indicates that it was. These documents, as previously discussed, present ambiguous descriptions and inconsistencies in dates. Williams and co-workers (1927:686) find the Native American linguistic evidence tenuous because of possible confusion of syphilis and yaws. The absence of the dental stigmata associated with congenital syphilis (with the possible exception of the child from Virginia) has been cited as proof that venereal syphilis did not exist in the New World. The etiological unity of the treponemal syndromes, however, renders such objections moot.

Despite Williams's (1932:977) assertion that the amount of New World skeletal evidence of trepo-

BAKER AND ARMELAGOS *The Origin and Antiquity of Syphilis* | 719

nematosis is "almost embarrassing" in comparison with the Old World data, Hackett (1976:111) is alarmed that few pre-Columbian American bones (about 1 in 500) exhibit the diagnostic criteria of treponematosis. It must be reiterated that bone lesions are expected in only 1–5% of individuals in skeletal series from areas in which yaws or endemic syphilis occurred. Furthermore, a considerable amount of material has come to light since Hackett's review. Investigations in the Midwestern and Southeastern United States (e.g., Cassidy 1980, 1984; Cook 1976, 1984; Powell 1988a, b) reveal treponemal infections involving up to half of the population. While these reports differentiate localized inflammatory lesions from the syndrome of diffuse periostitis suggestive of treponematosis, the reported frequencies are so high that attribution to a single infectious disease may be questionable. Hill (1986) cautions that "postcranial marrow hypertrophy associated with acute and chronic anemia in children is virtually indistinguishable from generalized periostitis indicative of infection" and that "postcranial periosteal lesions associated with cranial porotic hyperostosis have been treated as a separate entity, i.e., infection." While the synergism of infection and nutritional deficiencies (such as iron deficiency anemia) cannot be overlooked, the appearance of diagnostic changes in some individuals from these skeletal populations indicates that a treponemal infection was undoubtedly present in the eastern half of the United States from Late Archaic times (as early as 3000 B.C.) and contributed to the generalized periosteal involvement evident in these remains.

The nature of the skeletal evidence found in North and South America is explained by treponemal epidemiology. The apparent absence of congenital syphilis is not surprising, considering that most of the populations in pre-Columbian times were gatherer-hunters or horticulturalists residing in small camps or villages rather than large cities. The prevailing hygienic conditions would be insufficient to prohibit transmission of the treponeme by casual contact among children. Such a pattern probably characterized more populous areas prior to European contact as well. The high frequency of treponemal lesions reported in some skeletal series may reflect population nucleation, particularly where sociopolitical organization allowed for widespread exchange of material goods and infectious diseases, as among Middle Woodland and Mississippian groups (cf. Buikstra 1984:229–30; Cassidy 1980:137; 1984:334–35; Cook 1984:261–62; Larsen 1984:379–80; Perzigian, Tench, and Braun 1984:356–58; Rose et al. 1984:415–18). Skeletal series in the pre-Columbian New World would therefore be expected to display a pattern of pathological involvement more typical of nonvenereal than of venereal syphilis—a situation encountered in several large skeletal series from the eastern half of the United States. As Buikstra (1979:232) has indicated, "it appears that certain forms of intercourse are less important in explaining the archaeological record than previously suggested."

The absence of skeletal evidence of treponematosis in the Old World and the abundance of such evidence in the New necessitates revision of Hudson's thesis that treponematosis originated in Africa and was subsequently carried throughout the world in the course of human migrations. It appears, instead, that treponematosis is a relatively new disease that originated in the tropical or temperate zone of the Americas and was spread by casual contact. This nonvenereal infection is the disease that was initially contracted by Columbus's crew, but social and environmental conditions in Europe at that time were conducive to its venereal dissemination in urban areas. The transition of one treponemal syndrome to another under differing environmental and social circumstances has been frequently documented in modern populations (e.g., Grin 1961; Hudson 1965a:889; 1965b:743–44; Willcox 1974:174).

This contention will undoubtedly meet with much dissent. Although there is universal agreement that Native American populations were decimated by diseases introduced by Europeans to which they had no immunity, the possibility of a parallel introduction of American diseases into Europe is rejected. Nearly 30 years ago, Harrison (1959:7) suggested that "if one could test mummies for antibodies to *T. pallidum* . . . one might perhaps settle this eternal question of the birth-place of syphilis." He thought his suggestion far-fetched, but immunological tests have recently been attempted on skeletal materials. An effort to inoculate rabbits with an extract from a pathological Crow Creek specimen to produce an antibody titre indicative of the presence of treponematosis ended with the animals' death (due to *Clostridium* contamination) before any results could be obtained (Gregg et al. 1981). A method developed in Czechoslovakia has proved capable of determining the presence of *Treponema* in a recent case of yaws from an Australian bone sample and in European cases of syphilis from the 16th and 19th centuries (Smrcka 1985). The most recent and significant immunological test has demonstrated the presence of treponemal antigen in the remains of a Pleistocene bear from Indiana radiocarbon-dated to 11,500 ± 520 B.P. (Rothschild and Turnbull 1987). Skeletal lesions include gumma formation and periosteal reaction in the mandible, humeri, radii, and ulna and in three thoracic vertebrae. Immunofluorescence analysis of histological sections revealed the presence of treponemal antigens, while tests for *Neisseria gonorrhea*, *Streptococcus*, and *Legionella pneumophilia* were negative. The pursuit of similar immunological analyses in pre-Columbian remains with skeletal lesions suggestive of treponemal infection should eventually resolve the controversy.

Conclusion

Current attention is focused on the epidemic of AIDS, which is similar in some respects to the epidemic of syphilis nearly 500 years ago. Because of disease synergism and the numerous complications that may finally cause the death of an AIDS patient, the question arises how long AIDS was present in human populations before it was recognized as a distinct disease. The AIDS virus has been recently discovered in tissue saved after the puzzling death of a St. Louis teenager in 1969, a decade 'before AIDS was recognized elsewhere in the United States (Associated Press 1987). As with syphilis, it could be argued that the "epidemic" of AIDS is a result of its differentiation from an array of complications with which it was previously confused. Arguments as to its point of origin (e.g., African green monkeys, Haitians, homosexual males, etc.) have ensued.

Recent research reveals that a positive serological test for syphilis in men, a history of syphilis in men, and a history of genital warts in women are significantly associated with seropositivity for human immunodeficiency virus (HIV), which causes AIDS (Quinn et al. 1988). Thus, sexually transmitted diseases which disrupt epithelial surfaces (particularly syphilis) may increase the efficiency of HIV transmission (Quinn et al. 1988:201–2). In light of these findings and the recent report that syphilis is at its highest level in the United States since 1950 (NBC News, January 28, 1988), it is apparent that the attention accorded syphilis in the past is likely to be renewed.

This review of the documentary and skeletal evidence of treponematosis supports the Columbian hypothesis. The abundance of New World human skeletal material exhibiting lesions suggestive of treponemal infection, particularly when encountered in large skeletal populations, and the discovery of treponemal antigens in the remains of a Pleistocene bear from the Midwestern United States clearly demonstrate the presence of the disease prior to 1492. The paucity of possible treponemal lesions in the vast collections of pre-Columbian Old World skeletal remains is a telling contrast to the New World situation. Newly developed immunological analysis should finally lay the controversy regarding the origin of syphilis to rest.

Comments

MARSHALL JOSEPH BECKER
Department of Anthropology and Sociology, West · Chester University, West Chester, Pa. 19383, U.S.A. 21 VI 88

Baker and Armelagos provided us with an extremely useful updated review of the literature on the origins and antiquity of venereal syphilis in the Old World. By addressing specific problems concerned with the three dominant hypotheses and reviewing the evidence as it now stands, they conclude that the Columbian hypothesis best fits these data. This is approximately the view that I take—that in some way the voyages of Columbus brought to Europe the pathogen that became manifest as venereal syphilis. The crux of their argument is that the "transition of one treponemal syndrome to another under differing environmental and social circumstances" is the explanation for the sudden rise in the Old World of a disease not previously known. The prob-

lems that continue to face me regarding this conclusion and that are not covered by Baker and Armelagos are as follows:

T. pallidum appears to be the agent responsible for syphilis, yaws, and related treponemal infections manifesting diverse symptomatology (cf. Hudson 1965a). The variations in the symptoms appear to be the result of differing expressions of the disease resulting from the pathogen's operating in different environments, a phenomenon known widely in biology.

If, however, this is the case, what is the evidence that supports the Columbian hypothesis rather than Hudson's unitarian one?

If a New World disorder (venereal syphilis) spread with unusual virulence into the Old World, was it because the urban environment into which it was introduced provided the circumstances under which it would flourish? If so, then one would expect that the original New World distribution of the disease would correlate with urban populations. The skeletal record does not appear to suggest this but rather may reflect a random distribution. Conversely, if the disorder were a transformation of an infection already existing in the Old World, as Hudson suggests, one would expect that increases in the manifestation of syphilis would parallel the growth of post-medieval cities. The spread of what Baker and Armelagos demonstrate to have been a new disease simply appears to be strongly correlated with the years after 1492. On the other hand, if the disease were transformed only *after arriving in* the Old World, then the skeletal evidence from the preceding period in the two hemispheres might not differ at all. In fact, while Baker and Armelagos note how infrequently one might expect to find skeletal evidence for syphilis, we are not told how frequently it actually appears in the many collections in which they have found it. The rate appears to me to be extraordinarily high.

Several general matters noted in this paper should also be discussed further. Although the belief that European-introduced diseases ca. 1500 sharply reduced Native American populations has nearly "universal agreement" in the popular literature, a growing number of scholars (Ramenofsky 1982, Becker 1988) have noted situations in which this was certainly not the case. Such examples call into question the application of this idea to all of the New World. The idea of European diseases' devastating New World populations ignores contacts stretching back to the Norse settlements and continuing with the long 15th-century contacts by whaling and fishing fleets from England, France, and so on. These contacts, rapidly accelerating before 1500, would be just as likely to have served as disease vectors in both directions, a point that Cockburn (1961) has noted. Also of note in this same period is the not so coincidental expulsion of the Muslim and Jewish populations from Iberia in 1492, after what some people might call the last great barbarian invasion. The dispersal of these peoples, both of which are considered to have been considerably more cleanly than their neighbors, may be a still unexplored factor in this matter.

While Hudson's thesis is attractive, the situations that

he suggests developed during the process of late- and post-medieval urbanization are too poorly documented to provide any reliable support for it. We simply do not know if the cities of that period were growing at an unusual rate or if hygiene actually was changing at that time. One of the basic problems with Hudson's argument lies in speculation concerning improvements in personal and community hygiene in antiquity and his apparent ignorance (1965a:895) of the late invention of soap. To infer that child-to-child contacts may be reduced with improvements in hygiene suggests ignorance of present vectors for head lice, chickenpox, etc., among some well-washed modern groups.

The availability of extensive evidence for pre-Columbian treponemiasis in the New World may also reflect the concerns of Americanist archaeology. Careful recovery of skeletons, outstanding curation, and concern for analysis developed early in the New World. These efforts have been matched in England, Denmark, and other areas, but the regions of Europe in which the reports of syphilis first appeared are just those in which skeletal studies have become important more recently. As such studies become increasingly available, the additional information may give us new perspectives on this topic. At this point Baker and Armelagos's paper is a most welcome contribution.

DON BROTHWELL
Institute of Archaeology, University of London, 31–34, Gordon Square, London WC1H 0PY, England. 24 VI 88

It was good to read of current New World thinking on ancient treponematoses. I have pondered this problem for some years and have the following reactions:

1. While the mind boggles at potential treponeme transmission by Paleo-Indian bestiality (with bears!), I like the idea of the human treponematoses' being initially a mammal zoonosis. However, I confess to serious doubts about the reported immunological findings. At least the results emphasize again the need for a careful and critical appraisal of the treponemes in other vertebrates, especially as regards the emergence of our own pathogens.

2. Regarding possible human treponemal material from Mexico, the list has grown somewhat beyond that detailed by the authors (Brothwell 1978).

3. There is indeed remarkably little evidence of Old World treponematoses, but there are a tantalizing few data, and the dating is not shaky on all of them. While the New World origin is a hypothesis one can nearly embrace, it simply doesn't fit all the facts. There is, for instance, the pre-European material from Borneo (Brothwell 1976), and new material from Australia (Prokopec and Pretty, unpub.) can be added to the Marianas Island data (Stewart and Spoehr 1967 [1952]) to establish treponematoses in early South-East Asia.

Europe is indeed a puzzle, but the rarity of finds may be related to the possible late adaptation and survival of endemic syphilis in northern climates following greater contact with the Palestinian area during the Crusades

(Brothwell 1970). It is interesting to recollect that Baldwin IV, king of Jerusalem in the 12th century A.D., is regarded as having had a fast-developing form of "leprosy," perhaps now to be considered as possible endemic syphilis. In northern Europe, there appears to be a definite case of treponematosis from medieval York (Dawes and Magilton 1980), confirmed as pre-Columbian by radiocarbon dating. There is also a claim of endemic syphilis from late medieval Trondheim in Norway, suggesting that the medieval period really was critical to the northward movement of the condition (Anderson et al. 1986).

We do, then, have a small amount of Old World evidence, spread widely from South-East Asia to northern Europe and of pre-Columbian date, and it simply can't be ignored. My feeling is that Asia may still turn out to be the original homeland for the evolution of the pathogenic human treponemes and that the scheme of differentiation I have discussed elsewhere still seems to fit all the archaeological and historical facts most satisfactorily (Brothwell 1981).

ANDREA DRUSINI
Department of Biology, University of Padua, Padua, Italy. 47 VI 88

This article contains all the necessary ingredients for a modern view of the history of disease: historical background, palaeoepidemiology, a review of the osteological specimens, and the inevitable parallel between syphilis and AIDS. There are, however, some remarks to be made.

First, scant importance is attributed to Sudhoff's contribution to the history of syphilis. Against the hypotheses of Iwan Bloch (1901–11), one of the principal advocates of the New World origin of syphilis, Sudhoff noted that beginning in the 12th century, Italian surgeons especially used metallic mercury as an ointment to cure chronic diseases of the skin such as leprosy and scabies. Some varieties of scabies (*scabies grossa* or, in French, *grosse vérole, gros mal*) healed completely with mercurial treatment. The proceedings of the trial of Dijon in 1463 clearly show that such a disease was transmitted by sexual contagion.

Meanwhile, about 1440 the term *mal franzoso* appeared in Italy, and in 1489 some Swiss mercenaries were insulted as *Kriegsbuben und Frankricher*, meaning ill of *mal franzoso*. The idea that a disease that presents cutaneous symptoms, transmitted by sexual contagion and curable with mercury, could be considered syphilis therefore seems justified (Sigerist 1923, with a complete bibliography of and comment on Sudhoff's works).

Also, the Veronese physicians of the Renaissance Giorgio Sommariva and Natale Montesauro stated that the "new" disease was already known as *mal franzoso*; Trithenius detected the contagion on the banks of the Rhine in 1493; Jeronymus Braunschweig (or Brunschwig) recognized it in 1493–94; the Sicilian physician Niccolò Scillacio (15th–16th century) found it in Barcelona and called it "morbus novus, qui nuper a Gallia defluxit" (Sigerist 1923). It is important that these Renaissance physicians did not for the most part link syphilis with the discovery of the New World.

Another important omission regards a basic work of Guerra (1978), who says (p. 40) that "new understanding about the evolution of treponematoses, the clinical syndromes of human infection, and a much clearer view of the effect of the environment upon the disease have made obsolete the traditional setting for the discussion of the role of America in the history of syphilis." Together with the most important debates among the Renaissance physicians, Guerra cites two interesting Renaissance documents: the opera "Sylva in Scabiem," written by Angelo Poliziano (1450–94) about 1475, in which he described a disease called lues or morbo gallico, and an epistle to "Ario Lusitano grecas literas Salmanticae" from Pietro Martire d'Anghiera (1455–1526), dated April 9, 1489, that gives a good description of a diseased called bubas by the Spaniards, morbo gallico by the Italians, and elephantiasis by some physicians.

Guerra (1978:44) also emphasizes the words of Ruy Diaz de Isla (1539) at the close of his book: "ten years before the [venereal] disease appeared, women did not know a better way of cursing their children, stepchildren and servants than by saying 'May you die of nasty bubas.' . . . This indeed shows that 'bubas' were common in Spain before the discovery of the New World." Finally (p. 56), he states that "the import into Europe of new tropical treponematoses, such as yaws from America, does not affect the truth of Sudhoff's thesis about the existence of urban treponematoses in Europe, such as venereal syphilis, during the medieval period." We must bear in mind that the European explorers of Southeast Asia and the Pacific Islands from the Renaissance to the modern age have found yaws among natives of humid and hot areas (see, for example, Dampier 1703).

Another work of Holcomb (1941:167) could have been quoted: "The description of leprosy given by Bernard de Gordon about 1308 A.D. is not modern leprosy, but a circumstantial description of congenital and venereally acquired modern syphilis. . . . Syphilis in a congenital and acquired form certainly prevailed in Europe long before the discovery of America." But perhaps, as Ackernecht (1955, 1965) has pointed out, the question will remain controversial from both the historical and the palaeopathological point of view.

As far as the osteological evidence is concerned, there is great disproportion in the amount of documentation between Europe and America. Two other Old World discoveries are perhaps to be mentioned: Vorberg (1896) and Rokhlin (1965), the latter concerning syphilitic bones dated 3000–2000 B.C. in the trans-Baikal area of Siberia. The absence of evidence of pre-Columbian syphilis in Europe may simply mean that research in the area is still incomplete.

Only one certainty emerges from this debate: in ancient times urbanism, migrations, and travels created a "common market" for syphilis (Dubos 1965).[1]

1. I am deeply indebted to Maurizio Rippa Bonati, Institute of the History of Medicine, University of Padua, for his kind suggestions.

MARIE CLABEAUX GEISE
Department of Anthropology, State University College at Buffalo, Buffalo, N.Y. 14222, U.S.A. 23 VI 88

As researchers attempt to trace the origins of the newest of the sexually transmitted diseases, AIDS, it is appropriate to assess our progress in tracking the history of an older one. It is also appropriate to remember that syphilis once caused the same fear of the disease itself and of its victims that AIDS is producing today. AIDS has emerged (apparently) within our lifetime, a time of highly developed medical technology, rapid and widespread scientific communication, and a sophisticated framework of theory, yet we do not know where, when, or how it developed. To try to answer these questions for a disease whose origins date far back into antiquity is an ambitious undertaking. As Baker and Armelagos note, the debate on the origins of syphilis is virtually as old as its recognition as a separate disease.

Those familiar with the paleopathological literature know that there is even more evidence for the occurrence of treponemal infection in the pre-Columbian New World than Baker and Armelagos have chosen to include. Although they say that such evidence is lacking for northwestern North America, this is not the case. Jerome S. Cybulski has found evidence of treponemal infection at two Northwest Coast sites: the Boardwalk site on Prince Rupert Harbour and the Duke Point site in the Gulf of Georgia region. The Boardwalk site yielded an adult female with a radiocarbon date of 2,325 ± 90 B.P. with cranial lesions of caries sicca. The Duke Point site dates to 3,490 ± 125 B.P. and has produced four individuals with signs of treponemal infection and as many as six affected. The burials include a female with node lesions on the tibial shaft. Situated in her pelvis was a fetus with cortical osteoporosis. One of the juveniles has a mulberry molar. Cybulski suggests that these cases represent an endemic nonvenereal syphilis which was stimulated to venereal syphilis in the contact situation of fur trading (Cybulski, personal communication and n.d.).

I am in strong agreement with Baker and Armelagos's conclusions, in part because their arguments are persuasive and in larger part because I have encountered evidence suggestive of treponemal infection in skeletons from the Northeast. If "seeing is believing," I have seen and I do believe. The existence of treponemal infection in Europe prior to Columbus's voyages is problematic. It is extremely difficult to prove a negative—that syphilis did not exist in Europe prior to contact. Baker and Armelagos have come as close to doing so as is possible. While they feel that new immunological analyses will end this controversy, I do not think this will be so. The results, either negative or positive, will be questioned. The bear evidence is already being disputed. Western scientists see the origins of AIDS in Africa, African scientists in the Western world, especially the United States. Our attitudes towards diseases are deeply embedded in the culture and have an emotional context. We still remember the Black Plague, but the influenza pandemic that was responsible for more deaths than the

First World War during which it occurred is dismissed. People still die from flu and no longer die from syphilis, but a diagnosis of syphilis carries much more emotional impact. Syphilis is still a disease with a high level of cultural meaning. A dispassionate assessment of the data such as that presented here will probably not end the debate.

MARC A. KELLEY
Department of Sociology and Anthropology, University of Rhode Island, Kingston, R.I. 02881, U.S.A. 28 VI 88

Baker and Armelagos have presented an energetic review of the syphilis controversy. While it is quite similar in content and structure to Steinbock's (1976), it does augment the debate with the latest developments in immunological testing for the treponemal antigen. This tool will indeed probably lead to the resolution of this tired controversy. Continued attempts to interpret the voluminous and contradictory literature on the history of syphilis can only lead to speculative conclusions. As far as such speculation is concerned, the view outlined by Baker and Armelagos is nearly identical to the one I have advocated in the classroom and among my colleagues for the last five years.

The comparison of AIDS to syphilis is in my opinion superficial and appears "tacked on."

IWATARO MORIMOTO
Department of Anatomy, St. Marianna University School of Medicine, 2-16-1 Sugao, Miyamae, Kawasaki, Kanagawa 213, Japan. 17 VI 88

Baker and Armelagos's attention to syphilis in their invaluable paper is timely because the recent epidemic of AIDS seems similar in some respects to that of syphilis nearly 500 years ago and because sexually transmitted syphilis, which disrupts epithelial surfaces, may increase the efficiency of AIDS virus transmission to those who have not previously been exposed to this frightening disease and have no effective immunity against it. On the basis of a great abundance of documentary and skeletal evidence they advocate the hypothesis that syphilis originated in the Americas and was carried to Europe by the crew of Columbus in 1493. In Japan, it is a matter of record that the first epidemic of venereal syphilis occurred at Kyoto in 1512, about 30 years before the first European sailors came to this country. The new venereal disease swept the Japanese islands within several years of the first epidemic, much as it did in Europe during the final decade of the 15th century. Suzuki (1984a), from the viewpoint of paleoepidemiology, has estimated the prevalence of syphilis in the adult citizens of Edo (Tokyo) from the 17th to the 19th century at as much as 54.4% on the average. Since the occurrence of bone changes is clinically scanty in venereal syphilis, he estimates the incidence of cranial syphilis in the same citizens at 7.9%. There seems to be no evidence of syphilitic lesions in Japanese skulls dated before the 15th century. I am greatly inclined to agree with Baker and Armelagos.

ALAN G. MORRIS
Department of Anatomy and Cell Biology, University of Cape Town, Observatory 7925, Cape Town, South Africa. 22 VI 88

Baker and Armelagos have done an excellent job in their expert collation and consideration of the confusing mass of data about the origins of syphilis. The impact of syphilis on the European populations of the 16th century is well known, and speculations on the origin of the disease have occupied learned circles for generations. The evidence for the presence of the treponemal infection in the New World now seems beyond doubt, and the focus of research, as Baker and Armelagos suggest, must shift to the skeletal remains of the inhabitants of the Old World.

Southern Africa might present an interesting test region for the prehistoric presence of treponemal infection. Of the four clinical variants of treponemal disease, all but pinta are currently found in the region. The ecological model clearly explains the modern distribution of the disease—yaws in the humid north and east, endemic syphilis in the arid centre and south, and venereal syphilis in the urban situation.

The argument against the introduction of treponemal sicknesses to southern Africa is primarily based on the pattern of endemic syphilis. Researchers who have examined endemic syphilis in trans-Kalahari populations (Nurse and Jenkins 1977, Nurse et al. 1973, Truswell and Hansen 1968) have concluded that the disease has been present for a considerable length of time. One paper (Nurse et al. 1973) goes so far as to suggest that the desert dwellers represent the reservoir from which the disease filters to the settled agricultural populations to the east. Maingard (1937) has described a root that the southern San used for the curing of the *vuilsiekte* (endemic syphilis). This suggests a knowledge of the disease that has had some time in which to accumulate.

Despite this, historical reports are adamant that syphilis was introduced to southern Africa, especially in the arid regions of the southern Kalahari and the western Highveld. Wikar in 1775 (Mossop and van der Horst 1935) Somerville in 1799 (Bradlow and Bradlow 1979), and Smith in 1835 (Kirby 1940) specifically state that the venereal form of the disease is not present in the native populations, and their lists of common disorders of the people do not include symptoms that resemble the endemic treponemal infection. Yet some of the towns that they visited contained upwards of 10,000 people in conditions epidemiologically perfect for the spread of the venereal treponeme. The venereal form of the disease was present in the Cape Colony from at least the 1690s (Grevenbroek 1695 in Schapera 1933) and was rampant amongst slaves, sailors, and soldiers by the 1730s (Mentzel 1944).

In common with other parts of the Old World, southern Africa has not produced archaeological specimens

724 | CURRENT ANTHROPOLOGY Volume 29, Number 5, December 1988

which show clear signs of treponemal disease. Periostitis occurs at regular intervals but not in patterns suggestive of yaws or endemic or venereal syphilis. Since we have a good idea of the frequency of endemic syphilis infection in modern Kalahari populations, perhaps the new immunological techniques referred to by Baker and Armelagos might be used on archaeological samples from the same region to indicate infection in individuals who do not show signs of osteological involvement. This not only would test the presence of treponemal infection in a pre-Columbian Old World population but could also indicate the presence of a specifically endemic pattern of the disease.

GEORGE T. NURSE
Department of Community Medicine, University of Papua New Guinea, P.O. Box 5623, Boroko NCD, Papua New Guinea. 2 VI 88

This satisfyingly up-to-date account of what is known about the ecogenesis of the treponematoses answers many outstanding questions and provokes some further speculation, particularly in the context of non-venereal syphilis.

Even syphilis acknowledged to be venereal is occasionally transmitted by other than the venereal route. Weeping secondary rashes and especially condylomata lata teem with treponemata, and casual skin contact with them not infrequently results in the development of chancre. This could account for the cases reported from Vienna as "endemic syphilis" by Luger (1972). The usual characterization of non-venereal syphilis as a disease of hot, dry rural areas makes it hard to agree with the ascription of its spread to overcrowding as well as imperfect hygiene. Overcrowding is more a feature of urban than of rural life, and the majority of urban populations, at least in developing countries, are not notably more cleanly. This disease is more likely to be perpetuated by the huddling together of scantily clad children outside the dwellings than within them. I have observed this in the Kalahari (Nurse et al. 1973) and in the Nafud Desert, in which the disease has lately been recorded (Pace and Csonka 1984). It probably was largely responsible for the spread and persistence of treponematosis in pre-Columbian North America. In all three environments the winters can be remarkably cold, and young children are or could have been dependent on the warmth of the bodies of their playmates. This may have played a part also in the long-standing endemicity in Bosnia and Hercegovina, where the successful eradication campaign coincided with an improvement in the standard of living (Grin and Guthe 1973). In the Kalahari, where a similar campaign was unsuccessful (Murray, Merriweather, and Freedman 1956), no change in the life-style of the San occurred at or around the time of the treatment.

It is certainly legitimate to suggest, as Baker and Armelagos do and as Hudson (1958) came close to doing, that the difference between the two forms of syphilis is purely epidemiological. Some immunity against T. pallidum does develop; if this happens in childhood, it could prevent the venereal form of the disease from emerging later. When children are more effectively shielded from infection by clothing and hygiene, the opportunity for the disease to spread may not come until the apposition of infected with uninfected mucous membrane happens during sexual activity in adults. It is not at all rare for an infectious disease occurring for the first time in adulthood to manifest itself differently from the same infection acquired in childhood: good examples of this are mumps and hepatitis A. Here, the argument from the absence of congenital syphilitic stigmata in Amerindian skeletal remains is a powerful one. It has proved impossible to distinguish microbiologically between the causative organism of venereal syphilis and that of its non-venereal counterpart. The two are almost certainly the same disease.

One or two historical points may be mentioned: Bonser (1963), in his comprehensive description of medical knowledge in England before the Norman Conquest, does not describe any disease which could possibly be a treponematosis, and this gives at least some negative support to the Columbian hypothesis. He does not mention scabies, either, which somewhat inhibits my suspicion that anything called "button scurvy" is more likely to be that than endemic syphilis. Baker and Armelagos probably derive their interpretation of the term from Lancereux (1868), to whom, however, they do not refer. Lancereux also talks of radesyge (?rosary or necklace disease), as they do, and of "sibbens." The last-named, more properly "sivvens," derives from the Gaelic suibhean, "raspberry" (Latin framboesia), which of course recalls yaws. The descriptions quoted in the Oxford English Dictionary (1933) are more suggestive of yaws than of endemic syphilis; but could yaws as we know it ever have survived in Scotland or Scandinavia? Or could this have been another treponematosis, now extinct? It may not even have been a treponematosis at all, though Pennant in his Tour in Scotland of 1776, cited in the OED, calls it a venereal disease. Perhaps we see here again the lubricious tendency to classify any disease which can have such a mode of spread as venereal, irrespective of the other, commoner routes by which it may also propagate itself.

MARY LUCAS POWELL
Museum of Anthropology, University of Kentucky, Lexington, Ky. 40506, U.S.A. 24 VI 88

In their provocative reconsideration of the centuries-old question of whether venereal syphilis originated in the Eastern or the Western Hemisphere, Baker and Armelagos marshal an impressive array of historical, epidemiological, and paleopathological evidence that this deadly form of treponemal disease was America's gift to Europe's invading conquerers. Skeletal specimens from a multitude of New World sites display lesions that meet the key diagnostic criteria set forth for treponemal disease by Hackett (1976). While some of these may date from the early period of European contact and are therefore suspect in the present context, others (such as the cases cited from the Indian Knoll site in Kentucky) securely establish the existence of treponematosis on this side of the Atlantic Ocean several millennia before the voyages of Columbus. No human cases have been documented that rival in antiquity the supposedly syphilitic Pleistocene bear reported by Rothschild and Turnbull (1987). This absence is not surprising, given the lack of human remains from that early time, but the pathologic lesions in the animal skeleton could be more reasonably diagnosed as representing nonspecific osteomyelitis compounded by an opportunistic fungal infection. The possibility that the results of the immunofluorescence analysis in that case represent a "false positive" reaction to related saprophytic or free-living spirochetes immunologically similar to the genus Treponema (Cockburn 1963:153) should also be kept in mind.

Given the abundance of pre-Columbian New World skeletal evidence for treponemal disease as evaluated by modern paleoepidemiological standards, as compared with the virtual absence of convincing contemporaneous Old World cases, the authors' conclusion that the appearance of venereal syphilis in early 16th-century Europe represented the adaptive transmutation of an ancient New World nonvenereal disease in a novel epidemiological context does not seem unreasonable. The existence of anomalous cases of apparently congenital origin, such as the child from pre–A.D. 1400 Virginia described by Ortner and Putschar (1981:207–10), does not invalidate arguments for the essentially nonvenereal nature of the New World treponematosis. Given the profound similarities documented between the nonvenereal and venereal treponema strains (Hudson 1958, 1965a), Grin (1956) has noted that transplacental infection should theoretically be possible. He argues that the rarity of this occurrence in modern yaws and endemic syphilis probably results from the typically very low levels of pathogenic treponemes in the maternal bloodstream at the time of pregnancy because of the long period of time separating treponemal infection in childhood from the onset of pregnancy in adulthood.

The remainder of my comments will address the seeming contradiction noted by the authors between expected frequencies of bone lesions from nonvenereal treponematoses, based upon modern clinical studies (cf. Steinbock 1976), and the frequencies of bone involvement in prehistoric skeletal series reported by myself (Powell 1988a, b, c, d) and other researchers (Cassidy 1980, 1984; Cook 1976, 1984; Brues 1966). The studies cited by Steinbock (1976) relied upon radiographic or clinical evidence (e.g., descriptions of bone pain) of bone involvement, thereby insuring that only certain levels of bone involvement would be noted. Lesser levels (e.g., cortical striations indicative of minor periosteal elevation) or, more important, remodeled lesions in older individuals would tend to be systematically excluded. Conversely, direct observation of dry bone specimens, with emphasis upon examination of all elements present

from each individual in a series, would include a broader range of lesser degrees of bone involvement. Admittedly, many of these manifestations are nonspecific in nature and could not be used alone to diagnose treponematosis in the absence of other, more clearly pathognomonic lesions. Nonetheless, a close reading of Hackett's (1951) masterful discussion of bone lesions of yaws and Hudson's detailed descriptions of bone involvement in endemic syphilis (1958, 1965a) gives a vivid impression of the full range of associated pathology. Clinical and paleopathological studies alike that emphasize only the "classic" treponemal lesions will invariably overlook the less spectacular evidence that is more abundant in both living and skeletal populations afflicted with treponemal disease. The soundest approach from an epidemiological perspective is to focus upon the "classic" lesions for the initial diagnosis of the disease in a particular specimen or population and then describe the lesser forms of involvement to document the specific gradient of pathological involvement observed in that particular context. In the skeletal series from Moundville, Irene Mound, and Nodena that I have observed, only a few cases could be presented as "classic examples" of treponematosis, yet it would make no sense epidemiologically to assume that those few cases were the only individuals affected in those populations. Hence the "seeming contradiction" mentioned earlier stems more from differences in methodology of observation and perspective of interpretation than from any real differences between the disease variants in question. Surely not all of the periostitis observed at Moundville, Irene Mound, and Nodena represents treponemal involvement, but undoubtedly a great deal of it does even in cases that cannot be securely diagnosed. However, any comprehensive assessment of the biological costs of chronic endemic disease in a population must take into consideration not only the most severe cases but also the much larger number of minor cases that also exacted their toll in the form of pain, depleted energy, and decreased resistance to other diseases.

BRUCE M. ROTHSCHILD
Department of Medicine, Northeast Ohio Universities College of Medicine and St. Elizabeth Hospital and Department of Earth Sciences, The Carnegie Institute, Pittsburgh, Pa. 15213, U.S.A. 24 v 88

Baker and Armelagos are to be congratulated for a masterful review and analysis of the history of treponemal disease. Provenience of historical as well as skeletal information and the often nonspecific nature of the latter are well documented as previous sources of confusion. While the idea of 19,000 leprosaria (Steinbock 1976) strains credulity, Baker and Armelagos appropriately note skeletal pathologic confirmation of the diagnosis of leprosy in a leper cemetery (Weiss and Møller-Christensen 1971) apparently associated with one such asylum. While a number of Old World venereal diseases were apparently called leprosy, the available skeletal re-

726 | CURRENT ANTHROPOLOGY Volume 29, Number 5, December 1988

mains provide no convincing evidence for treponemal disease. Difficult to reconcile with the skeletal record is Holcomb's (1934) notation that one medieval physician changed the title of his chapter "Leprosy" to "Morbus Gallicus" (the 16th-century European name for syphilis) without altering the text. Contemporary reporting of endemic syphilis as leprosy in Iraq (Hudson 1958, Steinbock 1976) further documents the challenge of deciphering pathology in historic records.

The unitarian hypothesis of treponemal diseases as an environmental adaptation or subspecies phenomenon (Hudson 1965b) retains merit even if no pre-Columbian Old World treponemal disease is identifiable. While the organisms of venereal syphilis cannot be distinguished immunologically or grossly, they can biologically. In vivo cultures (natural infections) reveal distinguishable dermatologic and osseous changes. Although the individual skeletal lesions of the various treponemal diseases cannot be distinguished, their differing skeletal distributions afford an epidemiologic approach (Hudson 1928, Hunt and Johnson 1923). Examination of a single bone or individual does not allow epidemiologic assessment, but examination of well-defined skeletal populations for population frequency and skeletal distribution of lesions provides samples that can be statistically compared with known "modern" afflicted populations (Woods and Rothschild n.d.). As treatment may affect skeletal manifestations and distribution, the comparison "modern" populations should be drawn from the prepenicillin era.

Evidence of congenital lesions would be expected on sampling a population affected by venereal syphilis. The diseases therefore remaining to be distinguished are nonvenereal syphilis and yaws. Bone lesions are noted in 9–24% of venereal syphilis, 3–5% of endemic syphilis, and 10–15% of yaws (Hudson 1958, Moss and Bigelow 1922, Steinbock 1976, Whitney 1915). While venereal and endemic syphilis predominantly affect the lower extremities (Steinbock 1976), yaws has a predilection for the upper (Moss and Bigelow 1922, Steinbock 1976, Whitney 1915). Digits are commonly involved in yaws but only rarely in syphilis. Cranial involvement in yaws is much less severe than in syphilis (though more generalized when it does occur). Syphilis, producing saddle-nose deformity, more commonly affects the nasal bone than does yaws, which more commonly affects the palate and maxillary bones. Examination of the epidemiology of the *Hippelates pallipes* fly, the insect vector of yaws (Sanchez, Mazzotti, and Salensas 1961, Turner 1937), may also provide diagnostic insight for a given population. This approach is of course premised on the diseases' having retained their characteristics through the millennia. Although that premise is of course subject to scrutiny, correlation of pre-Columbian skeletal distribution with that observed in the preantibiotic era would strongly suggest the identity of the disease. Treponemal disease can now be immunologically confirmed (Rothschild and Turnbull 1987). The controversy regarding the origin of treponemal disease should be resolved as the gummatous lesions from all suspected pre-Columbian skeletons are subjected to immunologic analysis. Even the specific treponemal disease responsible may well be determinable by epidemiologic analysis of such verified skeletal populations.

SHELLEY R. SAUNDERS
Department of Anthropology, McMaster University, Hamilton, Ont., Canada L8S 4L9. 13 VI 88

The novice "syphilologist," sifting through a voluminous literature on the origin of the disease, must feel like the wind-blown sapling bending to each successive argument, pre-Columbian, Columbian, or unitarian. Hudson's charge that medical historians tend to choose the "right" witnesses and dates is apt. Baker and Armelagos's survey of the historical events surrounding the ca. 1500 epidemic raises several questions:

What evidence is there for Columbus's men's having contracted the disease in the Indies during the first and/or second voyages?

Were there Spanish troops in Charles VIII's army, and, if so, was there time for them to have picked up the disease from Columbus's Indian captives in Barcelona or through infected crewmen and transmitted it to Naples?

Do the several European edicts issued regarding the disease really postdate Columbus's return from the first and/or second voyages?

Baker and Armelagos mention possible ambiguities in dating Charles's Naples campaign because of the use of different calendars. Since the difference is on the order of three months, this might put Charles's arrival in France about a month before the Worms edict. One wonders that the disease would have become widespread in Germany in such a short time. Morison (1942) indicates that there is no evidence in any of the *local* chronicles of the time of an outbreak of syphilis in Naples during Charles's campaign. He also notes that the presence of Spanish troops in Charles's army is debated by historians. He finds no evidence for Columbus's men's having become severely ill during the first or second voyages either in Columbus's journal or in other contemporary accounts by observers less likely than Columbus, writing for Isabella, to be biased in this regard. Baker and Armelagos's comments on the date of publication of Diaz de Isla's account confirm what seems to me the near futility of attempting to unravel the documentary history. Morison (though himself a Columbian supporter) agrees with Holcomb's translation of Diaz de Isla's "*al presente*" to mean the idiomatic "at that time" rather than "at present," which would weaken the argument that the treatise was written before 1506.

As Baker and Armelagos point out, most telling is the apparent absence of skeletal evidence of syphilis in the Old World. I agree that the lack of syphilitic bones in pre-1492 leper cemeteries and the weakness of the proposed Old World skeletal cases are convincing, but, again, I have some questions and comments:

That 80–90% of European skeletal collections are skulls alone compromises attempts at conclusive skeletal diagnoses.

There is no mention here of evidence, or lack thereof, of pathological skeletal material from Africa. Is there any?

The exceedingly rapid geographic spread of the disease to different populations in the Old World so soon after the proposed 1493 date is incredible. Suzuki (1984a) reports the entry of syphilis into Japan from the east coast of China at about A.D. 1512. Can this be attributed solely to European sea exploration?

Although Baker and Armelagos's discussion of the New World skeletal evidence is extensive, there is only one reference to samples in Canada. Hartney (1978) has identified potential pre-Columbian and early historic cases (admittedly not thoroughly discussed in the literature) of treponemal disease amongst southern Ontario Iroquois. Recently, the recovery of a potential case of osseous syphilis in a skeleton from a 16th-century village has prompted me to reexamine the southern Ontario evidence. It is possible that treponemal disease became prevalent in this region as settlement intensified and population increased in the 15th century.

Finally, why the persistent fascination with the *origin* of syphilis? Certainly the unitarian theory was attractive when formulated because it made sense in terms of evolutionary biology (see also Hollander 1981). The opposition of Columbian and unitarian theories reflects a deeper dissension between logical determinism and chance. A hypothesis that postulates a unique past event as its basis should have some observable consequences for the present, and I don't see what these are from the Columbian theory. If it prompts researchers to explore the immunological testing of exhumed bone, so much the better, but I doubt that the controversy will be resolved to everyone's satisfacion in the near future. The current epidemic levels of syphilis and its association with AIDS emphasize the fact that infectious diseases are complex bioecological puzzles reflecting a range of interactions among biological, environmental, and social forces. Herein, and not in origins alone, lie the intriguing problems for experimental and historical researchers alike.

MILAN STLOUKAL
Národni Muzeum v Praze, tř. Vitězného února 74, 115 79 Prague 1, Czechoslovakia. 21 VI 88

This paper presents an interesting survey of the literature and arrives at a conclusion essentially expressing my long-time conviction. Baker and Armelagos weaken their conclusion that syphilis was brought to Europe by the participants in the Columbian expeditions, however, with the statement that European evidence authorizing this conclusion is lacking. Surprisingly, they seem not to be acquainted with the European literature on the subject. In the last 20 to 30 years over 10,000 skeletons from medieval cemeteries in "Czechoslovakia have been studied and published; the majority date to the 7th–11th century, but skeletons from the late Middle Ages are also available. In this very large collection no cases that

could be diagnosed as syphilis have been found. The differential diagnosis of types of treponematosis, though certainly a problem, is unimportant in this connection because in these medieval collections it is simply out of the question.

The number of modern skeletons available for study is much smaller. Because cemeteries from the 16th–18th century are less attractive to archaeologists, the discovery of such skeletons is exceptional. In spite of this, a number of them have been anthropologically studied and published, and in addition we have bones from ossuaries, as a rule of the same date. Here, in contrast, wherever we have a sizable set of remains at our disposal we almost always find traces of lesions on tibiae, fibulae, and skulls, some certainly of syphilitic origin and the rest possibly so. This contrast between the collections from before the end of the 15th century and those from later centuries is striking indeed.

Increasing urbanization and improved hygiene need not, I think, be closely connected. On the contrary, concentration of great numbers in medieval towns evidently produced a change for the worse in both hygiene and nutrition. But this fundamental change, with its increased potential for the diffusion of various epidemics, occurred earlier in Central Europe, very probably in the 13th century. The improvement of medicine at the end of the Middle Ages may not have been so substantial as to play a substantial role in the health of whole populations. Is it not possible to see the reason for the reduction in frequency of leprosy in the fact that it had passed its zenith and struck an immunological barrier in European populations? Moreover, traces of leprosy are rather rare in bone material, and therefore we can only rely on historical sources, untrustworthy with regard to diagnosis as they are.

REBECCA STOREY
Department of Anthropology, University of Houston, Houston, Tex. 77004, U.S.A. 22 VI 88

The effects of European contact with the New World were profound for both worlds, but the brunt of its disease and cultural disruption has fallen upon the Native American (Crosby 1972, Dobyns 1984, Denevan 1976). The idea that the Americas gave venereal syphilis to Europe has always seemed like a kind of rough justice. Because we are interested in the epidemiological aspects of the Columbian era, however, syphilis needs to be put in its proper place, at least as much as the evidence will allow.

It is in marshalling this evidence, both documentary and skeletal, that this article by Baker and Armelagos makes a real contribution. The development of paleopathological methods has made it finally possible for researchers, instead of depending on documentary sources, to look at the skeletal evidence that is the best we have for the origin of syphilis. Baker and Armelagos's review indicates that there is no good evidence of treponemal lesions on pre-Columbian skeletons in Europe and considerable such evidence from pre-Columbian times in the New World.

While I understand that one of the objectives of the article was a complete listing of the skeletons ever considered in the syphilis controversy, it would have been clearer if doubtful specimens had been grouped together and skeletons whose lesions are góod evidence for treponematosis presented more forcefully. The listing of skeleton after skeleton, many with questionable dates or lesions, tends to diffuse the argument that New World specimens are plentiful.

I agree that individuals with bone lesions will likely be rare. In my own work with the skeletons from an apartment compound in the preindustrial city of Teotihuacan (ca. A.D. 300–700) and the skeletal population from the Late Classic Maya center of Copan (ca. A.D. 700–1100), lesions diagnostic of treponematosis on skulls and especially tibiae are found in about 1% of individuals. Furthermore, there are no clear cases of congenital syphilis in these populations. The individuals affected are middle-aged to older adults. While postcranial periosteal lesions are common, they cannot necessarily be attributed to treponematosis, even "on trial."

Nevertheless, the lack of clear Old World pre-Columbian skeletal lesions of treponematosis should discredit the pre-Columbian hypothesis. I agree with Baker and Armelagos that, no matter what one feels about the documentary evidence, enough skeletal material is available from Europe alone to produce evidence of these lesions if the disease was present, and the fact that not even leper-colony material has yielded any such evidence is telling. The only controversy that may remain has to do with the transmission of nonvenereal and venereal treponematosis. Baker and Armelagos's epidemiological hypothesis may not explain everything. Preindustrial cities or other types of population nucleation are notorious centers of disease, where infections tend to cycle continually through the population (McNeill 1976). Hygiene may not have been much better in large population nucleations than in rural areas before modern sanitation systems, and water contamination is a health hazard even today. Better understanding of the epidemiology of treponematosis, especially the nonvenereal forms, will finally allow us to explain what happened at the Columbian contact and how syphilis was transferred from one world to another.

DAVID S. WEAVER
Departments of Anthropology and Comparative Medicine, Wake Forest University, Winston-Salem, N.C. 27109, U.S.A. 23 VI 88

Baker and Armelagos have compiled an impressive and very useful review of the propositions and data concerning the origin and antiquity of syphilis. In fact, they properly do not restrict the paper to syphilis, reflecting the likelihood that treponemal conditions have had a complex and convoluted evolutionary history. Their case against European pre-Columbian syphilis, although largely based on a lack of clear evidence, is well made. Particularly since various publications by Cook, Powell, and others, the skeletal evidence for pre-Columbian New World treponemal conditions has been accumulating rapidly. We have observed skeletal conditions consistent with a treponematal syndrome in our ongoing studies of ossuary material from coastal North Carolina (Bogdan and Weaver 1988) and since have seen similar and even more characteristic skeletal signs, including stellate bone lesions, cavitation, and radial scars, in other coastal ossuary material. The debate will soon be settled in favor of a New World Syndrome by skeletal evidence from a number of quarters.

Baker and Armelagos could clarify the theoretical implications of at least two epidemiological points: why a high frequency of skeletal signs of infection per se would be useful to exclude syphilis as a diagnosis and how they would have us distinguish venereal from nonvenereal treponemal infections. This last point may prove intractable.

A final aside may be of some interest. Since the zoonotic origin of the human HIV's (AIDS viruses), probably in African green monkeys, was proposed by Kanki et al. (1986), many of us have been confused by the lack of overt symptoms in most apparently infected nonhuman primates (especially African green monkeys) and by the lack of a clear mode of transmission for the virus. It now seems likely that the proposed HTLV-4 is a laboratory contaminant (STLV-III$_{mac}$) and not a strain or variety that is communicable to humans (Kestler et al. 1988). Of course, this does not alter the general points about disease/host coadaptation made by Baker and Armelagos, but it eventually may turn out to be of some comfort to those of us working with nonhuman primates on a daily basis.

AL B. WESOLOWSKY
Journal of Field Archaeology, Boston University, 675 Commonwealth Ave., Boston, Mass. 02215, U.S.A. 22 VI 88

When I was an undergraduate, one of the first series of prehistoric New World skeletons I was shown had a number of instances of "cortical swelling" on the tibiae. In subsequent years I noticed similar, characteristic occurrences in other series and wondered if perhaps treponematosis might be the culprit. I suspect that anyone with any amount of experience with New World materials has harbored similar thoughts.

Now we have this important and timely contribution to the debate on the origins of the treponematoses, and it should be read with care by historians of disease, historiographers, and archaeologists. It brings together an updated synthesis of several theories and strands of research and includes recent and older scholarship on an epidemic that, as the authors point out, has implications for the current concern with the spread of Acquired Immune Deficiency Syndrome.

The article is somewhat ambitious in its scope and tries to do several things, only one of which it does well. The necessary review of theories regarding the introduction of syphilis into Europe is less effective than it could have been. Its organization, so promising at first, becomes, finally, an obstacle to an appreciation of the wealth of information that the authors are trying to bring together. The political and medical status of Europe from 1494 through the first half of the 16th century is complex but explicable; this article does little to clarify matters. The putative role of the army of Charles VIII of France in the spread of syphilis is crucial to the Columbian hypothesis, but we are presented with only a patchy account of both the campaign and the chronology of the various edicts and proclamations that seem to have been issued in the wake of the siege of Naples.

The use of the early accounts of Columbus's voyages is heartening, and it is here, I think, that Baker and Armelagos are in more familiar surroundings and begin to speak with greater authority. The principal contribution of this article is its use of excavated skeletal remains to demonstrate the existence of treponematosis in the New World long before the European discovery of America. I *think* that the authors have demonstrated their main contention, but I am frustrated by three aspects of their presentation. (1) Since several direct quotations from articles that discuss skeletal materials are used, one surmises that the descriptions and diagnoses of the remainder are paraphrases of the original publications, but one cannot be certain. Also, it is not clear which, if any, of these materials the authors have themselves examined. (2) The review consists of an east-to-west, north-to-south presentation that has no bearing on the problem at hand. It merely forces the reader to construct a personal chart of the chronology and incidence, as seen in the excavated remains, of the disease in the Americas. (3) The most serious shortcoming in this otherwise most useful survey is the utter lack of illustrations of specimens. There are frequent citations to figures that appear in the original publications, so one may be assured that the specimens are shown in print, but how is the specialist to judge the accuracy of these observations and the resultant diagnoses?

The importance of this survey of excavated remains is not to be underestimated. It does appear that while Europe has no convincing evidence of syphilis prior to 1493, America has plenty. If we accept these diagnoses of treponemal infections in New World skeletons, and I see no reason we should not, it is clear that this disease (or diseases) developed in the New World long before 1492 and that the crews of Columbus's voyage are historically and epidemiologically the most likely vector for the introduction of syphilis into Europe.

It is a disappointment that no mention is made of McNeill's *Plagues and Peoples* (1976), especially since Baker and Armelagos, correctly, I am sure, point out in their closing argument that immunological analyses of diseased bone material should resolve the controversy. More than a decade ago, McNeill pointed out (p. 194) that "proof, one way or the other, awaits development of pre-

cise and reliable methods whereby the organisms causing lesions in ancient bones can be identified."

JOHN A. WILLIAMS
Department of Anthropology, University of North Dakota, Grand Forks, N.D. 58201, U.S.A. 23 VI 88

Like the question of the origin of New World tuberculosis (Buikstra 1981, Clark et al. 1987), that of syphilis has not been conclusively answered. As Baker and Armelagos point out, it is beneficial from time to time to summarize the evidence on such complex issues. While the reader unversed in diagnosis and interpretation may have difficulty understanding some sections of their article, they should be commended for their concise presentation of the wide range of information on the subject of syphilis. Although they favor a New World origin for venereal syphilis, they maintain an even hand in presenting all sides of the argument.

The conjecture that New World treponematoses, like tuberculosis, may have experienced an expansion with the appearance of sedentary agriculture, as opposed to urbanization, is intriguing (Hudson 1965a). It is unfortunate that Baker and Armelagos do not expand on this hypothesis, probably one of the more important contributions of their synthesis. To a certain extent, the evidence for syphilis and tuberculosis in the New World is similarly ambiguous and equivocal. For example, an examination of several hundred prehorticulture Plains Indian skeletons ranging in age from Archaic to Late Woodland has yet to turn up a single case of treponemal infection (Gregg and Gregg 1987). To date only two cases of skeletal tuberculosis have been identified in this same series of samples (Williams 1985). Yet both diseases are documented on the Northern Plains by the early 19th century, prior to any significant Euro-American contact but after the adoption of a sedentary subsistence pattern (Reid 1947–48, Thwaites 1905).

Although this article does not end the controversy surrounding the origins of venereal syphilis, it brings us closer to formulating a more appropriate hypothesis.

Reply

BRENDA J. BAKER AND GEORGE J. ARMELAGOS
Amherst, Mass., U.S.A. 30 VII 88

It is gratifying to receive such a positive response to our paper. Our position that nonvenereal treponemal infection is a New World disease that spread to the Old World and became a venereal disease following European contact is accepted by most of the commentators. Kelley, however, sees the evolution of the syphilis as a "tired" topic and considers our paper similar in structure and content to Steinbock's (1976). We feel that active investigation of even a "tired" topic is likely to illuminate

730 | CURRENT ANTHROPOLOGY Volume 29, Number 5, December 1988

new facets of it. We did in fact rely extensively on Steinbock, as the frequency of citations indicates. He provides an exceptional analysis of the differential diagnosis of the treponemal infections and extensive discussion of the skeletal evidence of treponemal infection in the New and Old Worlds. Even with his thorough study, however, he sees a need for additional work: "The paucity of lesions and questionable dating and diagnosis of specimens has caused some authorities to doubt the presence of syphilis in the New World before European contact." He agrees with T. Dale Stewart's call for "a general survey of the New World material, particularly newly excavated material, to establish the prevalence and distribution of venereal and nonvenereal syphilis in well-dated specimens" (Steinbock 1976:96–97). Our paper is a response to this call.

Only Drusini strongly objects to our position, while Brothwell says that the hypothesis we offer is one that can nearly be embraced but suggests that there is tantalizing evidence of pre-Columbian treponemal infection in the Old World that does not fit it. Others, while in general agreement, question or comment on aspects of our interpretation.

Drusini believes that our analysis of the documentary evidence is skewed toward a New World origin and that we have not considered the osteological evidence from the Old World that supports the pre-Columbian origin of syphilis. He places great emphasis on the documentary evidence, arguing among other things that some varieties of scabies healed completely after mercury ointment treatment and that in the proceedings of a 1493 trial evidence was presented that showed the disease to be sexually transmitted. We do not dispute this interpretation and have presented similar ones of others. In fact, as we have reported, mercury ointment was prescribed for a variety of ailments, including headaches (for which it was rubbed on the inner arm). We do not find this or Drusini's other documentary evidence very compelling. The fact that Italian, Sicilian, and German physicians recognized a venereal disease before 1493 and made no link to the New World at the time is not sufficient to warrant the identification of the disease as syphilis.

Drusini considers our failure to cite Guerra (1978) a major omission. We have since read Guerra's work, and while it is an excellent treatment of the literary history of the controversy, it has significant shortcomings. It does not, for example, consider the osteological evidence that is essential for understanding the origin of treponemal infection, and we find little that is new in the interpretation of the documentary evidence. Guerra's case for pre-Columbian syphilis in the Old World is based on the argument that diseases described in the literature prior to 1493 are in fact syphilis. We continue to view these reports as ambiguous. Drusini quotes Guerra as saying that current understanding of the environmental effects on the disease has altered the context for discussion of the role of America in the history of syphilis. Guerra's approach (p. 57) is reminiscent of Hackett's:

There were in America the four types of human pathogenic treponematoses, pinta, yaws, venereal syphilis and probably endemic syphilis, in pre-Columbian times, while there existed in Europe at the same time venereal and endemic syphilis. The discovery of America brought the spread to Europe of American *bubas* or yaws, a new rural and tropical treponematosis; after several generations, yaws adapted itself to the temperate urban environment of venereal syphilis, changing the original violent epidemiological character, as corresponding to a new mutant of treponematoses.

We believe that our analysis of the documentary evidence is fair and evenhanded. Nurse cites additional (although negative) evidence that supports it. The material cited by Drusini does not alter the case. We do wish that there were more clear-cut evidence concerning the actual vector of transmission. Saunders asks if there is evidence that Columbus's sailors were infected with the treponemal pathogen. In the paragraph of Diaz de Isla's original manuscript cited earlier, Williams et al. (1927: 695) point to a report that the disease "was seen in the armada itself in a pilot of Palos who was called Pinçon and others." Saunders is also concerned about the timing of the transmission by Charles VIII's troops, but while the time is short there is no evidence that this rapid transmission could not have occurred.

As for the osteological evidence, Drusini would add Rokhlin (1965) on syphilitic bones from the trans-Baikal region of Siberia dated 3000–2000 B.C. We have in fact cited this material, but with the 1000–800 B.C. date for reported by Steinbock. Drusini suggests that the absence of other European examples is simply the result of a lack of research in the area. Becker, Saunders, and Brothwell raise similar issues of sampling.

Brothwell states that we cannot ignore the osteological evidence for pre-Columbian Old World treponemal infection. In addition to the reports he cites from the Marianas, Borneo, and Australia, we have since uncovered Pietrusewsky's (1971) publication of a possible case of yaws in precontact Tonga. Brothwell also points to reports of syphilis in medieval York and Trondheim. The evidence from Trondheim is provocative because the level from which it comes must be earlier than 1531, the burial being covered by a deposit of wood ash from a fire recorded at that time. There is no other evidence of treponemal infection from this period, but there is indication of it in the subsequent periods of occupation. The possibility that the disease was brought back by earlier Norse explorers of the New World ought to be considered.

Contrary to the impression conveyed in our paper, Steinbock, while recognizing problems with the dating of the Australian specimens, does state that there is a strong suggestion of precontact syphilis in Australia.

While we do not deny the importance of this osteological evidence, pre-Columbian examples from the Old World are sparse compared with those found in the New World. In addition, if the alleged venereal disease in pre-

Columbian Europe had in fact been syphilis, then we would expect to find widespread skeletal evidence of it. Even in those instances in which the dating of the osteological specimen is not in dispute, the evidence is meager; for example, on the York specimen the classic stellate scars are found on the fragmentary cranium of one individual, and there is diffuse osteitis on a tibia and a fibula of another.

Are these differences a matter of sampling? Becker suggests that the interest shown by Americans has been matched only in England and Denmark, and Saunders points out that European museum collections are mostly skulls, perhaps not the best part for identifying treponemal infection. Brothwell, who suggests that the original homeland of the treponemes may be Asia, implies a similar concern for sampling in that area. To prove that treponemal infection did not occur in pre-Columbian Europe is extremely difficult, since we are arguing from negative evidence. It is not that we were not familiar with the European evidence, as Stloukal implies, but that we were unwilling to report an absence of evidence unless this was specifically stated.

In responding to the question of sampling we should examine the areas in which there has been extensive excavation. The work on leper cemeteries in Denmark is especially critical, since many of those who claim that syphilis existed in pre-Columbian Europe believe that many individuals who were diagnosed as lepers were in fact suffering from syphilis. Examination of cemeteries associated with leprosaria has not revealed individuals with treponemal lesions. Furthermore, Stloukal notes that in the last 20–30 years over 10,000 skeletons have been excavated and studied from medieval Czechoslovakian cemeteries without producing any evidence of syphilis, whereas in the 16th–18th century cemeteries there is ample such evidence.

Saunders asks about the evidence from Africa. Steinbock (1976:97) states that Smith and Jones (1910) examined 25,000 Egyptian skeletons and found no indication of syphilis. A reexamination by Hussein (1949) describes two possible cases. Armelagos and colleagues found no evidence in an examination of 1,000 Meroitic, X-group, and Christian burials from the Republic of the Sudan. Morris confirms that there are no reports of treponemal infection in South Africa prior to European contact.

Morimoto points out that the first evidence of venereal syphilis in Japan comes from Kyoto in 1512, and Saunders inquires about the relationship of this date to the earliest arrival of Europeans in Japan. This occurrence pre-dates the arrival of European sailors by 30 years. Suzuki (1984b) states that shortly after that first occurrence there was a virulent outbreak. He also cites Koganei's (1894) description of a case of syphilis in an Ainu skeleton and his own 1963 report of evidence of syphilis in 3 of 23 skulls from the Muromachi period. He describes another case of syphilis from a burial associated with a medieval castle from Hokkaido (1984c).

Storey claims that the inclusion of doubtful specimens from the New World diffuses the argument that the New World specimens are plentiful. We saw a need, however,

to sort through all the material and present it as we resurrected the hypothesis of a New World origin. Geise, Saunders, Weaver, and Storey provide additional data on pre-Columbian treponemal infections in the New World. Storey points out, further, that there is no evidence of congenital syphilis at either Teotihuacan or Copan. Nor would we expect it, since venereal syphilis need not be present wherever there is urbanization. While not all periosteal involvement need be treponemal, Story might find it fruitful to reevaluate the proportion that is the result of treponemal infection. Allison et al. (1982) have reported evidence of treponemal infection in South America that is dated at 7,000 years ago. If the diagnosis and dating are confirmed, this discovery would suggest great antiquity for the treponemes in the New World.

Wesolowsky asks if we have seen the material that we report in the paper. Unfortunately, we have not seen much of the material discussed but have relied on the primary investigators' descriptions and illustrations. We apologize for the absence of illustrations here but have been careful to cite the relevant ones in the published material reviewed.

Our presenting this synthesis was made possible by the agreement that has developed among skeletal biologists as a result of the work of Hackett and others in defining the criteria for diagnosis. Workshops held at the annual meetings of the Paleopathology Association have been very effective in developing consensus on diagnostic criteria. In addition, Powell, Cook, and others have undertaken excellent studies using the most up-to-date methods of diagnosis and provided the epidemiological model for others to use in examining their material for evidence of treponemal infections.

Hackett (1976) was concerned that few pre-Columbian American bones exhibited diagnostic features of treponematosis, and we calculated that we would expect to find lesions in 1–5% of the individual skeletons if the disease were endemic. In contrast, researchers such as Powell, Cook, and others working in the East and Midwest find half of their populations showing the disease. Powell provides a reasonable resolution of this riddle in pointing to the difference between the earlier radiographic assessments and the most recent assessments based on the direct observation of dry bones. Powell also solves another problem of interpretation—that of the evidence for transplacental infection—by citing Grin (1956) to the effect that transplacental transmission is possible. Its rarity in modern yaws and endemic syphilis reflects the generally low level of pathogenic treponemes in the maternal bloodstream because of the length of time separating the onset of the treponemal infection and the occurrence of pregnancy.

Weaver asks if distinction between nonvenereal and venereal syphilis is intractable. As we have pointed out, the skeletal symptoms are similar, but the pattern of infection in the population is likely to be different. For example, nonvenereal syphilis is likely to infect younger individuals prior to reaching sexual maturity. If a population is exposed to nonvenereal syphilis, we would not

732 | CURRENT ANTHROPOLOGY Volume 29, Number 5, December 1988

expect to find any individuals with evidence of congenital transmission.

Rothschild suggests that immunological testing can confirm treponemal infection in prehistoric bone. He argues that once all the pre-Columbian bones with suspected treponemal infections have been analysed in this way, the controversy will be resolved, and Kelley echoes this view. Geise questions it, noting that doubts have already been raised about the immunological evidence of the treponemal infection in the Pleistocene bear. Powell suggests that it may represent a nonspecific osteomyelitis with an opportunistic fungal infection that gives a false positive result. On reflection, while we see tremendous possibilities for immunological testing, we agree that it will not present a quick solution. As Brothwell notes, the analysis of the treponemes in other vertebrates will be necessary to see if this is in fact a zoonosis.

Becker states that the crux of our argument is the transformation of the treponemal pathogen under differing environmental and social circumstances. While generally agreeing with our position, he asks if venereal syphilis spread with unusual virulence into the Old World from the New because the urban environment conduced to it and, if so, why the New World distribution is not associated with urban centers. We do not claim that venereal syphilis existed in the New World; rather, we argue that the endemic nonvenereal treponemal infection was present and was transformed into a sexually transmitted disease following its spread to Europe. We do not see a need for urban centers for the transmission of endemic treponemal infections. As Nurse points out, it is "the huddling together of scantily clad children" that is the most likely avenue for the transmission of the pathogen. We do agree with Hudson that urban centers are an ideal environment for the sexual transmission of treponemal disease. Hudson argues, however, that this is because of improved hygiene that delayed the transmission until it was spread sexually. We agree with Becker, Nurse, and others that improved hygiene is not a feature of urban life.

Several of the comments suggest that we deal more fully with the question of the impact of infectious disease in the New World. While this was not one of our objectives, we will respond. Storey and others mention the problems with the notion of depopulation cited by a number of researchers (Crosby 1972, Dobyns 1984, Denevan 1976). Becker argues that there is no evidence of a universal decline in population following contact. While we agree that depopulation was not universal, we would not want to minimize its impact in many areas.

Saunders argues that the postulation of a unique past event should have observable consequences for the present that do not seem to emerge from the Columbian hypothesis. We have elsewhere discussed the limitations of historical studies that are concerned only with establishing the chronological and spatial dimensions of a specific disease (Armelagos, Mielke, and Winter 1971). Paleopathology has in the past been hindered by the constant search for the earliest manifestation of a disease. We believe that biocultural and processual analysis that

goes beyond history is an important aspect of paleopathology as a science. We see our discussion of the treponemal infections in a broader context that considers methods of analysis, use of skeletal and documentary evidence, ecology, and the evolution of pathogen and host.

One of the pleasing aspects of presenting a review such as this is eliciting responses that suggest future research. Morris notes that yaws, endemic syphilis, and venereal syphilis coexist today in southern Africa. As he points out, this would be an ideal region in which to examine the ecological relationships between the pathogen and its physical and social environment in historical context.

While we realize that we have not had the last word in this interesting controversy, we hope that we have clarified the issues for the continuing debate.

References Cited

ACKERNECHT, ERWIN H. 1955. *A short history of medicine.* New York: Ronald Press. [AD]
———. 1965. *History and geography of the most important diseases.* New York: Hafner. [AD]
ALLISON, M. J., G. FOCACCI, E. GERSZETEN, M. FOUANT, AND M. CEBELIN. 1982. La sifílis: ¿Una enfermedad americana? *Chungara* 9:275–83.
ANDERSEN, J. G. 1969. Studies in the mediaeval diagnosis of leprosy in Denmark. *Danish Medical Bulletin* 16(suppl. 9):1–142.
ANDERSON, JAMES E. 1965. Human skeletons of Tehuacan. *Science* 148:496–97.
ANDERSON, T., C. ARCINI, S. ANDA, A. TANGERUD, AND G. ROBERTSEN. 1986. Suspected endemic syphilis (treponarid) in sixteenth-century Norway. *Medical History* 30:341–50. [DB]
ARMELAGOS, G. J., J. H. MIELKE, AND J. WINTER. 1971. *Bibliography of human paleopathology.* Department of Anthropology, University of Massachusetts, Research Reports 8.
ASSOCIATED PRESS. 1987. Report says AIDS surfaced in 1969. *Boston Globe,* October 25, p. 21.
BAKER, BRENDA J. 1985. Use of written documentation in diagnoses of pre-Columbian syphilis. Paper presented at the 12th annual meeting of the Paleopathology Association, Knoxville, Tenn.
BECKER, MARSHALL JOSEPH. 1988. "Lenape population at the time of European contact: Estimating native numbers in the lower Delaware Valley," in *Proceedings of the American Philosophical Society.* Edited by Susan E. Klepp. Philadelphia: American Philosophical Society. [MJB]
BLOCH, IWAN. 1901–11. *Der Ursprung der Syphilis.* Jena: Fischer. [AD]
BOGDAN, G., AND D. S. WEAVER. 1988. Possible treponematosis in human skeletons from a pre-Columbian ossuary of coastal North Carolina. *American Journal of Physical Anthropology* 75:187–88. [DSW]
BONSER, W. 1963. *The medical background of Anglo-Saxon England.* London: Wellcome Historical Medical Library. [GTN]
BRADLOW, E., AND F. BRADLOW. 1979. *William Somerville's narrative of his journeys to the eastern Cape Frontier and to Lattakoe 1799–1802.* Van Riebeeck Society, 2d series, 10. [AGM]
BRODY, SAUL N. 1974. *The disease of the soul: Leprosy in medieval literature.* Ithaca: Cornell University Press.
BROTHWELL, DON. 1961. The palaeopathology of early British man: An essay on the problems of diagnosis and analysis. *Journal of the Royal Anthropological Institute* 91:318–44.
———. 1970. The real history of syphilis. *Science Journal* 6:27–32. [DB]
———. 1976. Further evidence of treponematosis in a pre-Euro-

pean population from Oceania. *Bulletin of the History of Medicine* 50:435–42. [DB]

———. 1978. Possible evidence of the parasitisation of early Mexican communities by the micro-organism *Treponema*. *Bulletin of the Institute of Archaeology*, no. 15, pp. 113–30. [DB]

———. 1981. Microevolutionary change in the human pathogenic treponemes: An alternative hypothesis. *International Journal of Systematic Bacteriology* 31:82–87. [DB]

BROTHWELL, DON, AND RICHARD BURLEIGH. 1975. Radiocarbon dates and the history of treponematoses in man. *Journal of Archaeological Sciences* 2:393–96.

BROWN, WILLIAM J., JAMES F. DONOHUE, NORMAN W. AXNICK, JOSEPH H. BLOUNT, NEAL H. EWEN, AND OSCAR C. JONES. 1970. *Syphilis and other venereal diseases.* Cambridge: Harvard University Press.

BROWNE, S. G. 1970. How old is leprosy? *British Medical Journal* 3:640–41.

BRUES, ALICE M. 1966. "Discussion," in *Human palaeopathology.* Edited by Saul Jarcho, pp. 107–12. New Haven: Yale University Press.

BRÜHL, G. 1890. Pre-Columbian syphilis in the Western Hemisphere. *Cincinnati Lancet-Clinic* 63:275–80.

BUIKSTRA, JANE E. 1979. "Contribution of physical anthropologists to the concept of Hopewell: A historical perspective," in *Hopewell archaeology.* Edited by David S. Brose and N'omi Greber, pp. 220–33. Kent: Kent State University Press.

———. Editor. 1981. *Prehistoric tuberculosis in the Americas.* Northwestern University Archaeological Program Scientific Papers 5. [JAW]

———. 1984. "The lower Illinois River region: A prehistoric context for the study of ancient diet and health," in *Paleopathology at the origins of agriculture.* Edited by Mark N. Cohen and George J. Armelagos, pp. 215–34. Orlando: Academic Press.

BULLEN, ADELAIDE K. 1972. Paleoepidemiology and distribution of prehistoric treponemiasis (syphilis) in Florida. *Florida Anthropologist* 25:133–74.

CANNEFAX, GEORGE R., LESLIE C. NORINS, AND EUGENE J. GILLESPIE. 1967. Immunology of syphilis. *Annual Review of Medicine* 18:471–82.

CASSIDY, CLAIRE MONOD. 1980. "Nutrition and health in agriculturalists and hunter-gatherers," in *Nutritional anthropology.* Edited by Norge W. Jerome, Randy F. Kandel, and Gretel H. Pelto, pp. 117–45. Pleasantville: Redgrave.

———. 1984. "Skeletal evidence for prehistoric subsistence adaptation in the central Ohio River valley," in *Paleopathology at the origins of agriculture.* Edited by Mark N. Cohen and George J. Armelagos, pp. 307–45. Orlando: Academic Press.

CHAMBERLAIN, W. E., N. E. WAYSON, AND L. H. GARLAND. 1931. The bone and joint changes of leprosy: A roentgenologic study. *Radiology* 17:930–39.

CLARK, GEORGE A., MARC A. KELLY, JOHN M. GRANGE, AND M. CASSANDRA HILL. 1987. The evolution of mycobacterial disease in human populations: A reevaluation. CURRENT ANTHROPOLOGY 28:45–62. [JAW]

CLAY, ROTHA MARY. 1966 (1909). 2d edition. *The mediaeval hospitals of England.* New York: Barnes and Noble.

COCHRANE, R. G. Editor. 1959. *Leprosy in theory and practice.* Bristol: John Wright.

COCKBURN, T. A. 1961. The origin of the treponematoses. *Bulletin of the World Health Organization* 24:221–28.

———. 1963. *The evolution and eradication of infectious diseases.* Baltimore: Johns Hopkins Press.

COLE, HAROLD N., JAMES C. HARKIN, BERTRAM S. KRAUS, AND ALAN R. MORITZ. 1955. Pre-Columbian osseous syphilis. *Archives of Dermatology* 71:231–38.

COOK, DELLA COLLINS. 1976. Pathologic states and disease process in Illinois Woodland populations: An epidemiologic approach. Ph.D. diss., University of Chicago, Chicago, Ill.

———. 1984. "Subsistence and health in the lower Illinois Valley: Osteological evidence," in *Paleopathology at the origins of agriculture.* Edited by Mark N. Cohen and George J. Armelagos, pp. 235–69. Orlando: Academic Press.

———. 1985. Treponematosis in the Chirikof Island population.

Paper presented at the 54th annual meeting of the American Association of Physical Anthropologists, Knoxville, Tenn. (Abstracted in *American Journal of Physical Anthropology* 66:158.)

CORREAL URREGO, GONZALO. 1987. Paleopathology in preceramic bones from Colombia: Examples of syphilitic lesions from the site of Aguazuque, Soacha. Paper presented at the 14th annual meeting of the Paleopathology Association, New York, N.Y.

CREIGHTON, CHARLES. 1965 (1894). 2d edition. *A history of epidemics in Britain.* Vol. 1. *From A.D. 664 to the Great Plague.* New York: Barnes and Noble.

CROSBY, ALFRED W., JR. 1969. The early history of syphilis: A reappraisal. *American Anthropologist* 71:218–27.

———. 1972. *The Columbian exchange: Biological and cultural consequences of 1492.* Westport: Greenwood Press. [RS]

CYBULSKI, JEROME S. n.d. "Physical anthropology and paleopathology," in *Handbook of North American Indians,* vol. 7. In preparation. [MCG]

DAMPIER, WILLIAM. 1703. *A new voyage round the world.* London: James Knapton. [AD]

DAWES, J. D., AND J. R. MAGILTON. 1980. *The archaeology of York.* Vol. 12, fasc. 1. *The cemetery of St. Helen-on-the-Walls, Aldwark.* York: Archaeological Trust. [DB]

DENEVAN, W. M. 1976. "Introduction," in *The native population of the Americas in 1492.* Edited by W. M. Denevan, pp. 1–12. Madison: University of Wisconsin Press. [RS]

DENNIE, CHARLES C. 1962. *A history of syphilis.* Springfield: Thomas.

DENNINGER, HENRI S. 1938. Syphilis of Pueblo skulls before 1350. *Archives of Pathology* 26:724–27.

DOBYNS, H. F. 1983. *Their number become thinned.* Knoxville: University of Tennessee Press. [RS]

DOLS, MICHAEL W. 1979. Leprosy in medieval Arabic medicine. *Journal of the History of Medicine and Allied Sciences* 34:314–33.

DRUTZ, DAVID J. 1981. "Leprosy," in *The science and practice of clinical medicine,* vol. 8, *Infectious diseases.* Edited by Jay P. Sanford and James P. Luby, pp. 298–305. New York: Grune and Stratton.

EL-NAJJAR, MAHMOUD Y. 1979. Human treponematosis and tuberculosis: Evidence from the New World. *American Journal of Physical Anthropology* 51:599–618.

ELTING, JAMES J., AND WILLIAM A. STARNA. 1984. A possible case of pre-Columbian treponematosis from New York State. *American Journal of Physical Anthropology* 65:267–73.

ESGUERRA-GÓMEZ, GONZALO, AND EMILIO ACOSTA. 1948. Bone and joint lesions in leprosy. *Radiology* 50:619–31.

FAGET, G. H., AND A. MAYORAL. 1944. Bone changes in leprosy: A clinical and roentgenologic study of 505 cases. *Radiology* 42:1–13.

FIELDSTEEL, A. HOWARD. 1983. "Genetics of *Treponema,*" in *Pathogenesis and immunology of treponemal infection.* (Immunology Series 20.) Edited by Ronald F. Schell and Daniel M. Musher, pp. 39–55. New York: Marcel Dekker.

FULDAUER, A., A. H. BRACHT, AND W. R. K. PERIZONIUS. 1984. Difficulties in scoring syphilis: The limits of systematic diachronic paleopathology. Paper presented at the 5th European Members' Meeting of the Paleopathology Association, Siena, Italy.

GANN, THOMAS. 1901. Recent discoveries in Central America proving the pre-Columbian syphilis in the New World. *Lancet* 2:968–70.

GOFF, CHARLES W. 1963. New evidence of syphilis(?), yaws(?) from Cueva de la Candelaria, Mexico. (Abstract.) *American Journal of Physical Anthropology* 21:402.

———. 1967. "Syphilis," in *Diseases in antiquity.* Edited by Don Brothwell and A. T. Sandison, pp. 279–93. Springfield: Thomas.

GOLDSTEIN, MARCUS S. 1957. Skeletal pathology of early Indians in Texas. *American Journal of Physical Anthropology* 15:299–311.

GORDON, BENJAMIN L. 1959. *Medieval and Renaissance medicine.* New York: Philosophical Library.

GREGG, JOHN B., MARVIN J. ALLISON, AND LARRY J. ZIMMER-

MAN. 1981. Possible treponematosis in fourteenth-century Dakota Territory: A progress report. *Paleopathology Newsletter*, no. 34, pp. 5–6.

GREGG, JOHN B., AND P. S. GREGG. 1987. *Dry bones: Dakota Territory reflected.* Sioux Falls: Sioux Printing. [JAW]

GRIN, E. J. 1956. Endemic syphilis and yaws. *Bulletin of the World Health Organization* 15:959–73. [MLP]

———. 1961. Endemic treponematoses in the Sudan. *Bulletin of the World Health Organization* 24:229–38.

GRIN, E., AND T. GUTHE. 1973. Evaluation of a previous mass campaign against endemic syphilis in Bosnia and Herzegovina. *British Journal of Venereal Diseases* 49:1–19. [GTN]

GUERRA, FRANCISCO. 1978. The dispute over syphilis: Europe versus America. *Clio Medica* 13:39–61. [AD]

GUMERMAN, GEORGE J., AND EMIL W. HAURY. 1979. "Prehistory: Hohokam," in *Handbook of North American Indians*, vol. 9, *Southwest.* Edited by Alfonso Ortiz. Washington, D.C.: Smithsonian Institution.

GUTHE, T, AND R. R. WILLCOX. 1954. Treponematoses: A world problem. *Chronicle of the World Health Organization* 8:37–113.

HACKETT, C. J. 1951. *Bone lesions of yaws in Uganda.* Oxford: Blackwell Scientific Publications.

———. 1963. On the origin of the human treponematoses. *Bulletin of the World Health Organization* 29:7–41.

———. 1967. "The human treponematoses," in *Diseases in antiquity.* Edited by Don Brothwell and A. T. Sandison, pp. 152–69. Springfield: Thomas.

———. 1976. *Diagnostic criteria of syphilis, yaws, and treponarid (treponematoses) and of some other diseases in dry bones.* Berlin: Springer-Verlag.

HALTOM, W. L., AND A. R. SHANDS, JR. 1938. Evidences of syphilis in Mound Builders' bones. *Archives of Pathology* 25:228–42.

HANSEN, KLAUS, KELD HVID-JACOBSEN, HELLE LINDEWALD, PER SOELBERG SORENSEN, AND KAARE WEISMANN. 1984. Bone lesions in early syphilis detected by bone scintigraphy. *British Journal of Venereal Diseases* 60:265–68.

HARRISON, L. W. 1959. The origin of syphilis. *British Journal of Venereal Diseases* 35:1–7.

HARRISON, WILLIAM O. 1986. "Gonorrhea," in *Sexually transmitted diseases.* Edited by Yehudi M. Felman, pp. 51–63. New York: Churchill Livingstone.

HARTNEY, PATRICK C. 1978. Paleopathology of archaeological aboriginal populations from southern Ontario and adjacent regions. Ph.D. diss., University of Toronto, Toronto, Canada. [SRS]

HILL, M. CASSANDRA. 1986. Postcranial periostitis: A problematic in the differential diagnosis of porotic hyperostosis and infection. Paper presented at the 55th annual meeting of the American Association of Physical Anthropologists, Albuquerque, N.M. (Abstracted in *American Journal of Physical Anthropology* 69:214.)

HOLCOMB, RICHMOND C. 1934. Christopher Columbus and the American origin of syphilis. *United States Naval Medical Bulletin* 32:401–30.

———. 1935. The antiquity of syphilis. *Medical Life* 42:275–325.

———. 1940. Syphilis of the skull among Aleuts and the Asian and North American Eskimo about Bering and Arctic Seas. *United States Naval Medical Bulletin* 38:177–92.

———. 1941. The antiquity of syphilis. *Bulletin of the History of Medicine* 10:148–77.

HOLLANDER, DAVID C. 1981. Treponmatosis from pinta to venereal syphilis revisited: Hypothesis for temperature determination of disease patterns. *Sexually Transmitted Diseases* 8:34–37. [SRS]

HOOTON, EARNEST A. 1930. *The Indians of Pecos Pueblo.* New Haven: Yale University Press.

HOVIND-HOUGEN, KARI. 1983. "Morphology," in *Pathogenesis and immunology of treponemal infection.* (Immunology Series 20.) Edited by Ronald F. Schell and Daniel M. Musher, pp. 3–28. New York: Marcel Dekker.

HUDSON, ELLIS HERNDON. 1928. Treponematosis among the Bedouin Arabs of the Syrian desert. *United States Naval Medical Bulletin* 26:817–24. [BMR]

———. 1958. *Non-venereal syphilis: A sociological and medical study of bejel.* Edinburgh: E. and S. Livington. [MLP, BMR]

HUDSON, ELLIS HERNDON. 1961. Historical approach to the terminology of syphilis. *Archives of Dermatology* 84:545–62.

———. 1963a. Treponematosis and anthropology. *Annals of Internal Medicine* 58:1037–49.

———. 1963b. Treponematosis and pilgrimage. *American Journal of the Medical Sciences* 246:645–56.

———. 1964. Treponematosis and African slavery. *British Journal of Venereal Diseases* 40:43–52.

———. 1965a. Treponematosis and man's social evolution. *American Anthropologist* 67:885–901.

———. 1965b. Treponematosis in perspective. *Bulletin of the World Health Organization* 32:735–48.

———. 1968. Christopher Columbus and the history of syphilis. *Acta Tropica* 25:1–16.

———. 1972. Diagnosing a case of venereal disease in fifteenth-century Scotland. *British Journal of Venereal Diseases* 48: 146–53.

HULSE, E. V. 1975. The nature of biblical "leprosy" and the use of alternative medical terms in modern translations of the Bible. *Palestine Exploration Quarterly* 107:87–105.

HUNT, D., AND A. L. JOHNSON. 1923. Yaws: A study based on over 2,000 cases treated on American Samoa. *United States Naval Medical Bulletin* 18:599–607. [BMR]

HUSSEIN, M. K. 1949. Quelques specimens de pathologie osseuses chez les anciens egyptiens. *Bulletin de l'Institut d'Egypte* 32:11–17.

HYDE, JAMES N. 1891. A contribution to the study of pre-Columbian syphilis in America. *American Journal of the Medical Sciences* 102:117–31.

ISCAN, M. YASAR, AND PATRICIA MILLER-SHAIVITZ. 1985. Prehistoric syphilis in Florida. *Journal of the Florida Medical Association* 72:109–13.

JONES, JOSEPH. 1876. Explorations of the aboriginal remains of Tennessee. *Smithsonian Contributions to Knowledge* 22(259): 1–171.

KAMPMEIER, RUDOLPH H. 1984. "Early development of knowledge of sexually transmitted diseases," in *Sexually transmitted diseases.* Edited by King K. Holmes, Pers-Anders Mardh, P. Frederic Sparling, and Paul J. Weisner, pp. 19–29. New York: McGraw-Hill.

KANKI, P. J., F. BARIN, S. M'BOUP, J. S. ALLAN, J. L. ROMET-LEMONNE, R. MARLINK, M. F. MCLANE, T-H. LEE, B. AR-BEILLE, F. DENIS, AND M. ESSEX. 1986. New human T-lymphotropic retrovirus related to simian T-lymphotropic virus Type III (STLV-III_AGM). *Science* 232:238–43. [DSW]

KESTLER, H. W., Y. LI, Y. M. NAIDU, C. V. BUTLER, M. F. OCHS, G. JAENEL, N. W. KING, M. D. DANIEL, AND R. C. DESROSIERS. 1988. Comparison of simian immunodeficiency virus isolates. *Nature* 331:619–21. [DSW]

KIRBY, P. 1940. *The diary of Dr. Andrew Smith 1834–1836.* Van Riebeeck Society 21. [AGM]

KOGANEI, Y. 1894. *Beiträge zur physischen Anthropologie der Ainu.* Vol. 1. *Untersuchungen am Skelete.* Tokyo.

LAMB, D. S. 1898. Pre-Columbian syphilis. *Proceedings of the Association of American Anatomists* 10:63–69.

LANCEREUX, E. 1868. *A treatise on syphilis.* Vol. 1. London: New Sydenham Society. [GTN]

LANGDON, F. W. 1881. The Madisonville prehistoric cemetery: Anthropological notes. *Journal of the Cincinnati Society of Natural History* 4:237–57.

LANNING, EDWARD P. 1967. *Peru before the Incas.* Englewood Cliffs: Prentice-Hall.

LARSEN, CLARK SPENCER. 1984. "Health and disease in prehistoric Georgia: The transition to agriculture," in *Paleopathology at the origins of agriculture.* Edited by Mark N. Cohen and George J. Armelagos, pp. 367–92. Orlando: Academic Press.

LU, GWEI-DJEN, AND JOSEPH NEEDHAM. 1967. "Records of diseases in ancient China," in *Diseases in antiquity.* Edited by Don Brothwell and A. T. Sandison, pp. 222–37. Springfield: Thomas.

LUGER, A. 1972. Non-venereally transmitted "endemic" syphilis in Vienna. *British Journal of Venereal Diseases* 48:356–60. [GTN]

LUKACS, JOHN R., AND SUBHASH R. WALIMBE. 1984. "Paleodemography at Inamgaon: An early farming village in western India," in *The people of South Asia: The biological anthropology of India, Pakistan, and Nepal.* Edited by John R. Lukacs, pp. 105–32. New York: Plenum Press.

MAC CURDY, GEORGE G. 1923. Human skeletal remains from the highlands of Peru. *American Journal of Physical Anthropology* 6:217–329.

MCNEILL, W. H. 1976. *Plagues and peoples.* Garden City: Doubleday Anchor. [RS, ABW]

MADRID, ALFONSO. 1986. Work in historical osteology at the National Museum of Antiquities in Sweden. *Museum* 38(3): 155–57.

MAINGARD, J. F. 1937. Some notes on health and disease among the Bushmen of the southern Kalahari. *Bantu Studies* 11:285–94. [AGM]

MATTHEWS, WASHINGTON, J. L. WORTMAN, AND JOHN S. BILLINGS. 1893. Human bones of the Hemenway collection in the United States Army Medical Museum. *Memoirs of the National Academy of Sciences* 6:141–286.

MEANS, H.J. 1925. A roentgenological study of the skeletal remains of the prehistoric Mound Builder Indians of Ohio. *American Journal of Roentgenology* 13:359–67.

MEER, R. M. 1985. Health and disease in protohistoric Alaska. Paper presented at the 84th annual meeting of the American Anthropological Association, Washington, D.C.

MILES, JAMES S. 1966. "Diseases encountered at Mesa Verde, Colorado. II: Evidences of disease," in *Human palaeopathology.* Edited by Saul Jarcho, pp. 91–97. New Haven: Yale University Press.

———. 1975. Orthopedic problems of the Wetherill Mesa populations, Mesa Verde National Park, Colorado. National Park Service Publications in Archeology 7G.

MILLS, WILLIAM C. 1906. Baum prehistoric village. *Ohio Archaeological and Historical Publications* 15:45–136.

MENTZEL, O. F. 1944. *A geographical and topographical description of the Cape of Good Hope.* Van Riebeeck Society 25. [AGM]

MØLLER-CHRISTENSEN, VILHELM. 1952. Case of leprosy from the Middle Ages of Denmark. *Acta Medica Scandinavica* 142 (suppl. 266):101–8.

———. 1967. "Evidence of leprosy in earlier peoples," in *Diseases in antiquity.* Edited by Don Brothwell and A. T. Sandison, pp. 295–306. Springfield: Thomas.

MØLLER-CHRISTENSEN, VILHELM, AND BORGE FABER. 1952. Leprous changes in a material of mediaeval skeletons from the St. George's Court, Naestved. *Acta Radiologica* 37:308–17.

MØLLER-CHRISTENSEN, VILHELM, AND R. G. INKSTER. 1965. Cases of leprosy and syphilis in the osteological collection of the Department of Anatomy, University of Edinburgh. *Danish Medical Bulletin* 12:11–18.

MOORE, CLARENCE B. 1907. Moundville revisited. *Journal of the Academy of Natural Sciences of Philadelphia* 13:337–405.

MORANT, G. M., AND M. F. HOADLEY. 1931. A study of the recently excavated Spitalfields crania. *Biometrika* 23:191–248.

MORISON, SAMUEL ELIOT. 1942. *Admiral of the ocean sea: A life of Christopher Columbus.* Boston: Little, Brown. [SRS]

MORSE, DAN. 1967. "Two cases of possible treponema infection in prehistoric America," in *Miscellaneous papers in paleopathology,* vol. 1. Edited by William D. Wade, pp. 48–60. Museum of Northern Arizona, Technical Series 7.

———. 1973. "Pathology and abnormalities of the Hampson skeletal collection," in *Nodena: An account of 75 years of archeological investigation in southeast Mississippi County, Arkansas.* Edited by Dan F. Morse, pp. 41–60. Arkansas Archeological Survey Research Series 4.

———. 1978. 2d revised edition. *Ancient disease in the Midwest.* Illinois State Museum Reports of Investigations 15.

MORSE, DAN F. 1973. "The Nodena phase," in *Nodena: An account of 75 years of archeological investigation in southeast Mississippi County, Arkansas.* Edited by Dan F. Morse, pp. 65–85. Arkansas Archeological Survey Research Series 4.

MORTON, R. S. 1967. The sibbens of Scotland. *Medical History* 11:374–80.

MOSS, W. L., AND G. H. BIGELOW. 1922. Yaws: An analysis of 1,046 cases in the Dominican Republic. *Bulletin of the Johns Hopkins Hospital* 33:43–47. [BMR]

MOSSOP, E. E., AND A. W. VAN DER HORST. 1935. *The journal of Hendrik Jacob Wikar (1779).* Van Riebeeck Society 15. [AGM]

MURDOCK, J. R., AND H. J. HUTTER. 1932. Leprosy: A roentgenological survey. *American Journal of Roentgenology* 28:598–621.

MURRAY, J. F., A. M. MERRIWEATHER, AND M. L. FREEDMAN. 1956. Endemic syphilis in the Bakwena Reserve of the Bechuanaland Protectorate: A report on mass examination and treatment. *Bulletin of the World Health Organization* 15:1975. [GTN]

MUSHER, DANIEL M., AND JOHN M. KNOX. 1983. "Syphilis and yaws," in *Pathogenesis and immunology of treponemal infection.* (Immunology Series 20.) Edited by Ronald F. Schell and Daniel M. Musher, pp. 101–20. New York: Marcel Dekker.

NURSE, G. T., AND T. JENKINS. 1977. *Health and the huntergatherer.* Basel: Karger. [AGM]

NURSE, G. T., N. TANAKA, G. MACNAB, AND T. JENKINS. 1973. Non-venereal syphilis and Australia antigen among the G/wi and G//ana San of the Central Kalahari Reserve, Botswana. *Central African Journal of Medicine* 19:207–13. [AGM, GTN].

OLANSKY, SYDNEY. 1981. "Treponematosis," in *The science and practice of clinical medicine,* vol. 8, *Infectious diseases.* Edited by Jay P. Sanford and James P. Luby, pp. 298–305. New York: Grune and Stratton.

ORTNER, DONALD J. 1986. Skeletal evidence of pre-Columbian treponemal disease in North America. Paper presented at the 6th European Members' Meeting of the Paleopathology Association, Madrid.

ORTNER, DONALD J., AND WALTER G. J. PUTSCHAR. 1985. Reprint edition. *Identification of pathological conditions in human skeletal remains.* Washington, D.C.: Smithsonian Institution Press.

ORTON, S. T. 1905. A study of the pathological changes in some Mound Builder's bones from the Ohio Valley, with especial reference to syphilis. *University of Pennsylvania Medical Bulletin* 18:36–44.

PACE, J. L., AND G. W. CSONKA. 1984. Endemic non-venereal syphilis (bejel) in Saudi Arabia. *British Journal of Venereal Diseases* 60:293–97. [GTN]

PARROT, M. J. 1879. The osseous lesions of hereditary syphilis. *Lancet* 1:696–98.

PATERSON, D. E. 1959. "Radiographic appearances and bone changes in leprosy: Their cause, treatment, and practical application," in *Leprosy in theory and practice.* Edited by R. G. Cochrane, pp. 243–64. Bristol: John Wright.

———. 1961. Bone changes in leprosy: Their incidence, progress, prevention, and arrest. *International Journal of Leprosy* 29: 393–422.

PATRICK, ADAM. 1967. "Disease in antiquity: Ancient Greece and Rome," in *Diseases in antiquity.* Edited by Don Brothwell and A. T. Sandison, pp. 238–46. Springfield: Thomas.

PERZIGIAN, ANTHONY J., PATRICIA A. TENCH, AND DONNA J. BRAUN. 1984. "Prehistoric health in the Ohio River valley," in *Paleopathology at the origins of agriculture.* Edited by Mark N. Cohen and George J. Armelagos, pp. 347–66. Orlando: Academic Press.

PIETRUSEWSKY, M. 1971. An osteological study of cranial and infracranial remains from Tonga. *Records of the Auckland Institute and Museum* 6:287–402.

POWELL, MARY LUCAS. 1988a. *Status and health in prehistory: A case study of the Moundville chiefdom.* Washington: Smithsonian Institution Press.

———. 1988b. Endemic treponematosis and tuberculosis in the prehistoric southeastern United States: The biological costs of

736 | CURRENT ANTHROPOLOGY Volume 29, Number 5, December 1988

chronic endemic disease. Paper presented at the 12th International Congress of Anthropological and Ethnological Sciences, Zagreb, Yugoslavia.

———. 1988c. "On the eve of the conquest: Life and death at Irene Mound, Georgia," in *Postcontact biocultural adaptation of Native American populations on St. Catherines Island, Georgia.* Edited by David Hurst Thomas and Clark Spencer Larsen. New York: American Museum of Natural History. In preparation.

———. 1988d. "Health and disease at Nodena, a Late Mississippian community in northeast Arkansas," in *Towns and temples along the Mississippi.* Edited by David Dye. Birmingham: University of Alabama Press. In press.

PUTNAM, FREDERIC W. 1878. Archaeological explorations in Tennessee. *Report of the Peabody Museum* 2:305–60.

QUINN, THOMAS C., DAVID GLASSER, ROBERT O. CANNON, DIANE L. MATUSZAK, RICHARD W. DUNNING, RICHARD L. KLINE, CARL H. CAMPBELL, EBENEZER ISRAEL, ANTHONY S. FAUCI, AND EDWARD W. HOOK III. 1988. Human immunodeficiency virus infection among patients attending clinics for sexually transmitted diseases. *New England Journal of Medicine* 318:197–203.

RABKIN, SAMUEL. 1942. Dental conditions among prehistoric Indians of northern Alabama. *Journal of Dental Research* 21:211–22.

RAMENOFSKY, ANN F. 1982. *The archaeology of population collapse: Native American response to the introduction of infectious disease.* Ann Arbor: University Microfilms. [MJB]

REICHS, KATHLEEN J. 1987. Treponematosis: A possible case from the Late Woodland of North Carolina. Paper presented at the 14th annual meeting of the Paleopathology Association, New York, N.Y.

REID, R. 1947–48. *Lewis and Clark in North Dakota.* North Dakota History 14 and 15. [JAW]

RICHARDS, PETER. 1977. *The medieval leper.* Cambridge: D. S. Brewer.

ROKHLIN, D. G. 1965. *Diseases of ancient men: Bones of the men of various epochs, normal and pathological changes.* Moscow-Leningrad: Nauka. [AD]

RONEY, JAMES G., JR. 1966. "Palaeoepidemiology: An example from California," in *Human palaeopathology.* Edited by Saul Jarcho, pp. 99–107. New Haven: Yale University Press.

ROSE, JEROME C., BARBARA A. BURNETT, MARK W. BLAEUER, AND MICHAEL S. NASSANEY. 1984. "Paleopathology and the origins of maize agriculture in the Lower Mississippi Valley and Caddoan culture areas," in *Paleopathology at the origins of agriculture.* Edited by Mark N. Cohen and George J. Armelagos, pp. 393–424. Orlando: Academic Press.

ROSEBURY, THEODOR. 1971. *Microbes and morals.* New York: Viking.

ROTHSCHILD, BRUCE M., AND WILLIAM TURNBULL. 1987. Treponemal infection in a Pleistocene bear. *Nature* 329: 61–62.

RUBIN, STANLEY. 1974. *Medieval English medicine.* New York: Barnes and Noble.

SANCHEZ, F. G., L. MAZZOTTI, AND E. G. SALENSAS. 1961. *Hippelates pallipes* as the vector of yaws. *Salud Pública* 3:183–88. [BMR]

SAUL, FRANK P. 1972. *The human skeletal remains of Altar de Sacrificios.* Papers of the Peabody Museum of Archaeology and Ethnology, Harvard University, 63(2).

SCHAPERA, I. 1933. *The early Cape Hottentots.* Van Riebeeck Society 14. [AGM]

SIGERIST, HENRY E. 1923. L'origine della sifilide. *Archivio di Storia della Scienza* 4:163–70. [AD]

———. 1951. *A history of medicine.* Vol. 1. *Primitive and archaic medicine.* New York: Oxford University Press.

SMITH, E. G., AND F. W. JONES. 1910. *Report of the human remains.* (Archaeological Survey of Nubia, Report of 1907–1908.) Cairo: Ministry of Finance.

SMRCKA, VACLAV. 1985. Treponematosis. *Paleopathology Newsletter,* no. 50, p. 9.

STEINBOCK, R. TED. 1976. *Paleopathological diagnosis and interpretation.* Springfield: Thomas.

STEWART, T. D., AND LAWRENCE G. QUADE. 1969. Lesions of the frontal bone in American Indians. *American Journal of Physical Anthropology* 30:89–110.

STEWART, T. D., AND ALEXANDER SPOEHR. 1967 (1952). "Evidence on the palaeopathology of yaws," in *Diseases in antiquity.* Edited by Don Brothwell and A. T. Sandison, pp. 307–19. Springfield: Thomas.

SUSSMAN, MAX. 1967. "Diseases in the Bible and the Talmud," in *Diseases in antiquity.* Edited by Don Brothwell and A. T. Sandison, pp. 209–21. Springfield: Thomas.

SUZUKI, TAKAO. 1963. *Human skeletal remains of the ancient Japanese populations.* Tokyo: Iwanami Shoten.

———. 1984a. *Paleopathological and paleoepidemiological study of osseous syphilis in skulls of the Edo period.* Tokyo: University of Tokyo Press. [IM, SRS]

———. 1984b. Paleopathological study on osseous syphilis in skulls of the Ainu skeletal remains. *Ossa* 9–11:153–68.

———. 1984c. Typical osseous syphilis in medieval skeletal remains from Hokkaido. *Journal of the Anthropological Society of Nippon* 92:23–32.

TEMKIN, OWSEI. 1966. "Discussion," in *Human palaeopathology.* Edited by Saul Jarcho, pp. 30–35. New Haven: Yale University Press.

TENNEY, J. 1986. Possible treponemal bone lesions among early native Californians. Paper presented at the 6th European Members' Meeting of the Paleopathology Association, Madrid.

THWAITES, R. G. 1905. *Early Western travels, 1748–1846.* Vol. 15. Cleveland: Arthur Clark. [JAW]

TRUSWELL, A. S., AND J. D. L. HANSEN. 1968. Medical and nutritional studies of the !Kung Bushmen in northwest Botswana. *South African Medical Journal* 28:1338–39. [AGM]

TURNER, T. B. 1937. Studies on the relationship between syphilis and yaws. *American Journal of Hygiene* 254:477–506. [BMR]

VORBERG, G. 1896. *Uber den Ursprung der Syphilis: Quellen geschichtliche Untersuchungen.* Stuttgart: J. Puttmann. [AD]

WAKEFIELD, E. G., SAMUEL C. DELLINGER, AND JOHN D. CAMP. 1937. A study of the osseous remains of the "mound builders" of eastern Arkansas. *American Journal of the Medical Sciences* 193:488–95.

WALKER, ERNEST G. 1983. Evidence for prehistoric cardiovascular disease of syphilitic origin on the northern Plains. *American Journal of Physical Anthropology* 60:499–503.

WAUGH, M. A. 1982. Role played by Italy in the history of syphilis. *British Journal of Venereal Diseases* 58:92–95.

WEISS, D. L., AND V. MØLLER-CHRISTENSEN. 1971. Leprosy, echinococcosis, and amulets: A study of a medieval Danish inhumation. *Medical History* 15:260–67.

WHITNEY, J. L. 1915. A statistical study of syphilis. *Journal of the American Medical Association* 65:1986–89. [BMR]

WHITNEY, WILLIAM F. 1883. On the existence of syphilis in America before the discovery by Columbus. *Boston Medical and Surgical Journal* 108:365–66.

WILLCOX, R. R. 1949. Venereal disease in the Bible. *British Journal of Venereal Diseases* 25:28–33.

———. 1974. Changing patterns of treponemal disease. *British Journal of Venereal Diseases* 50:169–78.

WILLIAMS, HERBERT U. 1929. Human paleopathology with some original observations on symmetrical osteoporosis of the skull. *Archives of Pathology* 7:839–901.

———. 1932. The origin and antiquity of syphilis: The evidence from diseased bones, a review, with some new material from America. *Archives of Pathology* 13:799–814, 931–83.

———. 1936. The origin of syphilis: Evidence from diseased bones, a supplementary report. *Archives of Dermatology and Syphilology* 33:783–87.

WILLIAMS, HERBERT U., JOHN P. RICE, AND JOSEPH RENATO LACAYO. 1927. The American origin of syphilis, with citations from early Spanish authors collected by Dr. Montejo y Robledo. *Archives of Dermatology and Syphilology* 16:683–96.

WILLIAMS, J. A. 1985. Evidence of pre-contact tuberculosis

in two Woodland skeletal populations from the Northern Plains. Paper presented at the annual meeting of the American Association of Physical Anthropologists, Knoxville, Tenn. [JAW]

WONG, K. CHIMIN, AND WU LIEN-TEH. 1936. 2d edition. *History of Chinese medicine.* Shanghai: National Quarantine Service.

WOODS, ROBERT, AND BRUCE ROTHSCHILD. n.d. Population analysis of symmetrical erosive arthritis in Ohio Woodland Indians (1200 years before present). *Journal of Rheumatology.* In press. [BMR]

WORLD HEALTH ORGANIZATION. 1980. *A guide to leprosy.* Geneva: WHO.

WRIGHT, D. J. M. 1971. Syphilis and Neanderthal man. *Nature* 229:409.

2
Disease and the Depopulation of Hispaniola, 1492–1518

Noble David Cook

Shortly after the encounter of a handful of European venturers and native peoples on the shores of one of the small Bahama islands, larger and more populous land masses were found. Old World sailors first touched the coast of Hispaniola in December 1492. The leader of the expeditionary forces, the Genoese navigator Christopher Columbus, believed he had reached the edge of the Asian Indies, thereby proving that a westward sailing route to the Orient was feasible. Before the Pinta and Niña returned to the Iberian peninsula with the promising news of discovery, a small garrison was planted on Hispaniola. By this action in early 1493, the ecological isolation between the earth's two hemispheres was broken forever (Crosby 1972, 1986; Phillips and Phillips 1992; Rouse 1992).

Columbus carried back to Spain ten native Americans; they were captured to be displayed as proof of the discovery, and were to be trained as interpreters for a second mission. Columbus by word and pen extolled the new land's virtues; he hoped to secure investors for subsequent expeditions. The navigator's initial reports suggested large settlements, and a dense population. The fifteen hundred settlers that set out aboard the second expedition's seventeen ships did find a dense population on Hispaniola when they reached the island in late 1493, but within a half-century of contact, virtually no aboriginals remained. The paradise Columbus described upon returning to Europe from the first voyage was transformed into a graveyard for most Caribbean natives.

214   Colonial Latin American Review, Vol. 2, Nos. 1-2, 1993

Hispaniola's population at contact

The size of the population of the island of Hispaniola at the time of contact as well as the explanation for the tragic disappearance of its inhabitants has attracted the attention of many Americanists (Denevan 1976, 1992; Sauer 1966; Rosenblat 1967, 1976; Moya Pons 1971, 1987; Zambardino 1978; Borah and Cook 1971; Watts 1987; Rouse 1992; Lovell 1992). The experience of the peoples of the island with the outsiders, does help explain the nature of the entire venture of conquest and colonization of the Americas. Unfortunately, solid evidence for estimation of aboriginal population size of Hispaniola at time of first contact does not exist. No matter how hard scholars have searched for fresh data, or squeezed old accounts for new truth, they have been frustrated. The reason is simple: the Taino had no cultural reason to count themselves, and by the time the colonists found a "census" to be necessary, the major impact of the ecological exchange between the eastern and western hemispheres was well underway. Furthermore, the first Spanish colonial counts, when finally taken, were flawed. They were incomplete, encompassing only part of the peoples of part of the island, and they were conducted at a time of catastrophic political and ecological change.· The Amerindian's agricultural mounds (*conucos*) were first exploited, then abandoned, by the hungry outsiders in their search for foodstuffs. Almost simultaneously European crops and livestock were introduced. Furthermore, the foreigners were making increasingly rapacious demands for labor. By 1542, a half century after contact, all was over, in spite of importation of Indians taken in slaving raids from nearby islands and the mainland to replace the disappearing Taino; the native Americans of Hispaniola were virtually extinct.

What then caused the demise of the Taino? Traditional interpretations factor in the superior technology of the Europeans: their steel swords, the canon and arquebuz, the defensive armor, the effective use of ships. The form of warfare was also important. Spaniards were far from their homeland and fought to destroy any capability native peoples might have had to resist. Europeans used the horse, and fierce attack dogs. They tried to instill fear in the psyche of their enemies. Other factors include "culture shock." Carl Sauer, for example, remarked that depopulation stemmed from "societal disruption with resulting social and psychological malaise." The Taino failed to reproduce; they suffered high mortality from overwork. The breakdown of the conuco system caused starvation, and the introduction of Old World livestock and plants disrupted native agricultural patterns and practices.

Modern estimates of Hispaniola's native population, ca. 1492

Source	Year	Estimate
Verlinden (1973)	1492	60,000
Amiama (1959)	1492	100,000
Rosenblat (1954, 1976)	1492	100,000
Lipschutz (1966)	1492	100,000-500,000
Moya Pons (1987)	1494	377,559
Cordova (1968)	1492	500,000
N.D. Cook (1993)	1492	500,000-750,000
Moya Pons (1971)	1492	600,000
Zambardino (1978)	1492	1,000,000
Denevan (1992)	1492	1,000,000
Guerra (1988)	1492	1,100,000
Denevan (1976)	1492	1,950,000
Watts (1987)	1492	3,000,000-4,000,000
Borah and Cook (1971)	1492	7,975,000

All who have surveyed the Hispaniola experience admit disease was a contributing factor, but only AFTER the introduction of smallpox in 1518. Angel Rosenblat, for example, noted that "there is no doubt that the Europeans imported their microbes to Hispaniola very early, but it is odd that the first epidemic recorded is that of smallpox of 1517-18, when there were only some 30,000 Indians on the entire island" (Rosenblat 1976, 55-56). Since he could not persuasively explain massive depopulation of the island, Rosenblat was forced to conclude that the aboriginal population was low. Frank Moya Pons (1987, 189) explains that the demise of the islanders was "produced by mass suicides, homicides, abortions, and maltreatment, not including the illness that also should have affected part of the population, although it may not have been in the same measure that the aforementioned factors did it." Borah and Cook (1971, 409-10) did suggest the importance of disease for Hispaniola's depopulation, stating outright that:

> we disagree on relative lateness of the introduction of disease. From the men of the first voyage of Columbus on, there was disease among the Spaniards. A large proportion of the men were ill at any given time, and there was a steady loss through death. It seems most unlikely that the sick among the Spaniards would have been kept so isolated that the natives would not have picked up any disease of epidemic possibility.

216   Colonial Latin American Review, Vol. 2, Nos. 1-2, 1993

But David Henige (1978, 235), in a critique of high estimates of aboriginal population, especially by Borah and Cook, argued that the "early arrival of epidemics needs to be argued on the basis of some sort of evidence. To produce the specter of epidemiological disaster merely as a *deus ex machina* to explain the otherwise unaccountable results of a chosen statistical procedure simply fails to persuade."

Frank Moya Pons (1987) recently entered the debate on Hispaniola's contact population size. A lifetime specialist on the early colonial history of the Dominican Republic's two-thirds of the island, Moya Pons knows the early sources well. Moya Pons (1987, 182) approached the work of Borah and Cook with respect, yet concluded that: "I have been convinced that using the same materials that he and the deceased Professor Cook used, by varying the method, distinct results can be reached." Moya Pons believes that Rodrigo de Albuquerque's 1514 distribution provides the most complete and reliable early source for Taino population data: there were then 26,334 natives on the island under Spanish domination. Moya Pons took the 1508 figure of 60,000 of Miguel de Pasamonte, as reported by Bartolomé de las Casas; the 1509 "count" of 40,000; and finally the 1510 Diego Columbus report of some 33,523 Indians, and subjected the figures to relatively simple mathematical manipulations to calculate rates of decline for three sets of years: 1508-09; 1508-10; and 1508-14. He did not use the 1496 "count" of 1,130,000 that misled Sauer, Borah and Cook. Further, Moya Pons noted concurrently with indigenous depopulation of Hispaniola, 40,000 Indian laborers from nearby islands were introduced. The importation confuses final results, for indigenous depopulation must have been even greater than the figures suggest. He calculated the 1508-09 annual rate of change at -33 percent and the 1508-10 rate at -25 percent, and used these figures to project (standard formula for exponential change) the population in 1494, when the true impact of contact was first biologically manifest. The higher rate gave a result of over sixteen million; the lower slightly over 3.3 million. Moya Pons rejected his initial projection on the basis of the carrying capacity of the island.

Moya Pons then scrutinized conditions on the island in closer detail. The regime of encomienda really began to function with the arrival of Governor Ovando along with 2,500 settlers in 1502-03. By 1510, according to las Casas, there were 10,000 Europeans on the island. Moya Pons argues that depopulation pressure must have been greatest during these years, with the massive foreign population and its seemingly insatiable demands for a shrinking number of Indian laborers, especially for the mines. He suggests that the rate of population loss must have been very different in the earlier period, from 1494 to 1502, when

Disease and the Depopulation of Hispaniola, 1492-1518   217

the Spanish population oscillated between a mere 360 to 500. Here Moya Pons returns to the work of Las Casas (1:419) in the *Historia de las Indias*: "En su obra, Las Casas dice que durante los años 1494, 1495 y 1496 desapareció *un tercio* (emphasis mine) de la población del centro de la Isla debido al tremendo choque que produjo la llegada y penetración de los españoles en las comunidades indígenas de aquellos lugares en tiempos de la Factoría colombina" (Moya Pons 1987, 185). Unfortunately, Moya Pons misread Las Casas. The friar actually wrote that only one-third of the natives remained (Las Casas 1956, 1:419): "*no quedaron* en las multitudes que en esta isla de gentes había desde el año de 94 hasta el de 6, segun se creía, *la tercera parte* de todas ellas." In spite of the fact that the results of Moya Pons' calculations are thrown off, let us follow his arguments to their conclusion. He asked, how do we measure the shock, and the fact that only a part of Hispaniola was under effective European control? Here Moya Pons uses the 1514 count. The central part of the island held about one-third the native population in 1514. He applies this ratio to the entire island and calculates on the basis of his 1503 projected population of 251,706 (on the -25 percent rate of decline), and the formula:

$$\text{Population 1503} = \text{2/3 Population 1494}$$
$$251{,}706 = \text{2/3 (1494 pop)}$$
$$X = 377{,}559$$

The fall in the population from 1494 to 1503 was of some 125,853 people, an annual rate of decline of 4.6 percent. Actually, if we correct for the misreading of Las Casas, and multiply his figure of 251,706 by three, the result is approximately 750,000.

Moya Pons also evaluated the ecological carrying capacity of the island. With the 377,559 estimate for the total population the resulting density was "relatively low . . ., 4.8 Indians per square kilometer, perfectly compatible with the degree of economic, social and political organization of the society of agriculturalists, collectors, fishers and hunters that lived in settlements of no more than four or five thousand inhabitants, sharing a kinship structured by clan" (Moya Pons 1987, 189). In a critique of the high population estimates for the island, Moya Pons (1987, 184) argued that the maximum demographic density could not exceed 20 to 30 inhabitants per square kilometer in digging stick (coa) agriculture, complemented with collection, hunting and fishing activities. If his real figure were 750,000, densities would still be below his maximums.

There is almost unanimous agreement that the native population of the island of Hispaniola reached virtual extinction a scant half century after

218   Colonial Latin American Review, Vol. 2, Nos. 1-2, 1993

Christopher Columbus first touched its northern shores. The magnitude of that population when the encounter of European and native American began continues to be debated, and estimates range from 100,000, posited by Angel Rosenblat to eight million proposed by Borah and Cook. The latter estimate has been challenged by a number of specialists, and largely rejected as unsustainable on a variety of grounds. Oftentimes census projections based on a set of reliable counts can be made. We do have relatively, but not absolutely, reliable figures of 1508, 1510, 1514, 1538, 1540. But in the case of the island of Hispaniola, census projection is problematic. Given the abnormal nature of contact and conquest of the New World, standard projections based on a normal long term exponential growth curves hardly replicates the reality of the demographic experience of aboriginal inhabitants. Zambardino's use of the standard formula and Borah and Cook's manipulations both presume a continuous curve. Hispaniola's reality is a normal and relatively stable preconquest situation, followed by sudden catastrophe. The curve is not continuous; it is a jagged collapse, much as a sea wave builds to a crest as it nears shore, then collapses in on itself as it expends its force in the surf. A once relatively stable population of Hispaniola collapsed as Old World pathogens took root and wiped out the island's populace. Age and sex selective factors also must have been important with the first epidemic waves. An epidemic that infected community elders would have little long term biological impact on a population, but one that especially decimated women of child-bearing age, would be devastating. An epidemic that recurred every twenty years with heavy mortality for children under five would take its toll, but the population could still survive. In the case of Hispaniola waves of conquest and disease were too quick and pronounced for the population to recover and survive. Hence, in the example of the island, the population became biologically extinct so rapidly that normal census projections based on adjusted counts produce results with a very wide margin of error. The "best" results probably range from a low of perhaps 200,000 through the 380,000 of Moya Pons, to Zambardino's potential million approaching the 1,130,000 "oral" version believed by some early island settlers. The range from low to high is in the magnitude of 1:5 or 1:6.

Given the difficulty of applying modern demographic analysis to the flawed and incomplete data for Hispaniola, the historian must return to the corpus of history: written evidence. Nicolas Federman, a German associated with the Welser attempt of settlement of Venezuela, was in Santo Domingo for a brief period in 1529-30 and again 1531-32. He provides an interesting observation on the size of the aboriginal population that must have been based on conversations with long-term insular residents. Federman in fact gives a figure that is remarkably close to some modern estimates:

> it is hopeless to speak of its natives, because forty years have already elapsed since the conquest of the island, and . . . almost all are gone. Of five hundred thousand inhabitants of various nations and languages that existed on the island forty years ago, there remain fewer than twenty thousand living; a large number died from the smallpox, others perished in the wars, still others in the gold mines where Christians forced them to work against their nature, because they are weak peoples, and poor workers. (Rodríguez Demorizi 1971, 19; from Federman, *Narraciones*)

It would be difficult to find a more dispassionate, perceptive description of the magnitude and demise of the island's native peoples than that provided by Federman who saw personally the results of the disaster.

About a decade before Federman's visit to Hispaniola, the licentiate Alonso de Zuazo penned an extensive report on conditions in the Caribbean that was sent to William of Croy (known in Spain as Monsieur de Xèrves), the Flemish minister of the young Charles V. The letter was dated 22 January 1518. Regarding "los repartimientos pasados desde el tiempo del Almirante viejo hasta hoy, se hallaron al principio que esta isla Española se descubrió, un cuento e ciento e treinta mill indios, e agora no llegan a once mill personas por las causas que arriba digo, y creese por lo pasado que de aquí a tres o cuatro años no habrá ninguno dellos si no se remedia" (Rodríguez Demorizi 1971, 253). The original source for Zuazo's number of 1,130,000 is not clear, nor is there a precise date that can be assigned. Suffice it to say that some colonists believed that there had been that many natives on the island when European settlement began. Pedro Mártir de Anglería (1944, 273), who probably collected the information by 1516, seems to refer to a similar tradition: "Se han disminuido inmensamente el número de aquellos infelices; muchos cuentan que alguna vez se hizo censo de más de un millón y doscientos mil; cuántos sean ahora, me causa horror el decirlo." Was there in reality an early count of the island Taino? Here opinion is divided. Rosenblat and Henige rejected the hypothesis, while Sauer and Borah and Cook accepted the possibility. Published documents are unlikely to provide more information, but some documentary evidence may be found, particularly in private Spanish collections, that will shed new light on the question. At the moment, caution is the best counsel.

Given the available data, estimation of the EXACT contact population of Hispaniola becomes largely an exercise in futility. Yet it seems likely that the population ranged from a minimum of 200,000 to perhaps a maximum of 1,200,000. My own inclination is to accept

220   Colonial Latin American Review, Vol. 2, Nos. 1-2, 1993

Federman's 1530 number of 500,000 at face value, along with a "corrected" Moya Pons figure of 750,000 to set a narrower range of 500,000-750,000. The Alonso de Zuazo-Pedro Mártir de Anglería figures of 1,130,000-1,200,000 may provide a conservative upper limit for estimates. Population estimates aside, the demographic experience of the Taino following European contact is tragic. The native population of the central Andes and Mesoamerica collapsed; the Taino became extinct.

The question of illness

The Caribbean disease environment between 1492 and the first great killer pandemic of smallpox that swept the Americas beginning in 1518 is the key to our understanding of the true nature of the demise of Hispaniola's peoples. That the Americas was not a disease-free paradise when Columbus arrived is a given fact (Denevan 1992; Stodder and Martin 1992); there was sickness throughout the hemisphere, and sickness led to death. There was leishmaniasis in restricted environmental niches in the New World, and Chagas disease. In all likelihood there was histoplasmosis and/or tuberculosis. Amoebic dysentery and intestinal worms weakened people and contributed to untimely death. Non venereal treponema (read endemic syphilis) existed over a wide area (Verano 1992). Yet a handful of Old World communicable diseases had not crossed the Atlantic or Pacific in any sustained fashion prior to 1492; these included smallpox, measles, typhus, the plague, cholera, and probably malaria and yellow fever (Henige [1992, 14] presents still inconclusive evidence for the presence of malaria and yellow fever in the Americas before 1492 [see ftn. 100]. Craton and Saunders [1992, 1:39] argue unsuccessfully that yellow fever and blackwater fever existed in the New World before Columbus).

Recent research on the impact of epidemic disease on the Amerindian population following 1518 suggests that, in spite of death precipitated by warfare, famine, exploitation, suicide, infanticide, and a drop in the birth rate, sickness was the predominant factor in the disappearance of native peoples (Alchon 1992; Cook 1981, 1982; Cook and Lovell 1992; Lovell 1985, 1992; and Whitmore 1992). Many experts believe epidemic disease appeared too late on Hispaniola to explain the extinction of the Taino. We have noted Henige's earlier (1978) arguments that there is no solid evidence for massive deaths stemming from Old World disease before 1518. Henige continues to argue against the disease link, and has made sharp critical thrusts against proponents—he calls them the "High Counters"—who have advocated such connections. It is with faltering steps that scholars have begun to review the evidence of Old World disease in the Americas before 1518, an undertaking that demands historiographical caution in the search for documentation. Accurate disease diagnosis is a major stumbling block; appropriate scientific identification has been possible only beginning in the twentieth century, and even at present misdiagnosis of contemporary sickness results in tragic consequences. Descriptions of disease symptoms in the fifteenth and sixteenth centuries are vague and often conflicting. Furthermore, pockets of people who have been isolated from exposure to a particular viral infection over several generations often experience symptoms, and morbidity and mortality levels, that vary significantly from what might be considered normal.

When, then, was Old World disease first introduced into the Americas? What was it, and what were the consequences? There is no current evidence that the first expedition of 1492 transported active viruses. Indeed, the number of men on the three vessels was small so that had there been a case of acute communicable disease on board one of the ships when they left Palos, the illness would have run its course before landfall. Further, the documentary record indicates that during the crossing the crew was healthy, including Columbus, who was frequently unwell. Phillips and Phillips (1992; 169), after careful reexamination of the available information on the first crossing, conclude that "no one had been sick or even had a headache on all three ships, except for one old man with a long-term problem with kidney stone." It should be noted, however, that if a vectored disease had been carried aboard, it could have easily made the initial trip, even with a small crew, if appropriate hosts were available.

The second expedition and the transfer of disease

Medical historian Francisco Guerra (1985, 1986, 1987, 1988) made the first modern case linking the introduction of Old World pathogens into the Caribbean with the massive second expedition of Columbus. For Guerra the infection was carried somewhere within one or more of the seventeen ships and 1,500 would-be colonists. The fleet left Cádiz on 25 September 1493, and reached the Canaries on 2 October. On board were Old World plants and animals the colonists planned to nurture in the new environment. Most significant, in the mind of Guerra, were eight sows that were loaded on ship on the island of Gomera in the Canaries between 5-7 October. One of the participants in the venture, Michele de Cuneo, wrote to a friend: "the Lord Admiral brought from Spain

222   Colonial Latin American Review, Vol. 2, Nos. 1-2, 1993

the ones most needed; and we found that *pigs, chickens, dogs and cats* reproduce there in a superlative manner, especially the pigs because of the huge abundance of the aforesaid fruits" (Morison 1963, 217). Several animals carry influenza, according to Pyle (1986, 23), "viruses identical or closely related to human pathogens infect ducks, turkeys, swine, horses, and other warm-blooded vertebrates." Humans probably acquired influenza when animals were first domesticated. Guerra postulates that both men and animals on board the second expedition quickly sickened. The voyage from the Canaries to the Caribbean was a swift one, with favorable winds the fleet reached the Caribbean island of Dominica on 3 November 1493. They stopped six days on Guadalupe and landed a force. On 13 November they disembarked on St. Croix in the Virgin Islands. On the 18th, they stopped at Puerto Rico to take on provisions, staying there until the 21st of November. They finally reached Hispaniola around 28 November. Guerra argued that almost immediately the illness that had come with the fleet of the second expedition spread across the island.

Guerra's account provides us with a descriptive exactness that seems missing in the documentary evidence he cites. He suggests that the foreign infection (influenza-swine flu) passed from pigs to horses, and by the time the animals and crew fled the ship as they disembarked on Hispaniola in December 1493, virtually all were infected. When the primary sources are reviewed, Guerra's positive statement of fact is more an inference based on epidemiological principles than a verified diagnosis. He states that illness debilitated the Spaniards, and many contemporary accounts confirm how difficult those first days and weeks were for the Europeans. Guerra argues that the highly contagious disease rapidly spread among native peoples as the foreigners fanned out across the island. Unfortunately, this statement seems more a supposition than a fact that can be documented. Furthermore, Guerra's (1988, 323) conclusion that all "sources coincide on the place, date, clinical manifestations and the mortality of the epidemic," is misleading, as is his observation that "symptoms were very high fever, ague, prostration, and excessive mortality." The actual accounts and terminology used are vague, and best apply to European settlers.

There is ample evidence to adduce high loss of life from starvation and accompanying sickness for the Europeans who attempted the first major settlement on Hispaniola. But information on native American illness or deaths in late 1493 and 1494 is scarce. Hence, it is necessary to use the tools of modern epidemiology, to work from the known biological behavior of homo sapiens, vectors, and disease organisms. One of the best, yet overlooked pieces of evidence comes from the experience of the ten native Americans captured during the first voyage, who were taken to Spain and trained as translators for the second venture. They were "lucayos y haitianos" and were baptised in Barcelona; the Admiral's purpose was to both train translators and to demonstrate to the monarchs the nature of the peoples of the newly discovered lands. In spite of inadequate food and an extremely difficult eastwardly passage to Spain in early 1493, all ten islanders survived. Seven of the ten re-embarked with the great Indies fleet as they left the Spanish coast for the Caribbean on 25 September 1493. Unfortunately, five of the seven men died before they reached land (Brau 1969, 32-33). Doctor Chanca wrote an extensive letter to the municipal authorities of Seville, that was sent back to the homeland with the fleet of Antonio de Torres in late January 1494. In one section of this missive he described the fate of the Indian interpreters. Of the seven who embarked in Andalusia, five died en route, and the other two escaped only by the skin of their teeth—"los cuales escaparon a uña de caballo" (Gil and Varela 1984, 171). One would expect that the Spaniards would have made every effort possible to secure the well-being of the trained translators, for they promised to be critical to the success of the new venture. The Amerindians had reached Spain healthy, and seven were healthy enough to reembark for their homelands with the 1493 fleet, but five-sevenths succumbed en route. What caused the death of these translators? Clearly, according to the text of Doctor Chanca, they fell ill from some type of illness and died. It is not surprising that Doctor Chanca did not label the sickness at this point. In the first place, he may not have seen them, and even if he did, symptoms may have been so vague as to prohibit anything more than a general statement that they fell "ill" and "died." Only in the twentieth century is it possible to make an accurate disease identification, yet even now medical misdiagnosis is frequent.

There is similar elevated mortality for the 550 native American slaves Columbus shipped off to Europe in lieu of treasure with the twelve ships in the Antonio de Torres fleet in January of 1494. Michele de Cuneo wrote describing the voyage after he returned to Europe in 1495. He participated with Columbus in the reconnaissance of Cuba and Jamaica during April-September 1494, and lamented bitterly how difficult the return passage with Torres was. Starting out from Puerto Rico, everything seemed to go wrong; as they neared the Spanish coast, two hundred of the Indians died. Michele de Cuneo (Gil and Varela 1984, 258; Morison 1963, 227) blamed the losses on the change of climate: "I believe because of the unusual air, colder than theirs [creo que por el aire insólito, mas frío que el suyo]." When they arrived in Cádiz illness still prevailed: "we disembarked all the slaves, who were half-sick. For

224   Colonial Latin American Review, Vol. 2, Nos. 1-2, 1993

your information they are not working people and they much fear the cold, neither have they long life [desembarcamos todos los esclavos, que estaban medio enfermos: para vuestro conocimiento, no son hombres de carga y temen mucho el frío y tampoco tienen larga vida]." What explains the high mortality on this trip? Might starvation or malnutrition been the primary factor, or disease, or more likely a combination of the two? Many native Americans taken to Seville in the first decades after the discovery of the New World did not live long. According to a letter of 11 June 1494 from Ferrara, addressed to the Marquesa of Mantua, one Morelletto Ponzone said that the Indians "are of such a weak constitution, that two of them became ill in Seville, so that the doctors were unable to treat the illness, and did not find their pulse, and they died [son de naturaleza tan débil, que enfermaron dos en Sevilla de suerte que los médicos no dieron con su enfermedad y no les encontraron el pulso, y han muerto]" (Gil and Varela 1984, 258, ftn. 42). Ponzone did not mention lack of food, the implication is that death was based on sickness, not starvation. Malnutrition, however, could have weakened their ability to ward off infection. Of the relation of malnutrition and mortality in early modern Europe, there continues much debate (Walter and Schofield 1989).

When Columbus reached Hispaniola during his second voyage, he ordered construction of a new headquarters east of Navidad, at a place he named Isabela. The site seemed excellent at first, but the work was hard, and the laborers lacked their accustomed European foodstuffs. Las Casas, who described the process, did not mention the use of a native labor force, and implied the Europeans did the bulk of the work. He noted (1:363) that "the men all of a sudden began to fall ill, and because of the little sustenance that was available for the sick, many of them began to die also, so that there did not remain a man among the hidalgos and plebeians no matter how robust he might have been, that did not fall ill from these terrible fevers [que de calenturas terribles enfermo no cayese]." Both Las Casas (1:363) and Columbus blamed the ill health of the settlers on the fact that "the men arrived greatly fatigued from such a long journey . . ., the change of the climate [aires] . . ., and the lack of foodstuffs . . ." Even the Admiral could "not escape falling ill as the others." Hernando Colón also recalled that his father had become ill: "Not only was the Admiral too pressed for time to chronicle events in his usual way, but he also fell ill and therefore left a gap in his diary from 11 December 1493 to 12 March 1494" (Cohen 1969, 158).

What illness did Columbus suffer from? Actually, he did write during this period. During his convalescence Columbus did pen a full report for the monarchs that was sent back with the fleet of twelve ships under

Antonio de Torres. Dated 30 January 1494, Christopher Columbus apologized that more gold had not been remitted to his sovereigns; the paltry amount was due to the fact that the greater part of the people employed fell suddenly ill ("yo deseaba mucho en esta armada poderles enviar mayor cuantidad de oro del que acá se espera poder coger, si la gente que acá está nuestra, la mayor parte subitamente no cayera doliente") (Major 1978, 72). Columbus failed to identify the illness; there are mere hints of the nature of the malady. He implied mortality might have been higher: "It was also extremely inconvenient to leave the sick men here in an open place and huts [era grande inconveniente dejar acá los dolientes en lugar abierto y chozas]" (Major 1978, 73). It seemed to make little difference where on the island one travelled, for, "the greatest part of those who have gone out to make discoveries have fallen sick on their return [los más cayeron dolientes después de vueltos]" (Major 1978, 74). Columbus enthusiastically reported that health of the settlers was being restored, indeed, "they speedily recover their health" (Major 1978, 75), and pointed out that fresh meat would help ("esta gente convalescerá presto, como ya lo hace, porque solamente les prueba la tierra de algunas ceçiones, y luego se levantan; y es cierto que si toviesen algunas carnes frescas para convalescer muy presto serían todos en pie"). Fresh red meat, rather than salted and dried, indeed would have probably assisted in shaking off infection, and speeding up restoration of health. Columbus, lacking a more accurate understanding of the sickness, concluded what many travelers to unknown lands long before and since have believed: "the cause of the sickness so general among us, is the change of air and water [las causas de las dolencias tan general de todos es de mudamiento de aguas y aires]" (Major 1978, 76). At the same time, there is the clear involvement of miasmastic theory, so prevalent in medical thought of the period (Cipolla 1992). Columbus requested Antonio de Torres to bring back with the next fleet raisins and almonds, and sugar and honey, as well as rice. These were foods long considered by the Spanish to have therapeutic effects aiding cure of illnesses (Phillips and Phillips 1992, 201-02). Furthermore, Columbus related that the major part of the medicines that had been brought were used up, "by the multitude of the many ill [por la muchedumbre de los muchos dolientes]" (Major 1978, 80).

The chief physician of the second expedition, Dr. Chanca, did his best to cure those who fell ill, indeed, Columbus lauded the good doctor's efforts in the report to the monarchs sent with Antonio de Torres: "you will inform their Highnesses of the continual labour that Doctor Chanca has undergone, from the prodigious number of sick and the scarcity of provisions: and that, in spite of all this, he exhibits the greatest zeal and

226   Colonial Latin American Review, Vol. 2, Nos. 1-2, 1993

benevolence in everything that relates to his profession" (Major 1978, 90). Doctor Chanca also sent a report back to Spain with the Torres fleet. He too indicates the impact of the illness on the first European settlers. So great was their fatigue, that "the admiral had at one time determined to leave the search for the mines until he had first dispatched the ships which were to return to Spain *on account of the great sickness* (my italics) which had prevailed among the men [después de una vez haber determinado el Almirante de dejar el descobrir las minas fasta primero enviar los navíos que se habían de partir a Castilla, por la mucha enfermedad que había seido en la gente]" (Major 1978, 66).

When the Antonio de Torres fleet departed from Hispaniola, "the Admiral improved from his indisposition and illness" and decided to conduct a brief survey of the island (Las Casas 1951, 1:366). By the time Christopher Columbus returned to Isabela on 29 March 1494, conditions had deteriorated markedly: "he found all the men very fatigued, because few escaped from illness and death, and those that still remained healthy, as a result of the little food, were flaccid" (Las Casas 1951, 1:376). The food shortage became critical, and rations were reduced time after time, with the result that more settlers fell ill and died (Las Casas 1951, 1:376-77). Unfortunately, when the second fleet had reached the Indies, they discovered that supplies loaded in Andalusia were damaged and spoiled. Columbus blamed it largely on the negligence of the ship's captains, but high humidity and heat on the island contributed to spoilage. Food ran so low that they "would purge five with one hen egg and with a kettle of cooked chick-peas" (Las Casas 1951, 1:377). A similar problem existed with the cure and medicines, given the fact that some had brought them, but not enough, "nor such that was necessary for so many, nor to suit all temperaments" (1:377). Furthermore, there was a lack of people to serve or care for the ill. Many died, "primarily of hunger, and without anyone to even give them a jar of water, and burdened with many painful aches . . ." (Las Casas 1951, 1:378).

In spite of the illness at Isabela, Columbus undertook a survey by sea (April to 29 September 1494) of the southern shore of the island of Cuba, and then Jamaica. His son Hernando wrote many years later that during the reconnaissance of Cuba, the "Admiral was utterly exhausted both by poor food and because he had not taken off his clothes or slept in his bunk from the day he left Spain to 19 May, and at the time when he wrote this he had been sleepless for eight nights on account of a severe illness" (Cohen 1969, 175). By the time he reached Puerto Rico, he was again too sick to keep record in the log book. His son Hernando related that "the reason for this was his exhaustion from the great hardships he had suffered and his weakness from lack of food. He was afflicted by a serious illness, something between an infectious fever and a lethargy, which suddenly blinded him, dulled his other senses and took away his memory" (Cohen 1969, 185). Las Casas chronicled that after Columbus returned to Isabela, he was "five months very ill, at the end of which Our Lord returned his health, for there still remained much for him to do . . ." (Las Casas 1951, 1:398). It is evident from the descriptions that sickness resulting in high mortality, and prolonged convalescence with frequent relapses, was the order following the arrival of the second expedition of Columbus to the Caribbean. The sickness was made more acute by malnutrition and poor water and hygiene. Guerra's guess that the Spaniards suffered from influenza-swine flu is appropriate, but it is also possible it was something else. Typhus, often associated with warfare and siege, was prevalent in Andalusia these years. For example, the fall of Granada was accompanied by typhus, which then lingered on in the area in endemic form.

During the Admiral's absence, Spanish abuses of islanders had led to violent retaliation. The cacique of Magdalena, Guatigana, "killed ten Christians and secretly ordered the firing of a house in which forty men lay sick" (Cohen 1969, 187). Columbus organized an expedition to punish the natives so severely that future rebellion would be unthinkable. According to Columbus, the Europeans faced 100,000 Indians with only 200 Christians, 20 horse, and about 20 ferocious attack dogs. Columbus later remembered that Divine Providence seemed to have saved them; he "thought it impossible that 200 men, ill-armed and half of them sick, would have been sufficient to conquer such a multitude" (Cohen 1969, 191). Even if the number of enemies faced by the Europeans was inflated, the consequence is the same. The native defeat was followed by a period of relative peace, so that the 630 mostly sick Spaniards then on the island, a number now including women and children could travel about without fear of reprisals. Columbus believed that during those difficult months God "had inflicted on the Christians shortage of food and severe illness, which reduced them to a third of their former strength" (Cohen 1969, 191). That is of a total of some 1,800, the number was reduced to about 630. Famine coincided with sickness, and all elements of the island's population, Europeans as well as the Taino, were afflicted, as is so often the case in the pre-modern era. Pedro Mártir, who had direct information from eyewitnesses of the events on Hispaniola, wrote that Columbus was informed by the Indians "that there was such hunger among the islanders that more than fifty thousand men had already died, and that they are falling each day, with every step, like cattle in an infected herd [le informaron que había tal hambre entre los insulares que habían muerto ya más de cincuenta mil hombres, y que caían todos los días a cada paso,

228   Colonial Latin American Review, Vol. 2, Nos. 1-2, 1993

como reses de un rebaño apestado]" (Mártir 1944, 45 [Decade 1, book 4, chapt. 2]). Mártir related that the primary cause for the famine was human. The natives had decided that the best way to rid themselves of the outsiders was to destroy their food, so they dug up crops and fled to the hillsides.

Yet disease also killed the islanders during this critical period. Bartolomé de las Casas relates that there

> came among them such illness, death and misery, that of fathers, mothers and children, an infinite number sadly died. Such that with the massacres of the wars and by the starvation and sicknesses that come because of them, and of the fatigues and oppressions that afterward took place, and miseries, and above all the great intimate pain, anguish and sadness, there did not remain of the multitudes of peoples that were on this island from the year of 1494 until that of 1496, it is believed, the third part of all them [vino sobre ellos tanta de enfermedad, muerte y miseria, de que murieron infelicemente de padres y mádres y hijos, infinitos. Por manera que con las matanzas de las guerras y por las hambres y enfermedades que procedieron por causa de aquéllas y de las fatigas y opresiones que después sucedieron y miserias y sobre todo mucho dolor intrínseco, angustia y tristeza, no quedaron de las multitudes que en esta isla de gentes había desde el año de 94 hasta el de 6, según se creía, la tercera parte de todas ellas. ¡Buena vendimia y hecha harto bien apriesa!]. (Las Casas 1951, 1:419-20)

Potential new infections of 1498-1500

Christopher Columbus had left his brother Bartolomé in charge of administration of the island in the capacity of adelantado when he returned to Spain in 1496. Columbus came back to Hispaniola on 31 August 1498 and found health conditions even worse than they were when he had departed for the homeland. Supplies were inadequate, even with reinforcements on board three ships under Pedro Niño that arrived in early July. As the capital was transferred to Santo Domingo on the south side of the island, native American resentment of the outsiders increased. Three hundred Spaniards had fallen victim to various illnesses (diversas enfermedades), the implication being SEVERAL illnesses were rampant, not a single one. Lacking supplies, especially food and medications, it was decided to distribute the remaining sick and emaciated (enfermos y flacos) settlers to the several forts and Indian villages that were scattered between Isabela and Santo Domingo (Mártir 1944, decade 1, book 5, chapt. 2). There they would not have doctors or medicines, but at least they might have food; they would therefore combat illness rather than a combination of sickness and starvation ("y así pelearían solamente con la enfermedad y no con ella y juntamente con la hambre" [Las Casas 1951, 1:444]). Sickness and hunger seemed general, and the distribution of the ill to various places provided the perfect vehicle for the spread of contagion.

Columbus unfortunately had delegated Francisco Roldán as *alcaide* and *justicia mayor* of Isabela. In May of 1497, during Columbus's absence is Spain, Roldán captained a group of malcontents who marched on Fort Concepción; it was only in the summer of 1499 that Bartolomé Columbus was able to subdue and capture Roldán and his followers. Roldán wrote to the archbishop of Toledo on 10 October 1499 defending his actions. He described the poor conditions the colonists had faced, including generalized sickness in·1498: "At that time the greatest part of the Christian people were sick of this general illness that is going around." Roldán suffered illness too, and the natives took advantage of the situation to rise up, and "kill the Christians who wère ill and scattered in many places and without healthy men to stand guard" (Gil and Varela, 271-72). Roldán said the Concepción garrison was in jeopardy, for the Indians there planned to rebel, and there were only eight men stationed at the post, "all sick [dolientes]." Roldán claimed that he had prepared defense for the settlers, concentrating at Concepción "the sick peoples," from all the estancias. He reported "they were dying of hunger, and there was nothing one could do about it." Gil and Varela (1984, 272) argue that "la sífilis se había apoderado de un 30 por 100 de la población." Oviedo had written that Isabela and Santo Tomás had to be abandoned because of loss of life, and attributed the loss to a combination of starvation and disease ("mal de buas," or syphilis [book 2, chapt. 12]).

The fleet of Francisco de Bobadilla, who had been sent to investigate the chaotic state of administration of the island, also brought renewed sickness and hunger. Bobadilla arrived in Santo Domingo in August 1500, and both Christopher and Bartolomé Columbus were dispatched to Spain in chains to face charges. Six Franciscans accompanied the Bobadilla fleet; in July of 1502 three of the friars sent letters back to Europe outlining conditions of the island. They too mention the deleterious consequences of illness. Friar Juan de Leudelle of Picardy wrote Cardinal Cisneros that they had landed well on October 1500, but "to a lesser or greater extent, all tested the effects of fevers [calenturas], in such fashion that when the caravels departed, we were already all well, except fray Rodrigo and I, who are still not free of them" (Gil and Varela 1984, 286-87). Friar Juan de Robles, who wrote in a similar vein, stated that more than 3,000 Indians had been baptised. He recalled that the land was extensive, and the population large. He concurred they all

230   Colonial Latin American Review, Vol. 2, Nos. 1-2, 1993

suffered ill health: "all of us became ill, some more, others less." In fact, the friar confesses, "here one finds oneself always somewhat ill" (Gil and Varela 1984, 288).

Thus from late 1493 to the end of the century there is frequent mention of sickness and food shortages on the "island paradise." The Europeans were obviously most interested in describing how illness afflicted their brethren, not native Americans. "Fevers" is most frequently listed as a symptom, with lethargy. The most devastation may have taken place as early as 1494, as Guerra suggests. Modern diagnosis of the 1494 crisis is impossible, but Guerra's educated guess that is was influenza may not far miss the mark. It could have been typhus or yet another unidentified disease. Whatever the case, illness and malnutrition went hand in hand. The diet of the Europeans was inadequate in the first place, and the newcomers found it difficult to adjust to native-American foodstuffs. Spanish mortality, caused by illnesses and outright starvation, may have approached two-thirds during the initial decade on Hispaniola. Taino mortality may have been even greater. Here we have only the very impressionistic observations of Mártir who wrote that 50,000 men had already come down at Hispaniola and that two thirds had succumbed. Perhaps mortality was even greater, as in the example of the five-sevenths of the small group of translators taken back to the islands with the second fleet of Columbus.

Each subsequent ship and fleet brought from southern Spain new settlers, animals, plants, and obviously pathogens. To argue that illness was not transported is to assume the highly improbable. During contemporary space probes, great efforts are made by scientists to avoid contamination of planetary objects with earth microbes. Disease arrived in the New World with the settlers on the second expedition of Columbus. The fifteenth-century Europeans lacked the medical knowledge and the means to prevent the spread of potentially harmful organisms from one part of the globe to another. The Spaniards realized that the closing of borders could help slow or deflect the spread of certain diseases, such as the plague. But even if the plague raged in Seville or Cádiz, ships set sail for the Indies. These fleets may have carried contagion, plague, influenza, typhus, at any time. Measles and smallpox would have been transported only when there were enough susceptible young people aboard to carry active cases. After the slave trade became fully developed, wave after wave of smallpox infection entering Brazil and the Caribbean can be traced to young people taken along the African coast (Alden and Miller 1987). The greater number of ships and people travelling to the Indies, the greater the chance for disease spread.

The 1502 series

The massive fleet of Governor Nicolás de Ovando carried 2,500 men and women aboard thirty vessels to Hispaniola. Leaving Sanlúcar de Barrameda in February 1502, they reached Santo Domingo in April. Bartolomé de las Casas sailed with the fleet, and his testimony is especially illuminating. Insufficient food and supplies had been transported to the New World; on landing a large group set out to try their luck in the search for precious metals. Quickly their food ran out and they returned to Santo Domingo for provisions; finding none "they were tested in this fashion with the new land giving them fevers [calenturas]." Las Casas lamented they lacked food, medicines and supplies. "They began to die in such number that it was impossible for the priests to bury all. More than 1,000 of the 2,500 died, and 500 of them, with great affliction, hunger, and needs, remained ill" (Las Casas 1951, 2:226). In 1503 the Hospital of San Nicolás was constructed in Santo Domingo to assist in curing the poor, but this did little to slow what Las Casas saw as a rapid die-off in the native population of the island during the administration of Governor Ovando. "The multitude of vecinos and peoples that there were on this island were being consumed, that according to the Admiral in a letter to the monarchs had been without number . . . and in the said eight years of that administration more than nine of ten parts perished. From here passed this drag-net to the island of San Juan (Puerto Rico) and to Jamaica, and afterwards to Cuba, and after that to Tierra Firme, and thusly spread and infected and devastated all this sphere" (Las Casas 1951, 2:257). The food shortages brought on by the poorly supplied foreigners had an immediate impact on the natives, who were forced to feed the outsiders. Clearly famine and disease were once again interconnected. Las Casas mentions fevers, but fails to describe other symptoms, so we cannot leap to a diagnosis of the illnesses of 1502 and early 1503.

The number of ships and people who made the crossing each year after the second expedition grew. The rough totals for registered shipping have been provided by the Chaunus, and Boyd-Bowman has given separate information. The total volume of possible contact between Amerindians and Eurasians in the Caribbean during these years was substantial. In 1508 alone, 45 vessels sailed from Spain to Hispaniola; according to the research of Huguette and Pierre Chaunu (1955-59: 2:20-23), approximately 185 ships crossed to the Indies between 1509 and 1515.

232   Colonial Latin American Review, Vol. 2, Nos. 1-2, 1993

The 1507-08 outbreaks

Although Old World disease was brought to the Americas with the second expedition of Columbus in 1493, and sickness came aboard many subsequent voyages, Floyd, in an examination of the "Columbus dynasty" in the Caribbean, postulated that the first bout of European disease that afflicted native Americans did not sweep the region until 1507.

> The Indian population had begun to decline especially in 1507-08, owing in all likelihood to the transmission to the Indies of the epidemic then raging in southern Spain. Since European diseases invariably affected the Indians more severely than the Spaniards, a considerable number of the Tainos, probably in the mines and at Santo Domingo where contact would be at its greatest, must have perished. (Floyd 1973, 95)

Later, in a more affirmative vein, Floyd recalled that "since Spain was ravaged by a pestilence that took many lives in 1507, I hold it likely that the first noticeable death rate among the Indians occurred as a result of the transmission of this unidentified disease by immigrants" (Floyd 1973, 243). Floyd did not attempt disease identification, yet other scholars have labelled smallpox for an "epidemic" of 1507. The 1507 smallpox diagnosis has been discredited by Henige (1986c), in a piece of excellent historical criticism. Although the existence of a 1507 New World smallpox epidemic, as Henige (1986c, 15) demonstrates, may be the consequence of "an illusion created by accident and perpetuated by carelessness," there was renewed sickness on Hispaniola that year.

Spain as reservoir of infection

Let us briefly review the "evidence" for severe epidemics in southern Spain in the years from 1502 to 1507, since these would be primary sources for any Old World disease that might be introduced into the Indies. Unfortunately few parish registers for burials for years prior to the seventeenth century can be found in Andalusia; such records would be of inestimable value in tracing epidemic disease that extracted high mortality. Epidemics are mentioned in ecclesiastical and secular chronicles of Spain in general and Andalusia in particular. The disease that most preoccupied the residents of the Iberian peninsula in the sixteenth century was plague, for the death it caused was horrific, and the levels of mortality were fearsome. Unfortunately, except in "classic" cases of fully developed bubonic plague, it was not always possible to identify the plague, or separate it from other prevalent killers such as typhus. In 1501 Barcelona was visited by what some have labelled the plague; in just the months of May to November 3,000 people died. The north of Spain seems generally afflicted that year. Pedro Mártir (1947, 24-26) travelled to Egypt representing the Catholic monarchs in 1501. In early September of 1501 he passed by Barcelona and Narbona, but was unable to enter either city because they were both infected by the "peste." Three old friends of the humanist fell victim to the contagion. As he continued through southern France and into northern Italy he had to prove he had not been in plague infected areas. The drought and ensuing famine of 1505-06 contributed to one of the most devastating plague years of the century, in fact mortality was so high that 1507 came to be referred to as "the year of the great peste." Some 3,500 people died in Barcelona; 3,000 in Madrid; 7,000 in Valladolid; 5,000 in Avila; 12,000 in Zaragoza; and most important for the purposes here, some 100,000 succumbed in Andalusia. Attempts at quarantine were rarely successful, and it would be surprising if this sickness did not make its way on board ships setting out from Andalusian ports such as Cádiz, Sanlúcar, Huelva and Palos (Ballesteros Rodríguez 1982, 42).

Andrés Bernáldez, the curate of the town of Los Palacios, in Andalusia, provides excellent insight into the hardship facing Spain during this entire seven year period: "From the year 1502 there began to be in Castilla . . . much hunger and many illnesses of pestilential *modorra* and pestilence . . . until the present year of 1507, when there began in the month of January . . ., in Jerez de la Frontera, and in Sanlúcar el Recio, and in Seville, and within all its jurisdiction, that ignited as a flame of fire at the end of February . . ." (Bernáldez 1962, 667; from Moreno Ollero 1984, 121). Bernard Vincent (1977, 351-58) found excellent information on this outbreak of disease in some deliberations of the city council, and in correspondence of the Count of Tendilla.

Illness in the circum-Caribbean, 1514-17

Disease was rampant on the isthmus of Panama shortly after the discovery of the "Southern Sea" by Blasco Núñez de Balboa in 1513. In the 1514-17 period, sickness was introduced into the narrow mainland by the men of the Pedro Arias de Avila (Pedrarias) expedition. Guerra argues it was a recurrence of swine flu, but other possibilities exist. Evidence on this illness comes from several sources, including a long report about the ill-fated group penned by Licentiate Zuazo. Some 1,500 men or so were collected in Seville, "all or most of the men had been in Italy with the Great Capitan." This also was a large expedition, that left Sanlúcar de Barrameda with up to seventeen ships on 12 April 1514.

234   Colonial Latin American Review, Vol. 2, Nos. 1-2, 1993

The crew spent sixteen days on the island of Gomera provisioning and repairing ships (Mártir 1944, 242); the voyage to Dominica required only 27 days. There they took on water and firewood, and sailed on to mainland Santa Marta. They continued to Cartagena, and reached Darién around the middle or end of June; illness struck quickly. Some 450 of the Blasco Núñez expedition resided in the area, and the 1,200 to 1,500 additional men of the Pedrarias group put a tremendous strain on the ability of settlers to provision them. The Pedrarias contingent included many hidalgos, as well as doña Isabel de Bobadilla, the leader's spouse. The settlement and surrounding district was swampy and wet; it was a place where "dense and sickly vapors rise, the men began to die and there died two-thirds of them, though dressed in silks and brocade" (Sauer 1966, 249). Andagoya, a participant, confirmed the account, writing that "the men began to sicken to such an extent that they were unable to care for each other and thus in one month seven hundred died of hunger and *modorra*" (Sauer 1966, 250).

The later historian Oviedo was a participant in the venture, and reported that "more had died or left than remained in the country" (Sauer 1966, 250). Oviedo also identified the malady as *modorra*. There is no mention of the previous Balboa party having experienced severe illness, nor the natives at the time, and it appears the sickness was introduced from Europe. One must note that once again starvation coincided with the passage of disease, for they had not brought enough food supplies with the fleet to support the settlement for more than a few days. Las Casas reported that hidalgos dressed in silk could be found begging in the streets for food. "So many died daily that in one pit they dug, many were interred together, and at times if they excavated a grave for one of them they did not want to close it, because they knew for certain that within a few hours another might die to accompany him" (Las Casas 1951, 3:38). Even Pedrarias, in spite of better food rations, fell ill. From the Darién base Pedrarias sent his nephew eastward with 200 men to explore the Cenú River, rumored to be rich in gold. The men were new and untried, and suffered molestations from "the large number of mosquitoes that attacked them . . . From all those accidents they began to fall ill and die." By the time the nephew returned to Darién he had lost half his expeditionary force (Las Casas 1951, 3:43).

There is much debate on identification of *modorra* that was so disastrous during the Pedrarias campaign. Rodrigo de Molina published a treatise on pestilence (Cádiz, 1554) and reported on a sickness "called modorra by the common people" (Sauer 1966, 250). But Molina failed to describe symptoms. Pérez Moreda (1980, 249) suggests that an epidemic described as *modorrilla* that swept Segovia in 1522 may have been the plague. John H. Parry (1976, 300) on the other hand, suggests *modorra* "may have been a deficiency disease" that hit those whose food on the voyage to the Indies had been inadequate. He argues that the supply of foodstuffs did not improve when the soldiers landed, for the "settlement which, though modestly flourishing, was too small to feed so great a force." but the description of the illness is more suggestive of influenza or typhus than a deficiency disease. People ill with influenza suffer lethargy for several days, their defenses become weakened, and they display a tendency to contract more deadly ailments. Inadequate food, frequently mentioned by contemporaries, exacerbates the problem.

López de Gómara provides a much more complete description of the symptoms of *modorra* in the following decade in his biography of Hernán Cortés. Licentiate Luis Ponce de León travelled to New Spain to conduct the *residencia* of Cortés. At last reaching Mexico City, the Licentiate attended Mass at the Convent of San Francisco, "and retired to his lodgings suffering from a high fever, occasioned by the *modorra*. He took to his bed and was unconscious for several days, his fever and drowsiness increasing the while. He died on the seventh day . . . Dr. [Cristóbal] de Ojeda, who attended him, treated him for *modorra*, and swore it was the cause of death." He had lost power of speech the day he died. "Of the hundred persons who had embarked with the Licenciado Ponce de León, most died at sea, or on the road within a few days of landing; of the Dominican friars, two. It was believed that a pestilence struck down and killed the others." L.B. Simpson, who translated and edited the edition of López de Gómara, said that modern *modorra* is a disease of sheep, but that it is "defined too vaguely for identification" (López de Gómara 1964, 382). Ernesto Schäfer (1947, 2:4, 254-55) described the symptoms of the illness of Ponce de León to G. Sticker, Professor of the History of Medicine of the University of Würzburg; he diagnosed epidemic meningitis. In retrospect, it is impossible to identify with certainty the malady, but the sickness labeled as modorra was often associated with travel, change of climate and diet, as well as malnutrition. Fever and lethargy, followed by prostration then coma strongly suggest that the malady was severe influenza, coupled with life threatening pneumonia. However, it might have been typhus, particularly when symptoms included macular and/or maculopapular eruptions, or another unidentified disease. European mortality was elevated in the worst episodes, and there is no reason why the infection would not be passed to anyone in the vicinity whose resistance was weak.

236   Colonial Latin American Review, Vol. 2, Nos. 1-2, 1993

The "first" epidemic: smallpox in 1518

Bartolomé de las Casas penned his description of the impact of the 1518 smallpox epidemic not long after he returned to the island in 1520, and must have interviewed both remaining natives and Europeans for his account. He suggested the original source was from someone who had arrived from Castile, and that although few Spaniards were touched, between one-third and one-half the Indians died. Las Casas (3:270) lamented the disappearance of the island Taino, for the illness left no more than one thousand "of the immensity of peoples that this island held, and that we have seen with our own eyes" (3:270).

More an historian than propagandist in his history of the Indies, Las Casas narrated the course and manifestations of the epidemic in some detail. He mentioned that quick death was often the consequence of natives bathing in the rivers while feverish. Lack of adequate food, nudity, and the custom of sleeping on the ground, as well as excessive labor and lack of attention to health all contributed to rapid demise, according to Las Casas. He pointed out that Spaniards, when they realized the devastation being caused by massive numbers of dead, sought to find cures, but

> they should have begun it many years earlier: [Finalmente, viendo los españoles que se les morían, comenzaron a sentir la falta que les hacían y habían de hacer, por donde se movieron a poner alguna diligencia en curallos, aunque aprovechó poco a los más, porque debieron de habello comenzado muchos años antes; no creo que quedaron vivos ni se escaparon desta miseria 1.000 ánimas, de la inmensidad de gentes que en esta isla había y vimos por nuestros ojos.]. (Las Casas 1951, 3:270)

Although it might appear from the text that the friar knew that native Americans were dying from disease "many years earlier" and the Spaniards should have been already searching for more adequate cures, Las Casas was really placing the blame primarily on overwork and exploitation. His use of the word "curallos" likely means the Spaniards should have mended their ways long before, only in this way could the Indians be saved.

Overview, 1492-1518

Other contemporaries identified the causes for depopulation of aboriginal Hispaniola. Hernando Gorjón, a vecino of the village of Azúa, penned a suggestive report around 1520. He recalled that he had come to the Indies in 1502. When he arrived, there were still many towns and people, but these had gradually disappeared over the years. He blamed the following factors: "la causa de esta despoblación es haber poca gente para trabajar e entender en grangerías." In addition "añade haberse ido muchos españoles, e la pestilencia de viruelas, sarampión e romadizo e otras enfermedades que han dado a los indios" (Rodríguez Demorizi 1971, 13-14; from CODOIN, 1:428). Hernando Gorjón confirms that prior to 1520 there passed through the population of the island several epidemics, not just the terrible and well known smallpox pandemic of 1518. Romadizo (influenza?), could he refer to 1493-94, or perhaps 1513-14, when it may have assaulted Tierra Firme? And the measles; there is fairly good evidence for an American measles outbreak in 1531, might there have been one earlier too? Gorjón forcefully confirms sickness in the Caribbean prior to the smallpox epidemic of 1518, and he clearly and succinctly establishes the link between disease and native American deaths.

Thus, there is evidence that in the quarter century between 1492 and 1518, not one, but several epidemics, coupled with hunger, overwork, and outright exploitation, swept the "paradise" described by Columbus, carrying away Tainos and European settlers. The consistent mention of disease by numerous contemporary eyewitnesses should put to rest the argument (Rosenblat 1976; Henige 1986, 1992) that it is difficult to blame massive mortality of the Amerindians on epidemics.

What of allegations that Las Casas failed to mention the disease factor? David Henige (1992, 6) argued that

> It must be a continual source of embarrassment that the redoubtable Bartolomé de las Casas, the godfather-by-acclaim of the movement [High Counters], had so little to say about the effects of disease, even though he wrote extensively, passionately, and extravagantly about the decline of the Indian population. Invariably, however, he attributed this to hunger, to famine, to mistreatment, or to a combination of these. To my knowledge no High Counter has ever addressed this awkward problem. Instead, they are content to use Las Casas' undocumented and implausibly high figures to hallow their enterprise.

Henige is wrong. Bartolomé de las Casas did establish a link between disease and depopulation of Hispaniola, both in the 1494-96 period, and subsequently. He noted that with the second expedition, there "came among them such illness, death and misery . . ., such that with the massacres of the wars and by the starvation and sicknesses that occur because of them . . . [vino sobre ellos tanta de enfermedad, muerte y miseria, de que murieron infelicemente de padres y madres y hijos, infinitos. Por manera que con las matanzas de las guerras y por las hambres y enfermedades que procedieron por causa de aquéllas y de

238   Colonial Latin American Review, Vol. 2, Nos. 1-2, 1993

las fatigas y opresiones que después sucedieron y miserias y sobre todo mucho dolor intrínseco, angustia y tristeza, no quedaron de las multitudes que en esta isla de gentes había . . .]" (Las Casas 1951, 1:419-20), only a third of those living in 1494 remained in 1496.

Disease raged among both Spaniards and the native peoples of Hispaniola, if not from 1492, then certainly beginning in November of 1493 with the arrival of the second expedition. Although we lack the data to identify accurately each illness, we can say that infectious disease became rampant. Given the devastating and documented impact Old World disease—smallpox, measles, typhus, plague, influenza, and later malaria and yellow fever—had on the native population of Mexico and Peru well into the nineteenth century, there is no reason that the equally virgin population of Hispaniola and the rest of the Caribbean should have been spared destruction in the first quarter century of contact. We suspect that influenza came early; strains of the virus mutate quickly, and a bout with one variety does not protect one against another strain. With over one thousand people on board the ships of the second fleet, influenza could have made the crossing easily. Malnutrition contributed to high mortality among the first European settlers. Gorjón suggested measles also made an early appearance in the New World. Measles, as influenza, is an acute communicable viral disease. Unlike influenza, a bout with measles confers strong immunity to the survivor. In Andalusia, measles was a childhood illness, endemic in cities as large as Seville. A number of susceptible passengers, probably youngsters, would have had to have been available for the disease to be carried to the Americas. We can identify an American outbreak in 1531, but one could have taken place earlier, as Gorjón suggests. Symptoms include a high fever, followed by a rash. Almost all native Americans who were exposed to the virus came down with the malady, and suffered a much higher rate of mortality than adult Europeans. Typhus also could have made an early crossing, since it is carried by the human louse, rather than an intermediate carrier as in the case of the plague. Typhus was prevalent in Spain in the late fifteenth century, and the *reconquista* of Granada had coincided with a particularly severe period of mortality. The Italian campaigns also saw serious outbreaks of typhus; as we have seen, many of the Pedrarias expedition had come from Italy. Conditions of malnutrition, human crowding, and poor hygiene, all common features of the transatlantic crossing, were ideal for the spread of typhus from one infected person to another. Native Americans who fell victim to any one of the most deadly killers, having had no previous exposure to the Old World diseases, died too quickly for symptoms to allow any diagnosis by the Spanish physicians resident in the Indies. So all too frequently, the first Europeans characterized Amerindians as weak, and quick to die.

Bartolomé de las Casas was a partisan. In his most polemical works in support of the native peoples of the Americas, especially the *Brevísima relación de la destrucción de las Indias*, the friar ignored the disease factor. To do otherwise would have destroyed the very foundation of his arguments for justice. Las Casas was an astute man; he had ample training in the law, and presented his case as any other solicitor of the sixteenth century. He chose his defense well, and disregarded evidence that might weaken his arguments. Las Casas knew the native Americans were dying of disease, and he did detail disease incidents in the massive *History of the Indies*. But he did not, nor could he, attribute the human catastrophe that he witnessed to disease alone. Instead, he emphasized exploitation and brutality.

In an attempt to understand the disaster that eliminated the Taino, the smallpox epidemic of 1518, Las Casas shifted the origin of both disease and the inhumane action of the Europeans to divine providence. Las Casas believed that devastating smallpox was brought on "by the will or permission of God, in order to free the few Indians who remained from so much torment and the anguished life that they suffered from, in all types of labor, especially in the mines, and at the same time in order to castigate those who oppressed them . . . [fue que por la voluntad o permisión de Dios, para sacar de tanto tormento y angustiosa vida que los pocos de indios que restaban padecían en toda especie de trabajos, mayormente en las minas, y juntamente para castigo de los que los oprimían, . . .]" (Las Casas 1951, 3:270-71). Las Casas argued that death gave freedom from European exploitation, and concluded that "no one who is Christian can doubt that although God in his secret judgments may have permitted such great inhumanity to have been inflicted on these peoples [ninguno que sea cristiano puede dudar que, aunque Dios por sus secretos juicios haya permitido así afligir estas gentes y con tanta inhumanidad]" (Las Casas 1951, 3:270-71), justice ultimately would be served. Friar Bartolomé de las Casas is not ambivalent regarding the hand of Providence; indeed, his response was shared by contemporary clerics who daily witnessed human frailty and the inevitability of death.

Note

*Research for this article, part of a longer project on disease in the Americas, was supported by a John Simon Guggenheim Memorial Foundation Fellowship

240   Colonial Latin American Review, Vol. 2, Nos. 1-2, 1993

in 1991-92. The author thanks the following for generous critical comments on an earlier version of the paper: Woodrow Borah, William M. Denevan, Henry F. Dobyns, Kenneth Kiple, W. George Lovell, Robert E. McCaa, David J. Robinson, and Mark Szuchman. Alexandra Parma Cook again helped clarify where obscurity initially prevailed. Any remaining errors are my own.

Bibliography

Alchon, Suzanne Austin. 1992.   Disease, population and public health in eighteenth-century Quito. In *"Secret judgments of God" : Old World disease in colonial Spanish America*, eds. Noble David Cook and W. George Lovell, 159-82. Norman: University of Oklahoma Press.

Alden, Dauril, and Joseph C. Miller.   1987a.   Out of Africa.   The slave trade and the transmission of smallpox to Brazil, 1560-1831. *Journal of Interdisciplinary History* 18:195-224.

———. 1987b. Unwanted cargoes: the origin and dissemination of smallpox via the slave trade, c. 1560-1830. In *The African exchange. Toward a biological history of Black people*, ed. Kenneth F. Kiple, 35-109. Durham: Duke University Press.

Amiama, Manuel A. 1959. La población de Santo Domingo. *Clio* 115:116-34.

Ballesteros Rodríguez, Juan. 1982. *La peste en Córdoba*. Córdoba: Diputación Provincial.

Bernáldez, Andrés.   1962.   *Memorias del reinado de los Reyes Católicos*. Madrid.

Borah, Woodrow.   1964.   America as model: the demographic impact of European expansion upon the non-European world. *Actas y memorias del XXXV Congreso Internacional de Americanistas*. México, D.F. 3:379-87.

———. 1976. The historical demography of aboriginal and colonial America: an attempt at perspective. In *The native population of the Americas in 1492*, ed. William M. Denevan, 13-34. Madison: University of Wisconsin Press.

Brau, Salvador. 1969. *La colonización de Puerto Rico*. San Juan: Instituto de Cultura Puertorriqueña.

Chaunu, Pierre, and Huguette Chaunu. 1956-60. *Seville et l'Atlantique (1504-1650)*. 12 Vols. Paris.

Chiappelli, Fredi, ed. 1976. *First images of America: the impact of the New World on the Old*. 2 vols. Berkeley: University of California Press.

Cipolla, Carlo M. 1973. *Christofano and the plague: a study in the history of public health in the age of Galileo*. Berkeley: University of California Press.

————. 1992. *Miasmas and disease. Public health and the environment in the pre-industrial age*. New Haven: Yale University Press.

Cohen, J. M., ed. *The four voyages of Christopher Columbus*. Baltimore, Md.: Penguin Books.

Colección de documentos inéditos relativos al descubrimiento, conquista, y organización de las antiguas posesiones españolas de América y Oceanía. 1864-84. 42 Vols. Madrid.

Cook, Noble David. 1981. *Demographic collapse: Indian Peru, 1520-1620*. New York: Cambridge University Press.

————. 1982. *People of the Colca valley: a population study*. Boulder: Westview Press.

————, and W. George Lovell, eds. 1992. *"Secret judgments of God": Old World disease in colonial Spanish America*. Norman: University of Oklahoma Press.

————, and W. George Lovell. 1992. Unraveling the web of disease. In *"Secret Judgments of God": Old World disease in colonial Spanish America*, eds. Noble David Cook and W. George Lovell, 215-44. Norman: University of Oklahoma Press.

Cook, Sherburne F., and Woodrow Borah. 1971-79. *Essays in population history: Mexico and the Caribbean*. 3 vols. Berkeley: University of California Press.

Córdova, Efrén. 1968. La encomienda y la desaparación de los indios en las Antillas mayores. *Caribbean Studies* 8:23-49.

Craton, Michael, and Gail Saunders. 1992. *Islanders in the stream: a history of the Bahamian people*. 2 vols. Athens: Unversity of Georgia Press.

Crosby, Alfred W. 1972. *The Columbian exchange: biological and cultural consequences of 1492*. Westport, Conn.: Greenwood Press.

————. 1976. Virgin soil epidemics as a factor in the aboriginal depopulation in America. *William and Mary Quarterly* 33:289-99.

————. 1986. *Ecological imperialism: the biological expansion of Europe, 900-1900*. Cambridge: Cambridge University Press.

Denevan, William M. 1992a. The pristine myth: the landscape of the Americas in 1492. *Annals of the Association of American Geographers* 82:369-85.

————, ed. 1976, rev. ed. 1992b. *The native population of the Americas in 1492*. Madison: University of Wisconsin Press.

Dobyns, Henry F. 1983. *Their number become thinned: native American population dynamics in eastern North America*. Knoxville: University of Tennessee Press.

Floyd, T. S. 1973. *The Columbus dynasty in the Caribbean, 1492 to 1526*. Albuquerque: University of New Mexico Press.

Gil, Juan, and Consuelo Varela, eds. 1984. *Cartas de particulares a Colón y Relaciones coetáneas*. Madrid: Alianza.

242   Colonial Latin American Review, Vol. 2, Nos. 1-2, 1993

————, eds. 1986. *Temas colombinos*. Sevilla: Escuela de Estudios Hispano-americanos.

Guerra, Francisco. 1966. The influence of disease on race, logistics, and colonization in the Antilles. *Journal of Tropical Medicine* 49:23-35.

————. 1975. The problem of syphilis. *First images of America: the impact of the New World on the Old*, ed. Fredi Chiapelli, 2:845-51. 2 Vols. Berkeley: University of California Press.

————. 1978. The dispute over syphilis: Europe versus America. *Clio Medica* (Netherlands) 13:39-62.

————. 1982. *Historia de la medicina*. 2 Vols. Madrid: Ediciones Norma.

————. 1985. La epidemia americana de influenza en 1493. *Revista de Indias* 45:325-47.

————. 1986. El efecto demográfico de las epidemias tras el descubrimiento de América. *Revista de Indias* 46:41-58.

————. 1988. The earliest American epidemic: the influenza of 1493. *Social Science History* 12:305-25.

Henige, David. 1978. On the contact population of Hispaniola: history as higher mathematics. *Hispanic American Historical Review* 58:217-37.

————. 1986a. If pigs could fly: Timucuan population and native American historical demography. *Journal of Interdisciplinary History* 16:701-20.

————. 1986b. Primary source by primary source? On the role of epidemics in New World depopulation. *Ethnohistory* 33:293-312.

————. 1986c. When did smallpox reach the New World (and why does it matter)? In *Africans in bondage: studies in slavery and the slave trade*, ed. Paul E. Lovejoy, 11-26. Madison: University of Wisconsin Press.

————. 1989. On the current devaluation of the notion of evidence: a rejoinder to Dobyns. *Ethnohistory* 36:304-7.

————. 1992. Native American population at contact: standards of proof and styles of discourse in the debate. *Latin American Population History Newsletter* 22:2-23.

Joralemon, Donald. 1982. New World depopulation and the case of disease. *Journal of Anthropological Research* 38:108-27.

Kiple, Kenneth F., ed. 1987. *The African exchange. Toward a biological history of Black people*. Durham: Duke University Press.

Las Casas, Bartolomé de. [bef. 1566] 1951. *Historia de las Indias*. 3 Vols. México: Fondo de Cultura Económica.

Lipschutz, Alejandro. La despoblación de los indios después de la conquista. *América indígena* 26:229-47.

López de Gómara, Francisco. [1552] 1964. *Cortés: The Life of the Conqueror by His Secretary*. Trans. by L. B. Simpson. Berkeley: University of California Press.

Lovell, W. George. 1985. *Conquest and survival in colonial Guatemala. A historical geography of the Cuchumatán highlands, 1500-1821*. Kingston and Montreal: McGill-Queen's University Press.

———. 1992. "Heavy shadows and black night": disease and depopulation in colonial Spanish America. *Annals of the Association of American Geographers* 82:426-43.

McNeill, William H. 1976. *Plagues and peoples*. Garden City, N.J.

Major, R. H., ed. 1978. *Christopher Columbus: four voyages to the New World*. Glouster, Mass.: Peter Smith.

Mártir de Anglería, Pedro. [bef. 1526] 1944. *Décadas del Nuevo Mundo*. Buenos Aires: Editorial Bajel.

———. [1511] 1947. *Una embajada de los Reyes Católicos a Egipto*. Valladolid: Consejo Superior de Investigaciones Científicas.

Moreno Ollero, Antonio. 1984. *Sanlúcar de Barrameda a fines de la edad media*. Cádiz: Diputación Provincial de Cádiz.

Morison, Samuel Eliot. 1963. *Journals and other documents on the life and voyages of Christopher Columbus*. New York: The Heritage Press.

Moya Pons, Frank. 1971. *La Española en el siglo XVI*. Santiago de los Caballeros: UCMM.

———. 1987. *Después de Colón. Trabajo, sociedad y política en la economía del oro*. Madrid: Alianza Editorial.

Newson, Linda. 1986. *The cost of conquest: Indian decline in Honduras under Spanish rule*. Boulder, Col.: Westview Press.

———. 1992. Old World epidemics in early colonial Ecuador. *"Secret Judgments of God": Old World disease in colonial Spanish America*, eds. Noble David Cook and W. George Lovell, 86-114. Norman: University of Oklahoma Press.

Parry, John H. A secular sense of responsibility. In *First images of America: the impact of the New World on the Old*, ed. Fredi Chiappelli, 1:287-304. Berkeley: University of California Press.

Pérez Moreda, Vicente. 1980. *La crisis de mortalidad en la España interior (siglos XVI-XIX)*. Madrid: Siglo Veintiuno.

Phillips, William D., and Carla Rahn Phillips. 1992. *The worlds of Christopher Columbus*. New York: Cambridge University Press.

Pyle, Gerald F. 1986. *The diffusion of influenza. Patterns and paradigms*. Totowa, N.J.: Rowman & Littlefield.

Ramenofsky, Ann F. 1987. *Vectors of death: the archaeology of European contact*. Albuquerque: University of New Mexico Press.

Reff, Daniel T. 1991. *Disease, depopulation, and culture change in northwestern New Spain, 1518-1764*. Salt Lake City: University of Utah Press.

Rodríguez Demorizi, Emilio. 1971. *Los dominicos y las encomiendas de indios de la isla Española*. Santo Domingo: Editora del Caribe.

244   Colonial Latin American Review, Vol. 2, Nos. 1-2, 1993

Rosenblat, Angel. 1954. *La población y el mestizaje en América*. 2 Vols. Buenos Aires: Editorial Nova.

─────. 1967. *La población de América en 1492: viejos y nuevos cálculos*. México: Colegio de México.

─────. 1976. The population of Hispaniola at the time of Columbus. In *The native population of the Americas in 1492*, ed. William M. Denevan, 43-66. Madison: University of Wisconsin Press.

Rouse, Irving. 1992. *The Tainos: rise and decline of the people who greeted Columbus*. New Haven: Yale University Press.

Sánchez-Albornoz, Nicolás. 1974. *The population of Latin America*. Berkeley: University of California Press.

─────. 1990. Demographic change in America and Africa induced by the European expansion, 1500-1800. In *The European discovery of the world and its economic effects on pre-industrial society, 1500-1800*, ed. Hans Pohl, 195-206. Stuttgart: Franz Steiner.

Sauer, Carl Ortwin. 1966. *The early Spanish Main*. Berkeley: University of California Press.

Schäfer, Ernesto. 1935-47. *El consejo real y supremo de las Indias*. 2 vols. Sevilla.

Stodder, Ann L. W., and Debra L. Martin. 1992. Health and disease in the Southwest before and after Spanish contact. In *Disease and demography in the Americas*, eds. John W. Verano and Douglas H. Ubelaker, 55-73. Washington: Smithsonian Institution Press.

Thornton, Russell. 1987. *American Indian holocaust and survival: a population history since 1492*. Norman: University of Oklahoma Press.

Verano, John W. 1992. Prehistoric disease and demography in the Andes. In *Disease and demography in the Americas*, eds. John W. Verano and Douglas H. Ubelaker, 15-24. Washington: Smithsonian Institution Press.

Verano, John W., and Douglas H. Ubelaker, eds. 1992. *Disease and demography in the Americas*. Washington: Smithsonian Institution Press.

Verlinden, Charles. La population de l'Amérique précolumbienne: une question de méthode. In *Méthodologie de l'histoire et des sciences humaines: mélanges en honneur de Fernand Braudel*, 453-62. Paris.

Villamarín, Juan A., and Judith E. Villamarín. 1992. Epidemic disease in the Sabana de Bogotá, 1536-1810. In *"Secret judgments of God": Old World disease in colonial Spanish America*, eds. Noble David Cook and W. George Lovell, 115-43. Norman: University of Oklahoma Press.

Vincent, Bernard. 1977. Las epidemias en Andalucía durante el siglo XVI. *Asclepio* 29:351-58.

Walter, John, and Roger Schofield, eds. 1989. *Famine, disease and the social order in early modern society*. New York: Cambridge University Press.

Watts, David. 1987. *The West Indies: patterns of development, culture and environmental change since 1492*. New York: Cambridge University Press.

Whitmore, Thomas M. 1992. *Disease and death in early colonial Mexico: simulating Amerindian depopulation*. Boulder, Col.: Westview Press.

Zambardino, Rudolph A. 1978. Critique of David Henige's "On the contact population of Hispaniola: history as higher mathematics." *Hispanic American Historical Review* 58:700-08.

3

New World Depopulation and the Case of Disease

Donald Joralemon

THERE ARE FEW WHO WOULD DOUBT that the indigenous population of the New World suffered a severe decline as a result of the arrival of European conquerors and settlers. How much of a decline, and its causes, remain subjects of controversy. In both cases debate arises from the simple fact that in the absence of reliable historical data, researchers must devise methods of retrospective projections. Beginning with a "known" (e.g., a well-documented census, evaluations of carrying capacity, etc.) demographers multiply by an assumed "constant" (e.g., a depopulation ratio), arriving thereby at an estimated figure for precontact population.

That the resulting estimates vary by as much as 104,153,750 (Table 1) is due to the use of radically different "knowns" and "constants." But it is more than basic data which causes such wide divergence in estimates. As Dobyns (1966) has suggested, the selection of projection material and the resulting conservative or liberal estimates often stem from uncritical assumptions about what the precontact New World must have looked like. Researchers, like Kroeber (1939), who imagined a sparsely settled hemisphere, would have chosen to leave out of the formula such factors as mortality from epidemics and ethnohistorical accounts of large populations. Given the opposite vision, as I think is true for Dobyns (1966), such evidence would weigh heavily in the calculation.

TABLE 1
New World Precontact Population Estimates

Source	Estimate
Alfred Kroeber (1939)	8,400,000
Angel Rosenblat (1954)	13,385,000
Paul Rivet (1924)	40,000,000 to 45,000,000
Karl Sapper (1924)	40,000,000 to 50,000,000
Herbert J. Spinden (1928)	50,000,000 to 75,000,000
Woodrow Borah (1964)	100,000,000
Henry F. Dobyns (1966)	90,000,000 to 112,553,750

An excellent example of divergent reasoning resulted in two very different estimates for precontact population in the Andean area of South America. In 1947 John Rowe reasoned from ethnohistorical records giving numbers of taxpayers in five provinces in 1525 (under the Inca) and in 1571 (under the Spanish) to total province figures at both points in time by assuming a 5:1 ratio of actual population to tribute payer. He then calculated a "depopulation ratio" for each province by comparing the total estimates for 1525 to those of 1571. The resulting ratios vary from a high of 25:1 on the coast to a low of 3:2 in the *sierra*. Rowe took the average ratio, 4:1, and applied it to a total Andean figure in 1571 of 1,500,000 persons to arrive at a precontact figure of six million persons living in the area as late as 1520 (Rowe 1947:184).

In 1966 Henry F. Dobyns chose to rely on what he called a "standard hemispheric depopulation ratio" of 20:1. This ratio suggested itself to him after a brief review of some area figures from various parts of the New World where such a drastic decline appeared to be the usual case. Applying this ratio to what he considered to be low points ("nadir") in area populations, he arrived at estimates for large sections of the two continents. The nadir figure he chose for the Andean area is 1,500,000, which, while the same as that chosen by Rowe, was placed as late as 1650. Multiplying by his depopulation factor of twenty, Dobyns came up with a precontact figure of thirty million (1966:415).

Thus, the two researchers arrived at figures which differ by a factor of five by accepting different depopulation ratios (their "knowns" being equal). That Rowe chose to average his ratios instead of taking the high coastal figure seems to reflect his conservative bias, just as Dobyns's selection of the highest ratio is reflective of a more liberal viewpoint. Likewise, Rowe's ethnohistorical accounts show less drastic depopulation, for the most part, than do those selected by Dobyns.

More recently other researchers have sought to improve Andean population estimates by using new sources of information (e.g., Cook 1977), as well as taking into account more geographic (e.g., Smith 1970) and demographic (e.g., Shea 1976) variables. These revisions are at least partially a response to criticisms leveled at anthropologists by demographers (e.g., Petersen 1975), but they have not significantly reduced the numerical variation of estimates. Although focused regional studies clearly improve historic population figures, the choice of mathematical operations in projecting back to periods without direct documentation still reflects subjective criteria.

What is often lost in these numerical calculations of population decline is a sensitivity to the range of precipitating factors. In Latin American demographic research this insensitivity has, in part, grown from a desire to free estimates from the assumed biases of early sources. The example of the well-known Indian advocate Bartolomé de Las Casas is often raised as an indication of the unreliability of the early chroniclers. It is widely assumed that the high mortality figures of Las Casas and others are broad exaggerations, generated to serve the particular vested interests of the author. This has led many researchers to dismiss the reports of the early chroniclers:

> Their characteristic methodology has included depreciation of all historical population figures. They deprecate the departure of historical witnesses from the "truth" for motives they intuitively impute, but which uniformly led said witnesses to overestimate, in their opinion, aboriginal populations (Dobyns 1966:398).

Unfortunately, not only is a potential first-hand source for numbers dismissed without evaluation for reliability, but also an awareness of the complex interplay of factors behind New World depopulation is lost when the witnesses are refused a hearing. An overconcern for numbers pure and simple has led many to ignore the reality those numbers reflect. A good example is Jehan Vellard's rejection of disease as a major cause of depopulation in Peru after the conquest (1956:85), an untenable position in the light of firm historical evidence (Polo 1913).

Many of the most widely recognized causes of depopulation are included in what has come to be known as the "Black Legend" (Carbia 1943; Hanke 1964), which records the loss of Indian lives by outright cruel practices on the part of the conquistadores. Early warfare and continued "pacification," mistreatment of Indians enslaved under the encomienda system, harsh labor practices, and general culture disruption resulting from the imposition of Spanish rule are all mentioned as contributing factors. Las Casas, who became protector of the Indians in 1515, ranks as the earliest and most eloquent spokesman to decry the conscious slaughter of Indians. While there remain questions as to the accuracy of his mortality figures, as well as to his having largely ignored disease as a causal agent, there is all too much evidence supporting his claim that a large proportion of Indian populations died at the hands of their captors (Sánchez-Albornoz 1974:51-54).

The mining communities in the province of Muzo, present-day Colombia, in the 1600s, highlight many of the factors mentioned above. In 1617 there were reported to be 9,127 Indians in the area; in 1629 there were only 4,261, a drop of 46.6 percent in just twelve years. In his analysis of the decline, Juan Friede (1967:343) used historical sources which give both total population and tributary population figures. The ratio between the two is 1:2.43, a proportion that indicates very small family size.

Assuming that such a ratio resulted from the decay of family structure in this labor community, Friede expands his vision of the impact of mining in colonial times to include high death rates for children and the old due to neglect, the increased need for a food surplus, the removal of adults, and family breakdown. All of this is in addition to extremely hard labor in the mines.

An unfortunate continuity is reflected in a more recent description of the mining community, at Corocoro, Bolivia, in 1914. Some thirteen thousand Indian workers, including women and children, labored there under conditions not very different from those of three hundred years earlier. In shafts so dangerous that even foremen would avoid descending, workers would climb down as much as 1500 feet on "chicken ladders"—inclined poles with notched steps.

> In one vertical shaft that was being sunk below the 1700 level it took so long for the miners to climb from the surface down and up again that they were required to stay underground 36 hours without a break. They alternately worked for an hour and sat down for ten minutes to eat a little dried meat and to chew dried coca leaves. These contained enough stimulant to keep the miners from collapsing. It was no wonder that the average length of life was about 25 years (Joralemon 1976:98).

It is all too easy to stop at this point and assume that high Indian death rates resulted solely from their treatment by Spanish overlords. Certainly the many accounts of Las Casas and other detractors bring these causes of depopulation into clear focus and suggest that herein lies sufficient explanation for population decline. However, a second major source of death has yet to be considered: epidemic diseases introduced to the New World by Europeans and Africans in the first century after contact contributed mightily to the loss of Indian lives.

The year 1492 initiated a biological interaction between European, New World, and, later, African epidemiological biospheres; the first two centuries after contact can be evaluated in terms of the biological impact of expansion into the New World. Two major questions are present from the start: what new disease agents were introduced into the New World at the point of contact, and how the initial impact of foreign disease differs from its repercussions in areas with prior exposure. Both questions have stirred great debate.

For the most part, the New World has been credited with a fairly clean bill of health prior to contact (Martin 1978:48). Few dispute the absence of smallpox, measles, and typhus in the New World before the arrival of Europeans, however much argument has arisen over the issue of syphilis, leprosy, and malaria. Evidence supporting New World origin of the latter is taken from the analysis of skeletons for characteristic bone lesions, references to native histories taken down by the Spanish soon after contact, and, in the case of syphilis, evaluations of European historical records for precontact outbreaks. Unfortunately, a lack of adequate criteria for judging the specific cause of various skeletal lesions, and ambiguous historical descriptions of diseases in both Europe and the New World make analysis very difficult.

While syphilis and leprosy have been significant factors in the health of Latin American Indians, neither has attained the status of mass killer. Malaria, however, has ranked as one of the most serious threats to life for as long as its presence has been known. Therefore, the issue of precontact presence of malaria deserves some further attention. The fact that the carriers of malaria, mosquitoes belonging to the subfamily Anophelinae, were almost certainly present in the aboriginal New World makes it more difficult to demonstrate that the disease was an import. Nevertheless, it is possible that the protozoan parasites (plasmodia) which are responsible for the disease were not present prior to the arrival of infected persons from Europe or, more likely, Africa.

Support for the postcontact introduction of malaria can be found in Boyd (1949), Jarcho (1964), Dunn (1965), and Coatney (1971); a good review of the arguments on both sides of the issue is offered by Bruce-Chwatt (1965). However, the argument made by Ashburn (1947:103-10) is perhaps the most appealing.

By comparing the reports of early travelers to more recent explorations in the same areas of South America, Ashburn noted a significant discrepancy. In reviewing the accounts of early trips into the Amazon, such as those of Gonzalo Pizarro in 1539, Francisco de Orellana in 1540, and Father Cristoval de Acuña in 1639, no reference to any illness identifiable as malaria is found. In fact the accounts describe thriving Indian villages all along the rivers, and ascribe what deaths as occurred to Indian attacks and starvation (Markham 1859). Compare this to the report of the 1926 Hamilton Rice Expedition into some of the same areas (Strong 1926:13, 69):

> Generally speaking, the inhabitants living upon the river banks show evidence of either acute or chronic disease, or the effects of having suffered from such disease. Portions of Amazonia today constitute some of the most unhealthy and most dangerous regions to reside in, from the standpoint of health, that exist in the tropics.
>
> Malaria is the most prevalent and most serious disease of Amazonia. The Oswaldo Cruz Commission, the members of which carried [out] investigations on the Rio Negro in 1913, reported that it was difficult to find a single individual who did not show signs of chronic malarial infection.

If malaria had developed in the New World prior to contact, then early Amazonian travelers almost certainly would have noticed the ravages of this disease. In the absence of any such report in their journals it may be assumed that the Amazon Basin had yet to be plagued by a malarial agent, and that overall it was a healthier environment than that described by travelers some three hundred years later. Both Scott (1939) and Ashburn (1947) are persuaded by this argument that malaria is a late introduction to the New World, probably originating in Africa and carried across the ocean by black slaves.

The second issue related to introduced disease is whether death rates reach higher levels in previously isolated areas than in areas where the disease is endemic. Most researchers agree that especially high mortality results from the occurence of disease on "virgin soil." C.W. Dixon (1962:189), for instance, suggests that both measles and smallpox "could produce a high mortality when occurring in a new population." George G. Ginglioli (1968:108) argues that "high susceptibility and reactivity in the Amerindian to malaria is without doubt related to recent introduction of the infection into the Western Hemisphere."

This claim, at least for malaria, is countered by Centerwall (1968:80), whose experience led him to conclude that there is "only very limited evidence for a greater innate susceptibility of the Indian to this disease." He argues that the presence or absence of nursing care is the greatest variable in differing mortality rates for malaria. His position is supported by the fact that excessive death rates have resulted from diseases to which a population has had prior exposure. The deadly outbreaks of smallpox in England in the late 1800s (Dixon 1962:200-13), even with vaccines in use, are a good example of this phenomenon.

The important point is that either position leads to the same conclusion: there were high Indian death rates from disease. Be it because of increased susceptibility or poor nursing care, there is no dispute that large numbers of Indians died as a consequence of epidemics started by contact with Europeans. It may be significant in this regard that some traditional Indian curing techniques, such as the well-known sweat house, may have aggravated an illness and caused death where better care might have prevented it.

For all of the debate over these issues it remains clear that epidemic disease must be considered a central factor in New World depopulation. As will be demonstrated, it is not as easy as some assume to dismiss early accounts that attribute many thousands of deaths to the ravages of a single epidemic. Ashburn's (1947:98) characterization of the interaction between European and African biospheres on one side, and that of the New World on the other, as a biological war is not far from the truth, at least as that truth is reflected in the historical record:

> Smallpox was the captain of the men of death in that war, typhus fever the first lieutenant, and measles the second lieutenant. More terrible than the conquistadores on horseback, more deadly than sword and gunpowder, they made the conquest by the whites a walkover as compared with what it would have been without their aid. They were the forerunners of civilization, the companions of Christianity, the friends of the invader.

DISEASE AND THE HISTORICAL RECORD

The most obvious source of evidence on the impact of epidemic disease is the historical record left behind by the earliest generations of conquerors and settlers. For Latin America these records come from a variety of persons, and range from outright histories to collections of letters between Spanish monarchs and the officials they appointed in the New World. The authors include Christian clerics and missionaries (e.g., Las Casas and Father Acuña), as well as companions of the conquerors (e.g., Díaz de Castillo).

Mention has already been made of one limitation of these sources, namely, the bias of the author. It is said that Las Casas ignored disease as a cause of Indian deaths because he wanted to impress the king of Spain with the cruelties being inflicted consciously by the conquistadores. The problems involved in such second guessing of motives, however, are manifold (Dobyns 1966:398). An example of a mistake resulting from such imputing of motives in the case of disease will clarify this point.

Juan Friede (1967) argues for an initial mistrust of all colonial reports mentioning epidemic outbreaks, suggesting that because many Spaniards viewed disease as either a selective mechanism or a result of sin, their reports of epidemics would necessarily be biased. He urges the use of supporting documents in a cross-checking analysis of any such report, claiming that real epidemics would leave many documented traces; one such trace would be a sudden increase in requests by *encomenderos* for more slaves. Applying this method, he demonstrates that a report of Cieza de Leon on a plague in the province of Cartago in New Granada cannot be trusted.

While cross-checking is absolutely essential to any use of the chronicles, Friede erred when he assumed that encomenderos would request large numbers of Indians after an epidemic. A well-documented epidemic occurred in Peru in 1546 (Dobyns 1966:499), but is not reflected in the collection of letters received by then-governor Gonzalo Pizarro (Laredo 1925). The number of requests for slaves found in the letters appears quite constant, and the only mention of disease in the time span covered by the collection (1532-60) is one in Arequipa, years later. An alternate motive could be suggested: those who owned slaves did not want the governor to know how quickly they were dying. One problem of assigning motives, then, is that far too often the opposite turns out to be just as feasible.

A much more significant limitation of the early chronicles for disease research stems from the dismal state of medical knowledge at the time, and the general inattention to symptom description. Frequently the accounts employ native terms that are difficult to interpret, and describe symptoms that could be attributed to many diseases. An epidemic in Mexico in 1545, for instance, was known by its Nahuatl name "matlazahuatl," while the Spanish simply called it "peste" (Dobyns 1963:499-500). The following description of the 1540 Peruvian epidemic mentioned above is supplied by Herrera and gives a good idea of what an especially good description of symptoms looks like (Palo 1913:9, my translation):

> A general plague from which innumerable people died occurred this year (1546) among Indians throughout the Kingdom of Peru, begining beyond Cuzco and extending through all the land; it was an illness that caused headaches and strong accompanying fever, and later the head pains passed to the left ear, so aggravating the sickness that they died in two or three days.[1]

Even when the description of symptoms is detailed, the diagnosis is often nothing more than guesswork. When Lozano, a Jesuit living in Paraguay in the early 1700s, describes the last throes of an epidemic disease, he mentions an occluded throat and death by suffocation (Helps 1966(4):259). One reasonable guess is diphtheria but a number of other possibilities, including fulminating smallpox (which shows no rash), might also be suggested. In only a few cases, usually when described symptoms are characteristic of only one disease, can an isolated account yield enough information for a retrospective diagnosis with any degree of certainty. With more than one account of a single disease outbreak the possibilities are far better.

But there is still a useful place for the accounts of early chronicles. No matter how poor their descriptions of symptoms, nor how underexaggerated their figures, they were still written by eyewitnesses, and can therefore supply information not otherwise attainable. Such accounts are useful in pinpointing in space and time occurrences of major epidemics, in generally describing which sectors of society were most seriously struck, and sometimes in providing reliable figures (through censuses, for instance) and helping to reduce to a minimum the number of possible diagnoses.

Not to be dismissed, either, are descriptions which convey more emotional responses to the results of epidemics, for this human factor is not adequately reflected in discussions of numbers and symptoms. The epidemic of smallpox which struck Meso-America on the eve of the conquest (1521) becomes real in the account of Bernal Díaz del Castillo, a foot soldier under Cortez (Ashburn 1947:84):

> The streets, the squares, the houses and the courts of Talteluco were covered with dead bodies: we could not step without treading on them and the stench was intolerable. Accordingly, they (the Indians) were ordered to remove to neighboring towns, and for three days and three nights all the causeways were full, from one end to the other, of men, women, and children, so weak and sickly, squalid and dirty, and pestilential that it was a misery to behold them.

The value of historical accounts is especially clear in the Andean area, where there is frequently enough material to cross-check accounts. In addition to the sources listed above, the Andean area also offers early newspaper stories, city annals, hospital records (e.g., the Santa Ana hospital for Indians), and letters from the region's viceroys. The pioneering work of José Torbio Polo (1913) and the more recent article by Dobyns (1963) serve as invaluable collections of relevant material, drawn from numerous sources. Such a wealth of information makes it possible to obtain a more vivid picture of the impact of epidemic diseases in the Andean area than in many other parts of Latin America, with the possible exceptions of Mexico (Borah and Cook 1960, 1963, 1967) and Colombia (Jaramillo Uribe 1964).

A particularly clear and well-documented account is that of the epidemic which struck the city of Arequipa in 1589, by the early historian Echeverria, quoted in Polo (1913:17-19) and paraphrased by Dobyns (1963:507):

> The onset of the disease brought severe headaches and kidney pains. A few days later, patients became stupified, then delirious, and ran naked through the streets shouting. Patients who broke out in a rash had a good chance to recover, reportedly, while those who did not break out seemed to have little chance. Ulcerated throat killed many patients. Fetuses died in the uterus. Even patients who broke out in a rash might lose chunks of flesh by too sudden movement . . . No count of victims was possible in Arequipa, where they had to be interred in open ditches in the public squares during the three month long episode.

This example will provide a base for further comment later, but at this point it is important to note that the description yields an unusually accurate picture of symptoms, as well as a vivid image of the chaotic state of a city undergoing a severe epidemic. If all accounts were this accurate, the image of epidemic disease in post-contact times would be far clearer.

The overall view Dobyns offers of Andean epidemic history from 1520 to 1720 is that of an initial severe drop in the first seventy years, due in part to an extension of epidemics arriving from Meso-America even before the Spanish. This was followed by a recovery period, in Dobyns's view, of just over 125 years, and then another drastic decline from 1718 to 1720. John Hemming (1970:350) takes a slightly different view, suggesting that while disease was an important contributor to decline in the first forty years of Spanish rule, more important was "profound cultural shock and chaotic administration." There is little doubt that the actual depopulation represented a complex of many factors, but what is significant is that disease is considered by both as a major influence on indigenous populations.

In these analyses of Andean epidemic history, as much as for those focusing on other parts of the New World, two valuable sources of evidence are insufficiently used. Little effort has been directed toward the utilization of detailed medical information on epidemic diseases, or of well-documented reports of analogous outbreaks in more recent times, in other parts of the world as well as in Latin America.[2]

The first step in using medical information is to consider the nature of the most important diseases in Latin American history (especially smallpox, measles, and malaria) in terms of disease agent, mode of transmission, and identifiable symptoms. Knowing these three variables will make it possible to evaluate ethnohistorical records in terms of diagnosis (where descriptions permit) and feasibility. Thus, if a source describes an illness that can be identified as malaria, but expands its range beyond the limits of the habitat of the anopheles mosquito, it would be possible to question the account.

It might be thought that this step is such an obvious check that scholars must already have employed it. In fact, with the exception of Ashburn (1947), who was a doctor himself, and Martin (1978), a remarkable inattention to medical details has characterized most analyses of depopulation trends in the New World. For the most part, the lack of medical knowledge has led researchers to underestimate the possible fatalities in reported epidemics. Kroeber's dismissal of high epidemic mortality figures for California Indians is a good example (Dobyns 1966:410).

Even when high death potential is granted to disease, there is seldom a careful weighing of medical information against historical accounts. Especially lacking is a sensitivity to the total disruption of community life in outbreaks of epidemics. While not directly reflected in mortality counts, this aspect of epidemics is certainly a significant factor, requiring treatment in any analysis of the effects of disease.

Aside from clearly defining diseases in medical terms, it is also extremely useful to employ information derived from well-documented outbreaks of the same sickness under similar conditions. It is necessary to insure comparability of cases by restricting analogues to outbreaks of introduced diseases in areas lacking medical care, and preferably under similar conditions of sanitation. Two other variables may also be significant, depending on the epidemiological characteristics of a given disease: population density and natural environment. For instance, if transmission of a specific disease occurs through the air, it may not be useful to compare an urban outbreak, where an infected individual can come in close contact with large numbers of people, with the more isolated conditions of a rural setting.

Alfred W. Crosby (1967:325), in his analysis of epidemics in early Latin American colonial history, demonstrates an unusual concern both for medical information and analogous cases, and yet he is also selective in his choice of data. Concerning smallpox he writes:

> Where it has struck isolated groups, the death rate has been awesome. Analysis of figures for some twenty outbreaks shows that the case mortality among an unvaccinated population is

about thirty percent. Presumably, in people who have had no contact whatever with smallpox, the disease will infect nearly every single individual it touches. When in 1707 smallpox first appeared in Iceland, it is said that in two years 18,000 out of the island's 50,000 inhabitants died of it.

Crosby's source for the thirty percent mortality figure in unvaccinated populations is Dixon (1962:325). Unfortunately, Dixon was referring to the death rate of only one major type of smallpox, variola major, which is the more severe but by no means most frequent form of the disease. For the other type, variola minor, Dixon gives a peak mortality figure of .6 percent (1962:326). The difference is best shown by comparing Iceland's outbreak, which may well have been variola major, with the following (Dixon 1962:203):

> Thomas Phillips describes the journey of a slaveship from Guinea to Barbados in 1694, during which apparently smallpox, although very prevelant, had a low mortality and an outbreak in Minorca in 1742 also produced very few deaths, but "every house a hospital."

Steam and Steam (1945) made a similar error in failing to distinguish between mild and severe forms of smallpox. Dobyns (1963:497) uses the same Iceland example to conclude that a 50 percent mortality might have occurred in the Andean area after 1520. The point is that greater care is needed in the use of medical information and analogous cases, lest the assumption be made that wherever a specific disease occurred among Latin American Indians a set percentage of people died. That diseases like smallpox have more than one manifestation, with corresponding differences in death rates, is enough reason to reject such an assumption.

As is always the case with reasoning by analogy, care must be taken in assuring that the comparison is valid, and unguided generalizing from the specific to the universal must be avoided. It is acceptable to use a well-documented mortality figure for a given disease to support a figure of equal magnitude in a specific, less well-documented outbreak; it is not acceptable to generalize that figure to all outbreaks of the disease. Thus, Crosby's Iceland example might be useful in substantiating a given outbreak where mortality is reported to have exceeded 30 percent of those afflicted, since such a high figure, assuming the presence of general smallpox symptoms in each outbreak, would suggest a diagnosis of variola major in both cases. The example is not useful as a general model for all outbreaks of smallpox, however.

Without attempting to connect each of the following to a specific historical example from Latin America, I would like to offer a few potential analogues, keeping in mind that their utility is proven only when such connections are made. They are presented in part to underline the potential severity of disease, as well as to provide evidence that indigenous and other isolated populations may be especially susceptible to drastic depopulation stemming from the introduction of foreign diseases. It becomes easier to place faith in the reports of the early chroniclers when the effects of epidemic disease in other places and in other times have been noted.

The Iceland example, where 36 percent of the total population died from an outbreak of smallpox in 1707-09, has already been mentioned. In 1713 the same disease was introduced into South Africa through the clothing of afflicted passengers of a ship from India. High death rates among the Hottentots contributed to a 35 percent case fatality (200 of 570 cases). Another outbreak in 1775 in the same area resulted in the deaths of 963 Europeans and more than 1,000 natives (Dixon 1962:207-8). Similar high mortality from smallpox was recorded among North

American Indians of the northern Plains and Upper Great Lakes in 1781-82, with perhaps as much as 60 percent of some groups succumbing to the disease (Martin 1978:131-33).

Measles also has been a significant killer. Various outbreaks in Peru, Chile, and Bolivia in the seventeenth century took thousands of Indian lives (Dobyns 1963:509-10). On the Faroe Islands an outbreak in 1846, after a sixty-five year isolation from the disease, resulted in a 77 percent infection rate (6,000 of 7,782) and over 100 deaths (Ashburn 1947:90). Similar high fatality in this century has plagued groups like the Yanomamö (Centerwall 1968), Tapirapé, and Kaingang (Wagley 1977:38, 136,277).

The effects of malaria have already been suggested by the earlier discussion of its introduction into the New World. It has been a steady killer of Indians as well as whites for centuries and is only recently being controlled in parts of Latin America (PAHO 1971:21).

To the above diseases should be added influenza, which alone and in combination with other sicknesses has been responsible for many Indian deaths since conquest. In 1918 a massive epidemic in Guatemala struck 325,220 persons, killing 13 percent of them (43,733, Shattuck 1933:350). A similar loss of life occured in a 1929 influenza outbreak among the Sabane of Brazil (Vellard 1956:80).

One last disease, cholera, had a late arrival in the New World, but once it had arrived it struck indigenous populations with special severity, since its transmission through contaminated water and food finds ideal ground in areas of low health standards, especially poor sanitation. An outbreak of cholera in Campeche, Yucatan, in 1833 is described in a sarcastic tone by a despairing Dr. Henry Perrine (Shattuck 1933:340-41):

> Officially we buried only about 4,000 in four weeks, and not more than 400 on the most fatal day. Estimating the whole population remaining in Campeche at 20,000, the mortality was nominally but 20%. In a village only five miles distant, along the coast, where there was no medical assistance, at least forty percent of the original number perished. Finally the living begin to envy the dead. Happy the dead, was the general remark, they had some aid during life, something like interment after death—but we must perish alone and be consumed by dogs and buzzards in our dwellings.

While accounts like these clearly demonstrate the potential magnitude of epidemic disease in terms of death counts, they fail to reveal adequately the extent of cultural disruption. The fact is that whole communities, as much as individual organisms suffer the impact of an epidemic. It is too simple to view an Indian child who survives disfiguring smallpox, or dies from malaria, as a statistic or a complex of symptoms. His or her illness develops in a cultural milieu with numerous institutions and beliefs that must also adapt to the presence of a deadly biological enemy. And the disease develops among living human beings intimately tied to each other in a complex of interpersonal relations, human beings who are involved in the course of the disease even if they suffer no symptoms.

In 1968, when a Brazilian boy sick with measles passed through Yanomamö Indian territory in southern Venezuela, an epidemic was started which within three months had spread over a hundred miles of waterways, striking more than fifteen villages. In three villages, where some medical care was available, there were 170 persons sick, of whom 29 died. Taking Chagnon's (1968:1) average of 80 persons per village, that means that nearly 70 percent of each community were sick, with 10 percent of them dying—and that with medical care. The situation is described by Centerwall, who along with others, joined Chagnon on a journey to the area that year (Centerwall 1968:79):

> We were particularly impressed with the devastating effect of measles in its near total involvement of the Indian community. When parents and children were simultaneously involved, there was a drastic breakdown of both the will and the means for necessary nursing care. We have even seen several instances where three generations of Indians were simultaneously ill with measles. The reaction of those not already prostrated in a fatalistic depression was usually one of panic. Sometimes the well members of the village even abandoned the sick, and normal community structure and function were lost. Village fragments often fled to other villages for haven, thus increasing the spread of the disease.

A similar mortality was the result of another measles epidemic, among the Xingu of Brazil in June of 1954. Where care was available, 9.6 percent of those afflicted died; where absent, the death rate rose to 26.8 percent (Nutels 1968:70). If this second figure is read back into the Yanomamö case, then where care was unavailable it is likely that fifteen individuals, or 18 percent of the total village died in the 1968 epidemic. The lasting effects of an epidemic can proceed in diverse directions, as is evidenced by an earlier (1940) Yanomamö measles outbreak that led an affected village to accuse another of having caused the disease by magic. The resulting sequence of revenge raids lasted into 1965, twenty-five years after the epidemic (Chagnon 1968:76).

From the Yanomamö there is also a fascinating insider's account of another epidemic, that sheds more light on this human side of the problem. In this case blame for the disease was laid by some on Shawara-wakeshi, a being that enters the body and kills the helping Hekura spirit. Others pinned it down to a more specific source (Biocca 1970:213):

> When the whites undress, they leave the illness in their clothes. We die because of Shawara-wakeshi; it is the whites. White men cause illness; if the whites had never existed, disease would never have existed either.

AREQUIPA, 1589—A TEST CASE

It has been suggested thus far that a careful blending of reliable historical accounts with medical information and analogous cases can be useful in presenting a more complete and accurate understanding of the impact of epidemic disease in Latin America after contact. Even without linking the analysis to specific historical epidemics, it has been possible to allow the latter two sources of evidence to sketch out potential scenarios.

The most obvious next step is to test the method in a specific historical epidemic, treating it in terms of what can be gathered about its total impact from the various sources of information. The Arequipa epidemic of 1589, to which reference was made earlier, will supply the test case. For reasons that will become clear as the discussion progresses, data on the epidemiological characteristics of smallpox, drawn mainly from Dixon (1962), will precede direct consideration of the epidemic itself.

Smallpox is an acute virus infection said to exist in two distinct variants, that causing variola major and that causing variola minor. The virus is most often transmitted through the air in droplets or dust, entering the victim through the respiratory tract. It is also possible for particles carrying the virus to be found on clothing, sheets, and even on food which has come in contact with an infected individual.

While some records claim that infection occurred through ingestion of contaminated substances (water, food), it is more likely that airborne particles are generally responsible for passage of the disease. Humans are the only source of the smallpox virus, and the period of infectiousness, beginning around the tenth day of the incubation stage, can last up to two weeks from the first appearance of symptoms. The corpse of a victim is highly contagious.

The survival of the virus outside of the body depends on the bearing agent, the temperature, and the humidity. On cotton, the virus can survive for 185 days at 30°C and 58 percent humidity. The higher the humidity, the shorter the survival time. On the scabs of a victim, and at room temperature with 55 percent humidity, the virus has been known to survive for eighteen months (Dixon 1962:304). With such a long survival time and with easy transmission through the air from contaminated articles, smallpox spread is due more to interaction networks than density of population.

For both varieties of smallpox there are ten possible classifications by symptoms, with varying mortality rates for each. In general, variola minor is believed to have a very low mortality rate in any of its manifestations. The same is true for five types of variola major (discrete, mild, abortive, variola sin eruptione, and miscellaneous). Thus, when high death rates occur they are likely to be caused by one of the first five types of variola major: fulminating (100 percent mortality), malignant confluent (70 percent), malignant semi-confluent (25 percent), benign confluent (20 percent), and benign semi-confluent (10 percent) (Dixon 1962:6-7).

Table 2 will demonstrate some of the confusions that occur in diagnosing smallpox at each stage of the development of the illness, even with current techniques. It is no wonder that the chroniclers had difficulty identifying what they saw.

On the question of susceptibility, Dixon (1962:318) argues that,

Racial predisposition probably does not exist as such, but a population that has experienced the disease for some generations, even if unvaccinated, appears to have a lower mortality than one that has never experienced it before.

It should be noted in this regard that normally high mortality among young and old can increase in areas of poor hygiene and poverty as a result of concomitant infections, particularly of the respiratory tract. Death is also especially high among pregnant women; up to 50 percent in cases of variola major. Even in the best of conditions, there are two types of smallpox that are devastating, virtually regardless of the extent of care (Dixon 1962:102):

The cases for which we are completely powerless to do anything are the fulminating and the malignant. In the fulminating the sledgehammer blow is so rapid and so devastating that it seems difficult to visualize any treatment having any effect, even assuming the diagnosis is made. With the malignant we have twelve to thirteen days from onset to death, but so far nothing has been of any value.

From the point of view of environmental factors there is little reason to believe that Peru would have presented smallpox with any major obstacles. The long life of the virus in dry air might have increased its spread during dry seasons in Peru's highlands and lowlands. At first one might believe that the coastal stretch, with densely populated river valleys isolated from each other by desert, might have impeded the progress of the disease. However, there is sufficient evidence of extensive interaction between valley populations during Inca times, in trade as well as through administrative and military networks, to eliminate any safety factor that geographic isolation might have produced.

TABLE 2
Diseases Confused with Smallpox at Different Stages*

Initial Stage

Influenza	Acute purpura
Acute septicemias	Acute leukemia
Toxic scarlet fever	Lumbago
Meningitis	Encephalitis
Appendicitis	Enteric fever
Pneumonia	

Early: Maculopapular and Erythematous Stages

Measles	Erythema multiforme
Rubella	Acne (modified cases)
Drug eruptions	Insect bites
Papular syphilides	

Late: Vesicular and Pustular Stages

Chickenpox	Impetigo
Vaccinia (generalized)	Drug eruptions
Erythema multiforme	Pustular syphilides
Stevens-johnson syndrome	Pemphigus
Scabies	Bullous impetigo

Secondary Causes of Death

Bronchopneumonia	Multiple staphyloccal abscesses
Streptococcal septicemia	Osteomyelitis
Staphylococcal septicemia	
Pyemia	Empyema

* From Dixon (1962:68, 88)

The increasing numbers of Spaniards in Peru after conquest would also have increased the potential spread of smallpox along their travel routes. Further impetus to the disease was surely provided through the encomienda system, with Indians from various regions being grouped together in labor communities. The mining work forces, representing forced labor drawn from as many regions as necessary, would have provided another interaction network for the spread of the smallpox virus.

It is not, however, the presence of interaction networks alone that would account for excessive death rates. As indicated in Table 2, a whole series of secondary causes of death is frequently involved in smallpox mortality figures. Some of these, especially bronchopneumonia, are more likely to occur under conditions of inadequate nursing care, poor health standards, and insufficient nutrition. There is good reason to believe that colonial Peru, with its disruption of Inca food distributional systems and its establishment of slavery, had the effect of drastically reducing overall health conditions among the indigenous peoples. Early warfare alone would have had this effect, since fields and towns were often burned to reduce the enemy's advantage. Such a reduction in health conditions would necessarily have increased the deaths due to complicating infections in any epidemic.

Inasmuch as there were few environmental factors in postconquest Peru that might have thwarted the spread of smallpox, and many social factors that could have intensified its movement and severity, it is likely that the disease had a most drastic impact once introduced. Exactly how much of an impact would have depended primarily on the strain of the disease, variola major or minor. For any given outbreak, careful attention should be given to symptomatic descriptions to see whether such an assessment can be made.

Where any one historical account fails to provide enough information to make a certain diagnosis, some cross-checks can be applied to ascertain the accuracy of stated figures. It would be useful not only to look for confirming reports from the same area, but also to see whether an isolated report could be tied in with others as part of a large-scale epidemic. If various accounts showed continuity in time and relative proximity (or interaction) in space, then their symptom descriptions might also be evaluated for continuity in the light of medical information. Thus, what one description left out, another might fill in so that a better diagnosis could be made. Having determined the likely disease, a final check could be made by ascertaining whether it is epidemiologically possible for it to have covered the assumed area.

In the historical account of the Arequipa epidemic of 1589, mention is made of severe head and kidney pains, a sort of delirium within a few days, ulcerated throat, and loss of flesh in sudden movement. Additionally, reference is made to a better prognosis in the presence of a rash, and to frequent miscarriages. There is little question that this epidemic was a combination of fulminating and malignant confluent (variola major) smallpox. Compare the following diagnostic statements made by Dixon (1962) with the description above (Dixon 1962:14, 97, 16, 17, 18):

Malaise, intense headache and general aching of the muscles occur. Backache may be very severe.

Loss of speech is a common phenomenon and probably the most constant symptom noticed. Personality changes, delusions, abnormal behavior are also quite common.

From about the seventh or eighth day of the disease there are complaints of increased difficulty in swallowing, and pain on talking, due to excessive lesions in the mucous membranes.

Uterine hemorrhages are common and may be severe; in pregnant women abortion or premature labor is almost certain to occur.

Slight rubbing of the bedclothes or movements of the arm by the nurse or doctor may cause a large piece of dead epidermis to become detached.

If the above comparison is not convincing, then the reference in the early source to the better prognosis when a rash occurs may be taken as a final persuasive point. While all of the above remarks apply to malignant confluent smallpox, many also hold true for fulminating smallpox; the difference is that in the latter there are seldom any focal lesions (rash), and death is virtually assured within twenty-four to thirty-six hours. A 25 percent difference in mortality reflects this point. It is also possible that the correlation of rash with a much higher chance for survival indicates the involvement of benign confluent smallpox, as well. Both the symptoms and fatality cancel the possibility of the epidemic having been variola minor.

Dobyns (1963:505-8) and Polo (1913:15-20) muster convincing evidence in the form of supporting accounts that this outbreak in Arequipa was part of an immense epidemic that must have involved most of Peru. Various symptom descriptions confirm that the epidemic was smallpox, almost undoubtedly a combination of the three most severe types of variola major. The following description taken from the letter of a Jesuit priest in Lima suggests the clarity of the accounts (Polo 1913:56, my translation):

> Virulent pustules erupted all over the body, deforming the miserable sick to the extent that they could be recognized only by name. The virus attacked in such a way that the skin, covered with prominent scabs, appeared burned by fire. The pustules obstructed the throat, impeding the passage of food and hardly permitting speech or respiration; and this caused many to die.[3]

This particular source puts the mortality of the 1589 epidemic at three million persons, a figure that sounds incredibly high. Having identified the disease, however, it is possible to offer a percentage figure from more reliable medical data (Dixon 1962:171):

> In natural smallpox, infection of a group of susceptibles with Variola major virus gives rise to a high proportion of severe cases with an overall case mortality of about thirty percent.

The first problem is to estimate how much of a population is likely to come down with the disease. Dixon (1962:310) presents a chart which suggests a 100 percent risk of infection in a community when there has been no prior exposure. The Iceland example seems to confirm such a strike rate for a virgin population, at least for what seems to have been variola major. Nevertheless, a lower percentage seems to be called for in Peru, due to greater geographic distribution and varying natural environment. Just to be conservative, an 80 percent infection rate will be accepted for the Andean case at hand.

Andean population estimates (see Figure 1) include those of Rowe (1947) and Smith (1970) for the population in 1570, both close to 1,500,000. Since no major epidemics broke out between then and the epidemic under consideration, it is possible to take this figure as a baseline for estimating how many were struck and how many died in the 1589 smallpox outbreak. If 80 percent contracted the sickness, then some 1,200,000 were sick during the epidemic. If 30 percent of those died, then around 360,000 Indians can be listed as casualties, a figure that works out to approximately 986 persons per day in all of Peru.

The other population estimate is Dobyns's (1966:415), also represented in Figure 1. Reading upward from 1589 to his line of population decline yields a figure of nearly 15,000,000. Calculating from that figure gives an infected population of 12,000,000 and a mortality of 3,600,000, or 9,863 per day for a year. While this estimate comes very close to that of the Jesuit priest, it represents an unprecedented mortality even for the most severe of the well-reported outbreaks. I have here accepted the previous estimate of 986 persons per day, not only because it is more feasible, but also because Rowe and Smith calculated their 1570 figure from an actual census count of tributary Indians, rather than from an estimated line of depopulation.

A brief medical note might be added at this point. It is important to recognize that for such a high death rate to have occurred there must not have been a general smallpox epidemic in the recent past, since such outbreaks yield a degree of immunity to survivors that Dixon calculates to be nearly ten times that of primary vaccination (1962:335-36):

> It would seem, therefore, that in most people this will give lifelong immunity. There are, however, the exceptions, who lose their immunity more quickly and therefore become susceptible to attack again.

NEW WORLD DEPOPULATION AND DISEASE   123

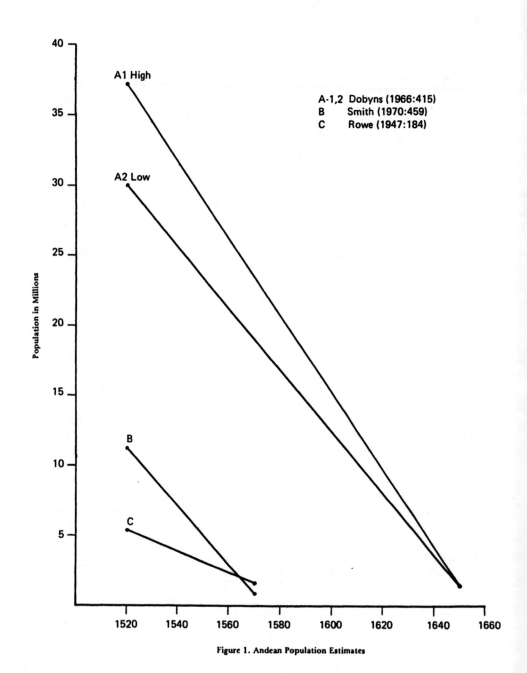

Figure 1. Andean Population Estimates

This fact suggests that the epidemic of 1558-59 (Polo 1913:11), which Dobyns (1963:500) identifies as smallpox, was either another strain or some other disease. Had it been the same strain of smallpox, it would have conferred substantial immunity to a large proportion of the surviving population, many of whom were probably alive just thirty years later when the 1589 epidemic struck. It is significant that no good symptom descriptions of this earlier epidemic have been found. Needless to say, there are many candidates other than smallpox for this outbreak.

It is exceedingly difficult to comprehend fully the conditions that must have prevailed during the smallpox epidemic of 1589-90. The situation in Cuzco was serious enough for the city council to cut the bridge over the Apurimac River in a vain attempt to isolate the community from the impending disaster (Dobyns 1963: 507). Translating such accounts and estimates into human terms is the last step in understanding the real impact of epidemic disease.

The first point that needs to be reaffirmed in this regard is that epidemics involve whole communities and can cause massive disruption of normal activities. Centerwall's (1968) experience among the Yanomamö clearly shows the extent of such a disruption, even in an epidemic that was less severe than the one being considered here. Undoubtedly, nursing care, food acquisition, and all other forms of labor were quick to collapse under the impact of a disease that struck eight out of every ten persons, and killed three of those afflicted.

However, the ramifications are even more widespread. The impact on a society's age structure must be considered, since death rates are much higher for young and old. As recently as 1885 the case mortality for ages 0-4 was 60 percent, and for ages over 40 the rate exceeded 40 percent (Dixon 1962:326), for variola major strains of smallpox. The results of a sudden shift in age-group proportions are likely to be far-reaching; perhaps the most serious demographic effect being a far smaller generation reaching reproductive age after the disease has passed.

Of equal importance is a whole series of psychological impacts that are likely to result from such an experience. Smallpox survivors must adjust, for instance, to a long-lasting disfigurement of face and body. In Europe up to the last century these facial marks were grounds for social ostracism, and even in the past decades it was recommended that mirrors be left out of smallpox wards in hospitals. If personal disfigurement is likely to have severe psychological repercussions, how much more severe would be the experience of a whole generation of children who watched parents, friends and siblings die of a disease that transformed loved ones into an unrecognizable mass of hideous pustules.[4] The following description, drawn from the Cakchiquel Maya who experienced the ravages of smallpox in 1520, shows how profound the impact can be (Crosby 1967:116):

> Great was the stench of the dead. After our fathers and grandfathers succumbed, half of the people fled to the fields. The mortality was terrible. Your grandfathers died, and with them died the son of the king and his brothers and kinsmen. So it was that we became orphans, oh, my sons! So we became when we were young. All of us were thus. We were born to die.

CONCLUSION

The utility of medical information and analogous, well-documented cases in the evaluation of postcontact Latin American epidemics has been clearly shown. The careful use of all historical accounts, through cross-checking wherever possible, supplies a base from which to proceed with external sources of evidence. Analyzing symptoms, combining isolated reports, and evaluating estimates of mortality all become possible through the use of such material as complements to the early chronicles. It is only by employing all relevant information that a full and accurate image of epidemic disease and its relation to demographic decline can be achieved.

The result of such a careful analysis is likely to be a rethinking of the Black Legend. Since the writings of Las Casas there has been a growing tendency towards the "weren't they awful" syndrome. Vivid accounts of Spanish brutalities are presented as the basis for self-righteous condemnations, and as sufficient explanation for the loss of many thousands, if not millions, of Indian lives. Without question the accounts of the activities of men like Pedro de Ursua and Lope de Aguirre (Bollaert 1861) are tragic documents for humanity to bear.

Nevertheless, we blind ourselves to what is a continuing tragedy if we seek only to assign responsibility to a particular nation at a particular place and time. Lewis Hanke (1964, 1965) clearly demonstrates that the issue is far more complex, and has to do with humans who are completely foreign to each other coming to grips with the reality of the other's existence. In the New World that process was complicated by religious concepts that initially denied the Indians human status, and by the avaricious dreams of men confronted for the first time with two whole continents of unknown possibilities. But these are human problems not peculiar to the Spanish of the fifteenth and sixteenth centuries.

In addition to the fact that all of human history, up to and including the present, is characterized by repeated failures in the process of coming to grips with the reality of others, the process has a biological as well as a social aspect. As this paper has shown, an uninvited third party accompanied the white man when he first met the natives of the New World. No question of responsibility is appropriate here; no blame can be ascribed. The tragedy appears to be a necessary outcome of human interaction across biological boundaries.

The process of adapting to the reality of others, socially and biologically, continues in Latin America's ongoing "Indian problem." Recent ethnographic literature is filled with reports of both consciously imposed disruption in Indian communities and high mortality from the ever-present threat of epidemic disease. If 1492 began the story, the last chapters are being written today. This is the reality that is missed when we focus our attention on retrospective condemnations.

NOTES

1. The Spanish text: ". . . hubo este Año (1546) entre los Indios una general pestilencia por todo el Reino del Perú, que comenzó, de mas adelante del Cuzco, i se extendió por toda la tierra, de la qual murieron gentes sin cuento: era el mal que daba un dolor de cabeza, i accidente de calentura mui recio, i luego se pasaba el dolor de la cabeza al oido izquierdo, i agravaba tanto el mal, que morían en dos ó tres días."

2. The work of Calvin Martin (1978) is a notable exception for North America. His analysis not only considers important epidemiological information, but also the cultural impact of epidemic disease, especially on native cosmology.

3. The Spanish text: "Salían en todo el cuerpo pústulas virulentas que deformaban á míseros enfermos, al punto que podían estos conocerse únicamente por el nombre. De tal modo los invadía el virus, que la piel misma, cubierta de costras sobresalientes, parecía

quemada por el fuego. Las pústulas obstruían las fauces, hasta impedir que se pasara la comida; dejando apenas hablar y respirar; y esto ocasionó á muchos la muerte."

4. Since we are not generally accustomed

to the effects of severe strains of smallpox, this may seem an exaggerated statement. However, a quick review of photos in Dixon (1962) will show it to be accurate.

REFERENCES CITED

Ashburn, P.M., 1947, The Ranks of Death: A Medical History of the Conquest of America. New York: Coward-McCann.

Biocca, E., 1970, Yanoáma: The Narrative of a White Girl Kidnapped by Amazon Indians. New York: E.P. Dutton.

Bollaert, W., tr., 1861, The Expedition of Pedro de Ursua and Lope de Aguirre in Search of El Dorado and Omagua in 1560-61. Translated from Fray Pedro Simon's "Sixth Historical Notice of the Conquest of Tierra Firme." London: Hakluyt Society.

Borah, W., 1964, America as Model: The Demographic Impact of European Expansion upon the Non-European World. Pp. 379-87 in Actas y Memorias del XXXV Congreso Internacional de Americanistas, vol. 3. México: Editorial Libros de México.

Borah, W., and S.F. Cook, 1960, The Population of Central Mexico in 1548. Ibero-Americana, no. 43. Berkeley: University of California Press.

Borah, W., and S.F. Cook, 1963, The Aboriginal Population of Central Mexico on the Eve of the Spanish Conquest. Ibero-Americana, no. 45. Berkeley: University of California Press.

Borah, W., and S.F. Cook, 1967, New Demographic Research on the Sixteenth Century in Mexico. Pp. 717-22 in Latin American History: Essays on its Study and Teachings, 1898-1965, vol. 2 (ed. by H.F. Cline). Austin: University of Texas Press.

Boyd, M.F., 1949, Malariology. 2 vols. Philadephia: W.B. Saunders.

Bruce-Chwatt, L.J., 1965, Paleogenesis and Paleoepidemiology of Primate Malaria. Bulletin of the World Health Organization 32:363-87.

Carbia, R.D., 1943, Historia de la leyenda negra hispano-americana. Buenos Aires: Ediciones Orientación Española.

Casas, B. de Las, 1552, Brevissima relación de la destruyción de las Indias. Sevilla: Seuilla en casa de Sebastian Trugillo.

Centerwall, W., 1968, A Recent Experience with Measles in a "Virgin-Soil" Population. Pp. 77-81 in Biomedical Challenges Presented by

the American Indian (Pan American Sanitary Bureau, Publicaciones Científicas 165). Washington, D.C.: World Health Organization.

Chagnon, N.A., 1968, Yanomamö: The Fierce People. New York: Holt, Rinehart and Winston.

Coatney, G.R., et al., 1971, The Primate Malarias. Bethesda: U.S. Department of Health, Education, and Welfare.

Cook, N.D., 1977, Estimaciones sobre la población del Perú en el momento de la conquista. Lima: Histórica 1:37-60.

Crosby, A.W., 1967, Conquistador y Pestilencia: The First New World Pandemic and the Fall of the Great Indian Empires. Hispanic American Historical Review 47:321-37.

Dixon, C.W., 1962, Smallpox. London: J. and A. Churchill.

Dobyns, H.F., 1963, An Outline of Andean Epidemic History to 1720. Bulletin of the History of Medicine 37:493-515.

Dobyns, H.F., 1966, Estimating Aboriginal American Populations: An Appraisal of Techniques with a New Hemispheric Estimate. Current Anthropology 7:395-416.

Dunn, F.L., 1965, On the Antiquity of Malaria in the Western Hemisphere. Human Biology 37:385-93.

Friede, J., 1967, Demographic Changes in the Mining Community of Muzo after the Plague of 1629. Hispanic American Historical Review 47:338-43.

Ginglioli, G.G., 1968, Malaria in the American Indian. Pp. 104-13 in Biomedical Challenges Presented by the American Indian (Pan American Sanitary Bureau, Publicaciones Científicas 165). Washington, D.C.: World Health Organization.

Hanke, L., 1964, The First Social Experiments in America: A Study in the Development of Spanish Indian Policy in the 16th Century. Gloucester, Mass.: Peter Smith.

Hanke, L., 1965, The Spanish Struggle for Justice in the Conquest of America. Boston: Little, Brown and Company.

Helps, A., 1966, The Spanish Conquest in

America. 4 vols. New York: AMS Press.

Hemming, J., 1970, The Conquest of the Incas. New York: Harcourt Brace Jovanovich.

Jaramillo Uribe, J., 1964, La población indígena de Colombia en el momento de la conquista y sus transformaciones posteriores. Anuario Colombiano de Historia Social y de la Cultura 1:239-93.

Jarcho, S., 1964, Some Observations on Disease in Pre-Historic North America. Bulletin of the History of Medicine 10:417-59, 568-92.

Joralemon, I.B., 1976, Adventure Beacons. New York: Society of Mining Engineers of American Institute of Mining Engineers.

Kroeber, A., 1939, Cultural and Natural Areas of Native North America. University of California Publications in American Archaeology and Ethnology, no. 38. Berkeley: University of California Press.

Laredo, S. De, ed., 1925, From Panama to Peru: The Conquest by the Pizarros, the Rebellion of Gonzalo Pizarro and the Pacification by La Gasca. London: Maggs Bros.

Markham, C.R., tr., 1859, Expeditions into the Valley of the Amazon: 1539 (Gonzalo Pizarro), 1540 (Francisco de Orellana), and 1639 (Cristoval de Acuña). London: Hakluyt Society, no. 24.

Martin, C., 1978, Keepers of the Game: Indian-Animal Relationships and the Fur Trade. Los Angeles: University of California Press.

Nutels, N., 1968, Medical Problems of Newly Contacted Indian Groups. Pp. 68-76 in Biomedical Challenges Presented by the American Indian (Pan American Sanitary Bureau, Publicaciones Científicas 165). Washington, D.C.: World Health Organization.

PAHO (Pan American Health Organization), 1971, Facts on Health Progress. Pan American Sanitary Bureau, Publicaciones Científicas, no. 227. Washington, D.C.: World Health Organization.

Petersen, W., 1975, A Demographer's View of Prehistoric Demography. Current Anthropology 16:227-45.

Polo, J.T., 1913, Apuntes sobre las epidemias en el Perú. Lima: Impresa Nacional de Federico Barrioneuvo.

Rivet, P., 1924, Langues americaines. Pp. 597-712 in Les langues du monde (ed. by A. Meillet and M. Cohen). Paris: Collection Linguistique, Société de Linguistique.

Rosenblat, A., 1954, La Población indígena y el mestizaje en América, vol. 1: La población indígena. Buenos Aires: Editorial Nova, Biblioteca Americanista.

Rowe, J.H., 1947, Inca Culture at the Time of the Spanish Conquest. Pp. 183-330 in Handbook of South American Indians, vol. 1 (ed. by J.H. Steward). Bureau of American Ethnology, Bulletin 143. Washington, D.C.: U.S. Government Printing Office.

Sánchez-Albornoz, N., 1974, The Population of Latin America: A History. Berkeley: University of California Press.

Sapper, K., 1924, Die Zahl und die Volksdichte der Indianischen Bevölkerung in Amerika von der Conquista und in der Gegenwart. Pp. 95-104 in Proceedings of the 21st International Congress of Americanists, The Hague, First Part. Leiden: E.J. Brill.

Scott, H.H., 1939, A History of Tropical Medicine. London: Edward Arnold.

Shattuck, G.C., 1933, The Peninsula of Yucatan: Medical, Biological, Meteorological and Sociological Studies. Washington, D.C.: Carnegie Institution, Publication No. 431.

Shea, D., 1976, A Defense of Small Population Estimates for the Central Andes in 1520. Pp. 157-80 in The Native Population of the Americas in 1492 (ed. by W.M. Denevan). Madison: University of Wisconsin Press.

Smith, C.T., 1970, Depopulation of the Central Andes in the 16th Century. Current Anthropology 11:453-64.

Spinden, H.J., 1928, The Population of Ancient America. Geographic Review 18:641-60.

Stearn, E.W., and A.E. Stearn, 1945, The Effect of Smallpox on the Destiny of the Amerindian. Boston: Bruce Humphries.

Strong, R.P., and G.C. Shattuck, 1926, Medical Report of the Hamilton Rice Seventh Expedition to the Amazon, in Conjunction with the Department of Tropical Medicine of Harvard University, 1924-1925. Cambridge, Mass.: Harvard University Press.

Vellard, J.A., 1956, Causas biológicas de la desaparición de los indios americanos. Lima: Pontífica Universidad Católica del Perú, Boletín del Instituto Riva-Agüero 2:77-93.

Wagley, C., 1977, Welcome of Tears: The Tapirapé Indians of Central Brazil. New York: Oxford University Press.

4

Conquistador y Pestilencia: The First New World Pandemic and the Fall of the Great Indian Empires

Alfred W. Crosby

THE MOST SENSATIONAL military conquests in all history are probably those of the Spanish conquistadores over the Aztec and Incan empires. Cortés and Pizarro toppled the highest civilizations of the New World in a few months each. A few hundred Spaniards defeated populations containing thousands of dedicated warriors, armed with a wide assembly of weapons from the stone and early metal ages. Societies which had created huge empires through generations of fierce fighting collapsed at the touch of the Castilian.

After four hundred years the Spanish feat still seems incredible. Many explanations suggest themselves: the advantage of steel over stone, of cannon and firearms over bows and arrows and slings; the terrorizing effect of horses on foot-soldiers who had never seen such beasts before; the lack of unity in the Aztec and Incan empires; the prophecies in Indian mythology about the arrival of white gods. All of these factors combined to deal to the Indian a shock such as only H. G. Wells' *War of the Worlds* can suggest to us. Each factor was undoubtedly worth many hundreds of soldiers to Cortés and Pizarro.

For all of that, one might have expected the highly organized, militaristic societies of Mexico and the Andean highlands to survive at least the initial contact with European societies. Thousands of Indian warriors, even if confused and frightened and wielding only obsidian-studded war clubs, should have been able to repel at least the first few hundred Spaniards to arrive.

The Spaniard had a formidable ally to which neither he nor the historian has given sufficient credit—disease. The arrival of Columbus in the New World brought about one of the greatest population disasters in history. After the Spanish conquest an Indian of Yucatán wrote of his people in the happier days before the advent of the Spaniard:[1]

---

[1] *The Book of Chilam Balam of Chumayel* (Washington, 1933), 83.

There was then no sickness; they had no aching bones; they had then no high fever; they had then no smallpox; they had then no burning chest; they had then no abdominal pain; they had then no consumption; they had then no headache. At that time the course of humanity was orderly. The foreigners made it otherwise when they arrived here.

It would be easy to attribute this lamentation to the nostalgia that the conquered always feel for the time before the conqueror appeared, but the statement is probably in part true. During the millennia before the European brought together the compass and the three-masted vessel to revolutionize world history, men at sea moved slowly, seldom over long distances, and across the great oceans hardly at all. Men lived at least in the same continents where their greatgrand-fathers had lived and rarely caused violent and rapid changes in the delicate balance between themselves and their environments. Diseases tended to be endemic rather than epidemic. It is true that man did not achieve perfect accommodation with his microscopic parasites. Mutation, ecological changes, and migration could bring the likes of the Black Death to Europe, and few men lived three-score and ten without knowing epidemic disease. Yet ecological stability did tend to create a crude kind of mutual toleration between human host and parasite. Most Europeans, for instance, survived measles and tuber-culosis, and most West Africans survived yellow fever and malaria.

Migration of man and his maladies is the chief cause of epidemics. And when migration takes place, those creatures who have been longest in isolation suffer most, for their genetic material has been least tempered by the variety of world diseases.[2] Among the major subdivisions of the species *homo sapiens* the American Indian prob-ably had the dangerous privilege of longest isolation from the rest of mankind. The Indians appear to have lived, died, and bred with-out extra-American contacts for generation after generation, develop-ing unique cultures and working out tolerances for a limited, native American selection of pathological micro-life.[3] Medical historians

[2] S. P. Bedson *et al., Virus and Rickettsial Diseases* (Baltimore, 1950), 50-51; Geddes Smith, *Plague on Us* (New York, 1941), 115-118.

[3] Solid scientific proof exists of this isolation. The physical anthropologist notes an amazingly high degree of physical uniformity among the Indians of the Americas, especially in blood type. Only in the Americas, and in no other large area, is there such a low percentage of aborigines with B-type blood or such a high percentage—very often one hundred percent—of O-type. The maps of blood type distribution among Indians suggest that they are the product of New World endogamy. Blood type distribution maps of the Old World are, in contrast, highly complex in almost all parts of the three continents. These maps confirm what we know to be true historically: that migration and constant mixing of genetic materials have characterized Old World history. There has also been a constant exchange of diseases and of genetically derived immunities. In the

guess that few of the first rank killers among the diseases are native to the Americas. (A possible exception is syphilis. It may be true, as Gonzalo Fernández Oviedo maintained four hundred years ago, that syphilis should not be called *mal francés* or *mal de Nápoles*, but *mal de las Indias*.)[4]

When the isolation of the Americas was broken, and Columbus brought the two halves of this planet together, the American Indian met for the first time his most hideous enemy—not the white man or his black servant, but the invisible killers which these men brought in their blood and breath. The fatal diseases of the Old World killed more effectively in the New, and comparatively benign diseases of the Old World turned killers in the New. There is little exaggeration in the statement of a German missionary in 1699 that "the Indians die so easily that the bare look and smell of a Spaniard causes them to give up the ghost." The process is still going on in the twentieth century, as the last jungle tribes of South America lose their shield of isolation.[5]

The most spectacular period of mortality among the American Indians occurred during the first century of contact with the Europeans and Africans. Almost all contemporary historians of the early settlements from Bartolomé de las Casas to William Bradford of Plymouth Plantation were awed by the ravages of epidemic disease among the native populations of America. We know that the most deadly of the early epidemics in the New World were those of the eruptive fevers—smallpox, measles, plague, typhus, etc. The first to arrive and the deadliest, said contemporaries, was smallpox.[6]

At this point the reader should be forewarned against too easy credulity. Even today smallpox is occasionally misdiagnosed as in-

Americas, on the other hand, there must have been almost no prophylactic miscegenation of this sort. A. E. Mourant, Ada C. Kopéc, and Kazimiera Domaniewska-Sobczak, *The ABO Blood Groups. Comprehensive Tables and Maps of World Distribution* (Springfield, Ill., 1958), 268-270.

[4] P. M. Ashburn, *The Ranks of Death. A Medical History of the Conquest of America* (New York, 1947), *passim;* Gonzalo Fernández Oviedo, *Historia general y natural de las Indias* (Madrid, 1959), I, 53; Henry H. Scott, *A History of Tropical Medicine* (London, 1939), I, 128, 283; Sherburne F. Cook, "The Incidence and Significance of Disease Among the Aztecs and Related Tribes," *HAHR*, XXVI (August 1946), 321, 335.

[5] Jehan Vellard, "Causas biológicas de la desaparición de los indios americanos," *Boletín del Instituto Riva-Agüero*, No. 2, 1956, 78-79; E. Wagner Stearn and Allen E. Stearn, *The Effect of Smallpox on the Destiny of the Amerindian* (Boston, 1945), 17.

[6] Ashburn, *Ranks of Death*, 80; Woodrow Borah, "America as Model: The Demographic Impact of European Expansion upon the Non-European World," *Actas y Memorias del XXXV Congreso Internacional de Americanistas* (México, 1964), III, 379-387.

fluenza, pneumonia, measles, scarlet fever, syphilis, or chicken pox, for example.[7] Four hundred years ago such mistakes were even more common, and writers of the accounts upon which we must base our examination of the early history of smallpox in America did not have any special interest in accurate diagnosis. The early historians were much more likely to cast their eyes skywards and comment on the sinfulness that had called down such obvious evidences of God's wrath as epidemics than to describe in any detail the diseases involved. It should also be noted that conditions which facilitate the spread of one disease will usually encourage the spread of others, and that "very rarely is there a pure epidemic of a single malady." Pneumonia and pleurisy, for instance, often follow after smallpox, smothering those whom it has weakened.[8]

Furthermore, although the Spanish word *viruelas*, which appears again and again in the chronicles of the sixteenth century, is almost invariably translated as "smallpox," it specifically means not the disease but the pimpled, pustuled appearance which is the most obvious symptom of the disease. Thus the generation of the conquistadores may have used *viruelas* to refer to measles, chicken 'pox, or typhus. And one must remember that people of the sixteenth century were not statistically minded, so that their estimates of the numbers killed by epidemic disease may be a more accurate measurement of their emotions than of the numbers who really died.

But let us not paralyze ourselves with doubts. When the sixteenth-century Spaniard pointed and said, *"Viruelas,"* what he meant and what he saw was usually smallpox. On occasion he was perfectly capable of distinguishing among diseases: for instance, he called the epidemic of 1531 in Central America *sarampión*—measles—and not *viruelas*.[9] We may proceed on the assumption that smallpox was the most important disease of the first pandemic in the recorded history of the Americas.

Smallpox has been so successfully controlled by vaccination and quarantine in the industrialized nations of the twentieth century that few North Americans or Europeans have ever seen it. But it is an old companion of humanity, and for most of the last millennium it was among the commonest diseases in Europe. With reason it was long thought one of the most infectious of maladies. Smallpox is usually communicated through the air by means of droplets or dust

---

[7] C. W. Dixon, *Smallpox* (London, 1962), 68.

[8] Franklin H. Top *et al.*, *Communicable and Infectious Diseases* (St. Louis, 1964), 515; Hans Zinsser, *Rats, Lice and History* (New York, 1960), 87-88.

[9] Raúl Porras Barrenechea (ed.), *Cartas del Perú, 1524-1543* (Lima, 1959), 22, 24, 33, 46.

particles, and its virus enters the new host through the respiratory tract. There are many cases of hospital visitors who have contracted the disease simply by breathing for a moment the air of a room in which someone lies ill with the pox.[10]

Because it is extremely communicable, before the eighteenth century it was usually thought of as a necessary evil of childhood, such as measles today. Sometimes the only large group untouched by it was also that which had been relatively unexposed to it—the young. Yet even among Spanish children of the sixteenth century smallpox was so common that Ruy Díaz de Isla, a medical writer, felt called upon to record that he had once seen a man of twenty years sick with the disease, "and he had never had it before."[11]

Where smallpox has been endemic, it has been a steady, dependable killer, taking every year from three to ten percent of those who die. Where it has struck isolated groups, the death rate has been awesome. Analysis of figures for some twenty outbreaks shows that the case mortality among an unvaccinated population is about thirty percent. Presumably, in people who have had no contact whatever with smallpox, the disease will infect nearly every single individual it touches. When in 1707 smallpox first appeared in Iceland, it is said that in two years 18,000 out of the island's 50,000 inhabitants died of it.[12]

The first people of the New World to meet the white and black races and their diseases were Indians of the Taino culture who spoke the Arawak language and lived on the islands of the Greater Antilles and the Bahamas. On the very first day of landfall in 1492 Columbus noted that the Tainos "are very unskilled with arms . . ." and "could all be subjected and made to do all that one wished."[13] These Tainos lived long enough to provide the Spaniard with his first generation of slaves in America, and Old World disease with its first beachhead in the New World.

Oviedo, one of the earliest historians of the Americas, estimated that a million Indians lived on Santo Domingo when the European arrived to plant his first permanent colony in the New World. "Of all those," Oviedo wrote, "and of all those born afterwards, there are not now believed to be at the present time in this year of 1548 five

[10] Dixon, *Smallpox*, 171, 299-301.

[11] Ashburn, *Ranks of Death*, 86.

[12] Dixon, *Smallpox*, 325; John Duffy, *Epidemics in Colonial America* (Baton Rouge, 1953), 20, 22; Stearn and Stearn, *Effect of Smallpox*, 14.

[13] Samuel Eliot Morison, *Admiral of the Ocean Sea. A Life of Christopher Columbus* (Boston, 1942), I, 304-305.

hundred persons, children and adults, who are natives and are the progeny or lineage of those first.''[14]

The destruction of the Tainos has been largely blamed on the Spanish cruelty, not only by the later Protestant historians of the ''Black Legend'' school but also by such contemporary Spanish writers as Oviedo and Bartolomé de las Casas. Without doubt the early Spaniard brutally exploited the Indians. But it was obviously not in order to kill them off, for the early colonist had to deal with a chronic labor shortage and needed the Indians. Disease would seem to be a more logical explanation for the disappearance of the Tainos, because they, like other Indians, had little immunity to Old World diseases. At the same time, one may concede that the effects of Spanish exploitation undoubtedly weakened their resistance to disease.

Yet it is interesting to note that there is no record of any massive smallpox epidemic among the Indians of the Antilles for a quarter of a century after the first voyage of Columbus. Indians apparently suffered a steady decline in numbers, which was probably due to extreme overwork, other diseases, and a general lack of will to live after their whole culture had been shattered by alien invasion.[15] How can the evident absence of smallpox be explained, if the American Indian was so susceptible, and if ships carrying Europeans and Africans from the pestilential Old World were constantly arriving in Santo Domingo? The answer lies in the nature of the disease. It is a deadly malady, but it lasts only a brief time in each patient. After an incubation period of twelve days or so, the patient suffers from high fever and vomiting followed three or four days later by the characteristic skin eruptions. For those who do not die, these pustules dry up in a week or ten days and form scabs which soon fall off, leaving the disfiguring pocks that give the disease its name. The whole process takes a month or less, and after that time the patient is either dead or immune, at least for a period of years. Also there is no non-human carrier of smallpox, such as the flea of typhus or the mosquito of malaria; it must pass from man to man. Nor are there any long-term human carriers of smallpox, as, for instance, with typhoid and syphilis. It is not an over-simplification to say that one either has smallpox and can transmit it, or one has not and cannot transmit it.

Consider that, except for children, most Europeans and their

[14] Oviedo, *Historia general*, I, 66-67.

[15] *Ibid.; Colección de documentos inéditos relativos al descubrimiento, conquista y colonización de las posesiones españolas en América y Oceanía. . . .* (Madrid, 1864-1884), I, 428.

slaves had had smallpox and were at least partially immune, and that few but adults sailed from Europe to America in the first decades after discovery. Consider that the voyage was one of several weeks, so that, even if an immigrant or sailor contracted smallpox on the day of embarkation, he would most likely be dead or rid of its virus before he arrived in Santo Domingo. Consider that moist heat and strong sunlight, characteristic of a tropical sea voyage, are particularly deadly to the smallpox virus. The lack of any rapid means of crossing the Atlantic in the sixteenth century delayed the delivery of the Old World's worst gift to the New.

It was delayed; that was all. An especially fast passage from Spain to the New World; the presence on a vessel of several non-immune persons who could transmit the disease from one to the other until arrival in the Indies; the presence of smallpox scabs, in which the virus can live for weeks, accidentally packed into a bale of textiles—by any of these means smallpox could have been brought to Spanish America.[16]

In December 1518 or January 1519 a disease identified as smallpox appeared among the Indians of Santo Domingo, brought, said Las Casas, from Castile. It touched few Spaniards, and none of them died, but it devastated the Indians. The Spaniards reported that it killed one-third to one-half of the Indians. Las Casas, never one to understate the appalling, said that it left no more than one thousand alive "of that immensity of people that was on this island and which we have seen with our own eyes."[17]

Undoubtedly one must discount these statistics, but they are not too far out of line with mortality rates in other smallpox epidemics, and with C. W. Dixon's judgment that populations untouched by smallpox for generations tend to resist the disease less successfully than those populations in at least occasional contact with it. Furthermore, Santo Domingo's epidemic was not an atypically pure epidemic. Smallpox seems to have been accompanied by respiratory ailments (*romadizo*), possibly measles, and other Indian killers. Starvation probably also took a toll, because of the lack of hands to work the fields. Although no twentieth-century epidemiologist or demographer would find these sixteenth-century statistics completely satisfactory, they probably are crudely accurate.[18]

[16] Bedson, *Virus*, 151-152, 157; Dixon, *Smallpox*, 174, 189, 296-297, 304, 359; Jacques M. May (ed.), *Studies in Disease Ecology* (New York, 1961), 1, 8.

[17] *Colección de documentos inéditos*, I, 367, 369-370, 429; *Colección de varios documentos para la historia de la Florida y tierras adyacentes* (London, 1857), I, 44; Bartolomé de las Casas, *Historia de las Indias* (Madrid, 1957), II, 484.

[18] *Colección de documentos inéditos*, I, 368, 397-398, 428-429; Dixon, *Smallpox*, 317-318, 325.

Thus began the first recorded pandemic in the New World, which was "in all likelihood the most severe single loss of aboriginal population that ever occurred."[19] In a matter of days after smallpox appeared in Santo Domingo, it leaped the channel to Puerto Rico. Before long, Tainos were dying a hideous and unfamiliar death in all the islands of the Greater Antilles.[20] Crushed by a quarter-century of exploitation, they now performed their last function on earth: to act as a reserve of pestilence in the New World from which the conquistador drew invisible biological allies for his assault on the mainland.

Smallpox seems to have traveled quickly from the Antilles to Yucatán. Bishop Diego de Landa, our chief sixteenth-century Spanish source of information on the people of Yucatán, recorded that sometime late in the second decade of that century "a pestilence seized them, characterized by great pustules, which rotted their bodies with a great stench, so that the limbs fell to pieces in four or five days." The *Book of Chilam Balam of Chumayel*, written in the Mayan language with European script after the Spanish settlement of Yucatán, also records that some time in the second decade "was when the eruption of pustules occurred. It was smallpox." It has been speculated that the malady came with Spaniards shipwrecked on the Yucatán coast in 1511 or the soldiers and sailors of Hernández de Córdoba's expedition which coasted along Yucatán in 1517. Both these explanations seem unlikely, because smallpox had not appeared in the Greater Antilles, the likeliest source of any smallpox epidemic on the continent, until the end of 1518 or the beginning of 1519. Be that as it may, there is evidence that the Santo Domingan epidemic could have spread to the continent before Cortés' invasion of Mexico. Therefore, the epidemic raging there at that time may have come in two ways—north and west from Yucatán, and directly from Cuba to central Mexico, brought by Cortés' troops.[21]

The melodrama of Cortés and the conquest of Mexico need no retelling. After occupying Tenochtitlán and defeating the army of his rival, Narváez, he and his troops had to fight their way out of the city to sanctuary in Tlaxcala. Even as the Spanish withdrew, an ally more formidable than Tlaxcala appeared. Years later Francisco de Aguilar, once a follower of Cortés and now a Dominican friar, recalled

[19] Henry F. Dobyns, "An Outline of Andean Epidemic History to 1720," *Bulletin of the History of Medicine*, XXXVII (November-December 1963), 514.

[20] Pablo Álvarez Rubiano, *Pedrarias Dávila* (Madrid, 1944), 608; *Colección de varios documentos para la historia de la Florida*, I, 45.

[21] Diego de Landa, *Relación de las cosas de Yucatán* (Cambridge, 1941), 42; *The Book of Chilam Balam*, 138.

the terrible retreat of the *Noche Triste*. "When the Christians were exhausted from war," he wrote, "God saw fit to send the Indians smallpox, and there was a great pestilence in the city. . . ."[22]

With the men of Narváez had come a Negro sick with the smallpox, "and he infected the household in Cempoala where he was quartered; and it spread from one Indian to another, and they, being so numerous and eating and sleeping together, quickly infected the whole country." The Mexicans had never seen smallpox before and did not have even the European's meager knowledge of how to deal with it. The old soldier-chronicler, Bernal Díaz del Castillo, called the Negro "a very black dose" for Mexico, "for it was because of him that the whole country was stricken, with a great many deaths."[23]

Probably, several diseases were at work. Shortly after the retreat from Tenochtitlán Bernal Díaz, immune to smallpox like most of the Spaniards, "was very sick with fever and was vomiting blood." The Aztec sources mention the racking cough of those who had smallpox, which suggests a respiratory complication such as pneumonia or a streptococcal infection, both common among smallpox victims. Great numbers of the Cakchiquel people of Guatemala were felled by a devastating epidemic in 1520 and 1521, having as its most prominent symptom fearsome nosebleeds. Whatever this disease was, it may have been present in central Mexico along with the pox.[24]

The triumphant Aztecs had not expected the Spaniards to return after their expulsion from Tenochtitlán. The sixty days during which the epidemic lasted in the city, however, gave Cortés and his troops a desperately needed respite to reorganize and prepare a counterattack. When the epidemic subsided, the siege of the Aztec capital began. Had there been no epidemic, the Aztecs, their war-making potential unimpaired and their warriors fired with victory, could have

[22] Patricia de Fuentes (ed. and trans.), *The Conquistadors. First-Person Accounts of the Conquest of Mexico* (New York, 1963), 159. For the argument that this was measles, not smallpox, see Horacio Figueroa Marroquín, *Enfermedades de los conquistadores* (San Salvador, 1955), 49-67.

[23] Bernal Díaz del Castillo, *The Bernal Díaz Chronicles: The True Story of the Conquest of Mexico* (Garden City, N.Y., 1956), 250; Diego Durán, *The Aztecs. The History of the Indies of New Spain* (New York, 1964), 323; Francisco López de Gómara, *Cortés, the Life of the Conqueror by his Secretary* (Berkeley, 1964), 204-205; Toribio Motolinía, *History of the Indians of New Spain* (Berkeley, 1950), 38; Bernardino de Sahagún, *General History of the Things of New Spain* (Santa Fe, 1950-59), Part 9, 4.

[24] *Anales de Tlatelolco, Unos anales históricos de la nación mexicana y códice de Tlatelolco* (México, 1948), 64; *The Annals of the Cakchiquels and Title of the Lords of Totonicapán* (Norman, Okla., 1953), 115-116; Bedson, *Virus*, 155; Díaz del Castillo, *Chronicles*, 289; Miguel León-Portilla (ed.), *The Broken Spears. The Aztec Account of the Conquest of Mexico* (Boston, 1962), 132; Top, *Communicable and Infectious Diseases*, 515.

330   HAHR | AUGUST | ALFRED W. CROSBY

pursued the Spaniards, and Cortés might have ended his life spread-eagled beneath the obsidian blade of a priest of Huitzilopochtli. Clearly the epidemic sapped the endurance of Tenochtitlán to survive the Spanish assault. As it was, the siege went on for seventy-five days, until the deaths within the city from combat, starvation, and disease—probably not smallpox now—numbered many thousands. When the city fell "the streets, squares, houses, and courts were filled with bodies, so that it was almost impossible to pass. Even Cortés was sick from the stench in his nostrils."[25]

Peru and the Andean highlands were also hit by an early epidemic, and if it was smallpox it most probably had to pass through the isthmus of Panama, as did Francisco Pizarro himself. The documentation of the history of Panama in the first years after the conquest is not as extensive as that of Mexico or the Incan areas, because the isthmus had fewer riches and no civilized indigenous population to learn European script from the friars and write its own history. We do know that in the first decades of the sixteenth century the same appalling mortality took place among the Indians in Central America as in the Antilles and Mexico. The recorded medical history of the isthmus began in 1514 with the deaths of seven hundred Darién settlers in a month, victims of hunger and an unidentified disease. Oviedo, who was in Panama at the time of greatest mortality, judged that upwards of two million Indians died there between 1514 and 1530, and Antonio de Herrera tells us that forty thousand died of disease in Panamá City and Nombre de Dios alone in a twenty-eight-year period during the century. Others wrote of the depopulation of four hundred leagues of land that had "swarmed" with people when the Spanish first arrived.[26]

What killed the Indians? Contemporaries and many historians blame the carnage on Pedrarias Dávila, who executed Balboa and ruled Spain's first Central American settlements with such an iron hand that he was hated by all the chief chroniclers of the age. It can be effectively argued, however, that he was no more a berserk butcher of Indians than Pizarro, for the mortality among Indians of the isthmus during his years of power is parallel to the high death rates

[25] Hernando Cortés, *Five Letters* (New York, 1962), 226; Díaz del Castillo, *Chronicles*, 405-406; Gómara, *Cortés*, 285, 293; León-Portilla, *Broken Spears*, 92; Sahagún, *General History*, XIII, 81.

[26] *Colección de documentos inéditos*, XXXVII, 200; Oviedo, *Historia general*, III, 353. For corroboration see M. M. Alba C., *Etnología y población histórica* (Panamá, 1928), *passim*; Porras Barrenechea, *Cartas del Perú*, 24; Juan López de Velasco, *Geografía y descripción universal de las Indias* (Madrid, 1894), 341; *Relaciones históricas y geográficas de América Central* (Madrid, 1908), 216-218.

among the Indians wherever the Spaniards went.[27] When charges against Pedrarias were investigated in 1527, his defenders maintained that the greatest Indian killer had been an epidemic of smallpox. This testimony is hard to reject, for another document of 1527 mentions the necessity of importing aboriginal slaves into Panama City, Nata, and "the port of Honduras," because smallpox had carried off all the Indians in those areas.[28]

The Spaniards could never do much to improve the state of public health in the audiencia of Panama. In 1660 those who governed Panama City listed as resident killers and discomforters smallpox, measles, pneumonia, suppurating abscesses, typhus, fevers, diarrhea, catarrh, boils, and hives—and blamed them all on the importation of Peruvian wine![29] Of all the killers operating in early Panama, however, smallpox was undoubtedly the most deadly to the Indians.

If we attempt to describe the first coming of Old World disease to the areas south of Panama, we shall have to deal with ambiguity, equivocation, and simple guesswork, for eruptive fever, now operating from continental bases, apparently outstripped the Spaniards and sped south from the isthmus into the Incan Empire before Pizarro's invasion. Long before the invasion, the Inca Huayna Capac was aware that the Spaniards—"monstrous marine animals, bearded men who moved upon the sea in large houses"—were pushing down the coast from Panama. Such is the communicability of smallpox and the other eruptive fevers that any Indian who received news of the Spaniards could also have easily received the infection of the European diseases. The biologically defenseless Indians made vastly more efficient carriers of such pestilence than the Spaniards.[30]

[27] Antonio de Herrera, *Historia general de los hechos de los castellanos en las islas y Tierra Firme del Mar Océano* (Madrid, 1936), V, 350; *Relaciones históricas y geográficas de América Central,* 200.

[28] Álvarez, *Pedrarias Dávila,* 608, 619, 621, 623; *Colección de documentos para la historia de Costa Rica* (Paris, 1886), IV, 8.

[29] Pascual de Andagoya, *Narrative of the Proceedings of Pedrarias Dávila* (London, 1865), 6; *Colección de documentos inéditos,* XVII, 219-222; Herrera, *Historia general,* IV, 217; Scott, *History,* I, 129, 288.

[30] Garcilaso de la Vega, *First Part of the Royal Commentaries of the Yncas* (London, 1871), II, 456-457; Fernando Montesinos, *Memorias antiguas historiales del Perú* (London, 1920), 126; Pedro Sarmiento de Gamboa, *History of the Incas* (Cambridge, 1907), 187. It has been suggested that the source of the great epidemic in question was two men, Alonso de Molina and Ginés, left behind by Pizarro at Tumbez on the reconnaisance voyage of 1527. Victor W. von Hagen (ed.), *The Incas of Pedro de Cieza de León* (Norman, 1959), n. 51. If the epidemic was smallpox or measles this explanation is unlikely because these diseases are of short duration and have no carrier state. The expedition of which these men were members had had no contact with pestilential Panama for some time before it returned there from Tumbez. If these two men caught smallpox or measles, it must have been already present among the Indians.

332   HAHR | AUGUST | ALFRED W. CROSBY

Our evidence for the first post-Columbian epidemic in Incan lands is entirely hearsay, because the Incan people had no system of writing. Therefore, we must depend on secondary accounts by Spaniards and by mestizos or Indians born after the conquest, accounts based on Indian memory and written years and even decades after the epidemic of the 1520s. The few accounts we have of the great epidemic are associated with the death of Huayna Capac. He spent the last years of his life campaigning against the people of what is today northern Peru and Ecuador. There, in the province of Quito, he first received news of an epidemic raging in his empire, and there he himself was stricken. Huayna Capac and his captains died with shocking rapidity, "their faces being covered with scabs."

Of what did the Inca and his captains die? One of the most generally reliable of our sources, that of Garcilaso de la Vega, describes Huayna Capac's death as the result of "a trembling chill . . . , which the Indians call *chucchu*, and a fever, called by the Indians *rupu*. . . ." We dare not, four hundred years later, unequivocally state that the disease was not one native to the Americas. Most accounts call it smallpox, or suggest that it was either smallpox or measles. Smallpox seems the best guess because the epidemic struck in that period when the Spaniards, operating from bases where smallpox was killing multitudes, were first coasting along the shores of Incan lands.[31]

The impact of the smallpox pandemic on the Aztec and Incan Empires is easy for us of the twentieth century to underestimate. We

[31] Felipe Guamán Poma Ayala, *Nueva corónica y buen govierno* (Lima, 1956), 85-86; Cieza de León, *Incas*, 52, 253; P. Bernabé Cobo, *Obras del P. Bernabé Cobo* (Madrid, 1956), II, 93; Garcilaso de la Vega, *Royal Commentaries*, II, 461; Martín de Murúa, *Historia general del Perú, origen y descendencia de los Incas* (Madrid, 1962), I, 103-104; Clements R. Markham (trans.), *Narratives of the Rites and Laws of the Incas* (London, 1873), 110; Pedro Pizarro, *Relation of the Discovery and Conquest of the Kingdoms of Peru* (New York, 1921), I, 196-198; Sarmiento de Gamboa, *History*, 167-168; Miguel Cabello Valboa, *Miscelánea antártica una historia del Perú antiguo* (Lima 1951), 393-394. Did smallpox exist in the Incan lands before the 1520s? Fernando Montesinos, writing in the seventeenth century, claimed that Capac Titu Yupanqui, a pre-Columbian Peruvian, died of smallpox in a general epidemic of that disease. Also, some examples of the famous naturalistic Mochica pottery show Indians with pustules and pocks which bear a very close resemblance to those of smallpox. But Montesinos is regarded as one of the less reliable historians of Incan times, and there are several other diseases native to the northwestern section of South America, such as the dreadful *verrugas*, which have a superficial dermatological similarity to smallpox. Furthermore, the aborigines of the Incan Empire told Pedro Pizarro that they had had no acquaintance with smallpox in pre-Columbian times. Montesinos, *Memorias*, 54; Pizarro, *Relation*, I, 196; Victor W. von Hagen, *Realm of the Incas* (New York, 1957), 106; see also Raoul and Marie D'Harcourt, *La medicine dans l'ancien Pérou* (Paris, 1939), *passim*.

have so long been hypnotized by the derring-do of the conquistador that we have overlooked the importance of his biological allies. Because of the achievements of medical science in our day we find it hard to accept statements from the conquest period that the pandemic killed one-third to one-half of the populations struck by it. Toribio Motolinía claimed that in most provinces of Mexico "more than one half of the population died; in others the proportion was little less." "They died in heaps," he said, "like bedbugs."

The proportion may be exaggerated, but perhaps not as much as we might think. The Mexicans had no natural resistance to the disease at all. Other diseases were probably operating quietly and efficiently behind the screen of smallpox. Add too the factors of food shortage and the lack of even minimal care for the sick. Motolinía wrote: "Many others died of starvation, because as they were all taken sick at once, they could not care for each other, nor was there anyone to give them bread or anything else." We shall never be certain what the death rate was, but, from all evidence, it must have been immense. Woodrow Borah and Sherburne F. Cook estimate that, for one cause and another, the population of central Mexico dropped from about 25,000,000 on the eve of conquest to 16,800,000 a decade later, and this estimate strengthens confidence in Motolinía's general veracity.[32]

South of Panama, in the empire of the Inca, our only tool for estimating the mortality of the epidemic of the 1520s is the educated guess. The population there was thick, and it provided a rich medium for the transmission and cultivation of communicable diseases. If the malady which struck in the 1520s was smallpox, as it seems to have been, then it must have taken many victims, for these Indians probably had no more knowledge of or immunity to smallpox than the Mexicans. Most of our sources tell us only that many died. Cieza de León gives a figure of 200,000, and Martín de Murúa, throwing up his hands, says "infinite thousands."[33]

We are reduced to guesswork. Jehan Vellard, student of the effect of disease on the American Indian, states that the epidemics in Peru and Bolivia after the Spanish conquest killed fewer than those in Mexico and suggests the climatic conditions of the Andean highlands as the reason. But smallpox generally thrives under dry, cool conditions. Possibly historians have omitted an account of the first and,

[32] Woodrow Borah and Sherburne F. Cook, *The Aboriginal Population of Central Mexico on the Eve of Spanish Conquest* (Berkeley, 1963), 4, 89; Motolinía, *History*, 38; Sahagún, *General History*, XIII, 81.

[33] Ashburn, *Ranks of Death*, 20; Cieza de León, *Incas*, 52; Murúa, *Historia general*, 104; Pizarro, *Relation*, I, 196.

therefore, probably the worst post-Columbian epidemic in the Incan areas because it preceded the Spanish conquest.[34] A half century or so after the Conquest, Indians in the vicinity of Lima maintained that the Spanish could not have conquered them if, a few years before Pizarro's invasion, respiratory disease (*romadizo y dolor de costado*) had not "consumed the greater part of them."[35] Was this the great killer of the 1520s in the Incan Empire? Perhaps future archaeological discoveries will give us more definite information.

The pandemic not only killed great numbers in the Indian empires, but also affected their power structures, striking down the leaders and disrupting the processes by which they were normally replaced. When Moctezuma died, his nephew, Cuitláhuac, was elected lord of Mexico. It was he who directed the attacks on the Spaniards during the disastrous retreat from Tenochtitlán, attacks which nearly ended the story of Cortés and his soldiers. And then Cuitláhuac died of smallpox. Probably many others wielding decisive power in the ranks of the Aztecs and their allies died in the same period, breaking dozens of links in the chain of command. Not long afterwards Bernal Díaz tells us of an occasion when the Indians did not attack "because between the Mexicans and the Texcocans there were differences and factions"[36] and, of equal importance, because they had been weakened by smallpox.

Outside Tenochtitlán the deaths due to smallpox among the Indian ruling classes permitted Cortés to cultivate the loyalty of several men in important positions and to promote his own supporters. Cortés wrote to Charles V about the city of Cholula: "The natives had asked me to go there, since many of their chief men had died of the smallpox, which rages in these lands as it does in the islands, and they wished me with their approval and consent to appoint other rulers in their place." Similar requests, quickly complied with, came from Tlaxcala, Chalco, and other cities. "Cortés had gained so much authority," the old soldier Bernal Díaz remembered, "that Indians came before him from distant lands, especially over matters of who would be chief or lord, as at the time smallpox had come to New Spain and many chiefs died."[37]

Similarly in Peru the epidemic of the 1520s was a stunning blow to the very nerve center of Incan society, throwing that society into

[34] Jehan Vellard, *Boletín del Instituto Riva-Agüero*, No. 2, 1956, 85; Bedson, *Virus*, 157, 167; Dixon, *Smallpox*, 313.

[35] Reginaldo de Lizárraga, *Descripción colonial por Fr. Reginaldo de Lizárraga* (Buenos Aires, 1928), I, 136.

[36] Díaz del Castillo, *Chronicles*, 282, 301; Gómara, *Cortés*, 238-239.

[37] Cortés, *Five Letters*, 136; Díaz del Castillo, *Chronicles*, 289, 311.

a self-destructive convulsion. The government of the Incan Empire was an absolute autocracy with a demigod, the Child of the Sun, as its emperor. The loss of the emperor could do enormous damage to the whole society, as Pizarro proved by his capture of Atahualpa. Presumably the damage was greater if the Inca were much esteemed, as was Huayna Capac. When he died, said Cieza de León, the mourning "was such that the lamentation and shrieks rose to the skies, causing the birds to fall to the ground. The news traveled far and wide, and nowhere did it not evoke great sorrow." Pedro Pizarro, one of the first to record what the Indians told of the last days before the conquest, judged that had "this Huayna Capac been alive when we Spaniards entered this land, it would have been impossible for us to win it, for he was much beloved by all his vassals."[38]

Not only the Inca but many others in key positions in Incan society died in the epidemic. The general Mihcnaca Mayta and many other military leaders, the governors Apu Hilaquito and Auqui Tupac (uncle and brother to the Inca), the Inca's sister, Mama Coca, and many others of the royal family all perished of the disease. The deaths of these important persons must have robbed the empire of much resiliency. Most ominous loss of all was the Inca's son and heir Ninan Cuyoche.[39]

In an autocracy no problem is more dangerous or more chronic than that of succession. One crude but workable solution is to have the autocrat, himself, choose his successor. The Inca named one of his sons, Ninan Cuyoche, as next wearer of "the fringe" or crown, on the condition that the *calpa,* a ceremony of divination, show this to be an auspicious choice. The first *calpa* indicated that the gods did not favor Ninan Cuyoche, the second that Huascar was no better candidate. The high nobles returned to the Inca for another choice, and found him dead. Suddenly a terrible gap had opened in Incan society: the autocrat had died, and there was no one to take his place. One of the nobles moved to close the gap. "Take care of the body," he said, "for I go to Tumipampa to give the fringe to Ninan Cuyoche." But it was too late. When he arrived at Tumipampa, he found that Ninan Cuyoche had also succumbed to smallpox pestilence.[40]

Among the several varying accounts of the Inca's death the one just related best fits the thesis of this paper. And while these

[38] Cieza de León, *Incas,* 53; Pizarro, *Relation,* I, 198-199.
[39] Ayala, *Nueva corónica,* 86; Cobo, *Obras,* 93; Sarmiento de Gamboa, *History,* 167-168; Valboa, *Miscelánea,* 393.
[40] Sarmiento de Gamboa, *History,* 167-168, 197-199. For corroboration see Cieza de León, *Incas,* 253; Valboa, *Miscelánea,* 394.

accounts may differ on many points, they all agree that confusion over the succession followed the unexpected death of Huayna Capac. War broke out between Huascar and Atahualpa, a war which devastated the empire and prepared the way for a quick Spanish conquest. "Had the land not been divided between Huascar and Atahualpa," Pedro Pizarro wrote, "we would not have been able to enter or win the land unless we could gather a thousand Spaniards for the task, and at that time it was impossible to get together even five hundred Spaniards. . . ."[41]

The psychological effect of epidemic disease is enormous, especially of an unknown disfiguring disease which strikes swiftly. Within a few days smallpox can transform a healthy man into a pustuled, oozing horror, whom his closest relatives can barely recognize. The impact can be sensed in the following terse, stoic account, drawn from Indian testimony, of Tenochtitlán during the epidemic.[42]

It was [the month of] Tepeilhuitl when it began, and it spread over the people as great destruction. Some it quite covered [with pustules] on all parts—their faces, their heads, their breasts, etc. There was a great havoc. Very many died of it. They could not walk; they only lay in their resting places and beds. They could not move; they could not stir; they could not change position, nor lie on one side; nor face down, nor on their backs. And if they stirred, much did they cry out. Great was its [smallpox'] destruction. Covered, mantled with pustules, very many people died of them.

In some places in Mexico the mortality was so great that, as Motolinía recorded, the Indians found it impossible to bury the great number of dead. "They pulled down the houses over them in order to check the stench that rose from the dead bodies," he wrote, "so that their homes became their tombs." In Tenochtitlán the dead were cast into the water, "and there was a great, foul odor; the smell issued forth from the dead."[43]

For those who survived, the horror was only diminished, for smallpox is a disease which marks its victims for the rest of their lives. The Spanish recalled that the Indians who survived, having scratched themselves, "were left in such a condition that they frightened the others with the many deep pits on their faces, hand, and bodies." "And on some," an Indian said, "the pustules were widely separated; they suffered not greatly, neither did many [of them] die. Yet many people were marred by them on their faces; one's face or nose was pitted." Some lost their sight—a fairly common aftereffect of smallpox.[44]

[41] Pizarro, *Relation*, I, 199.
[42] Sahagún, *General History*, XIII, 81.
[43] Motolinía, *History*, 38; Sahagún, *General History*, IX, 4.
[44] Sahagún, *General History*, XIII, 81; Gómara, *Cortés*, 204-205; Dixon, 94;

The contrast between the Indians' extreme susceptibility to the new disease and the Spaniards' almost universal immunity, acquired in Spain and reinforced in pestilential Cuba, must have deeply impressed the native Americans. The Indian, of course, soon realized that there was little relationship between Cortés and Quetzalcóatl, and that the Spaniards had all the vices and weaknesses of ordinary men, but he must have kept a lingering suspicion that the Spaniards were some kind of supermen. Their steel swords and arquebuses, their marvelously agile galleys, and, above all, their horses could only be the tools and servants of supermen. And their invulnerability to the pox—surely this was a shield of the gods themselves!

One can only imagine the psychological impact of smallpox on the Incan peoples. It must have been less than in Mexico, because the disease and the Spaniards did not arrive simultaneously, but epidemic disease is terrifying under any circumstances and must have shaken the confidence of the Incan people that they still enjoyed the esteem of their gods. Then came the long, ferocious civil war, confusing a people accustomed to the autocracy of the true Child of the Sun. And then the final disaster, the coming of the Spaniards.

The Mayan peoples, probably the most sensitive and brilliant of all American aborigines, expressed more poignantly than any other Indians the overwhelming effect of epidemic. Some disease struck into Guatemala in 1520 and 1521, clearing the way for the invasion shortly thereafter by Pedro de Alvarado, one of Cortés' captains. It was apparently not smallpox, for the accounts do not mention pustules but emphasize nosebleeds, cough, and illness of the bladder as the prominent symptoms. It may have been influenza;[45] whatever it was, the Cakchiquel Mayas who kept a chronicle of the tragedy for their posterity, were helpless to deal with it. Their words speak for all the Indians touched by Old World disease in the sixteenth century:

Great was the stench of the dead. After our fathers and grandfathers succumbed, half of the people fled to the fields. The dogs and vultures devoured the bodies. The mortality was terrible. Your grandfathers died, and with them died the son of the king and his brothers and kinsmen. So it was that we became orphans, oh, my sons! So we became when we were young. All of us were thus. We were born to die![46]

C. E. van Rooyen and A. J. Rhodes, *Virus Diseases of Man* (New York, 1948), 289.

[45] F. Webster McBryde, ''Influenza in America During the Sixteenth Century (Guatemala: 1523, 1559-1562, 1576),'' *Bulletin of the History of Medicine*, VIII (February 1940), 296-297.

[46] *Annals of the Cakchiquels*, 116.

5
An Outline of Andean
Epidemic History to 1720
Henry F. Dobyns

One of the great values of encyclopedic works such as the *Handbook of South American Indians* [2] is that they generate new research. By summarizing what is known in ways that stimulate scientific responses, these works reveal what is not known. The present paper attempts to deal briefly with one of the lacunae the *Handbook of South American Indians* revealed in scientific understanding of historic population trends in South America.

In the *Handbook's* comprehensive compendium of facts, George Kubler [3] stated that "not until 1720 did any great losses through pestilence occur in Peru," so that the population was not threatened with extinction as in Mexico. [4] Following the lead of the *Handbook*, Jehan Vellard [5] more recently also claimed that "epidemics as strong as occurred in Mexico" did not strike the people of Peru and Bolivia "after the conquest."

[1] This is a Cornell Perú Project publication made possible by a grant to Cornell University from the Carnegie Corporation of New York.

[2] Julian H. Steward, ed., Bulletin 143, Bureau of American Ethnology, vols. 1-6, 1946-1950.

[3] George Kubler, "The Quechua in the Colonial World," in *ibid.*, vol. 2, *The Andean Civilizations*, 1946, p. 334.

[4] *Ibid.*, p. 336.

[5] Jehan Vellard, "Causas biológicas de la desaparición de los indios americanos," *Boletín del Instituto Riva-Agüero* (Pontífica Universidad Católica del Perú) No. 2, 1956, p. 85.

494   HENRY F. DOBYNS

The thesis of the present paper is simply stated: great losses of Indian population did in fact occur in the Andean region prior to 1720 because of epidemic disease. Juan B. Lastres, in his monumental study of the history of Peruvian medicine,[6] counted seventeen "great plagues" in eighty years of the sixteenth century. So great was epidemic mortality in the Andean area that the native population declined rapidly and tremendously. Louis Baudin[7] had called attention to this population trend as had many historic writers, yet Kubler ignored it.

Whosoever gazes upon the massive and extensive systems of agricultural terraces lying unused today on the Andean eastern slope in the Cuzco area, in the Paucartambo River valley and elsewhere, on the flanks of the *Cordillera Negra* on both the coastal and *Callejon de Huaylas* sides, and in many other places, must perceive that human pressure on land resources has never been so great during historic times as it was prior to Spanish conquest and the introduction of Old World diseases.

The First New World Smallpox Epidemic. Discussing the disease environment of the Andean region only "after conquest" begs the question of the total impact of epidemic Old World diseases upon the aboriginal Andean population. For aboriginal disease environment conditions terminated in the Andes several years prior to Spanish conquest. As a result, full accounts of the initial impact of Old World disease agents on a virgin population of susceptible individuals lacking immunities do not exist. Most analysts have apparently confused the concept of "aboriginal times" with "pre-conquest" in the Andean area without realizing that aboriginal times terminated somewhat prior to conquest, at least in biological terms. The Inca Empire conquered by Pizarro's few hundred adventurers probably numbered less than half as many subjects then as it had a decade earlier.

Smallpox was carried from Europe to the Caribbean Island native populations early in the sixteenth century. It began among the Indians on the island of Hispañola (Santo Domingo) during December of 1518.[8] By late May royal officials reported it had killed "the greater part" of

[6] Juan B. Lastres. *Historia de la medicina peruana.* Vol. II: *La medicina en el virreinato.* Lima: Universidad Nacional Mayor de San Marcos, 1951, p. 77.

[7] Louis Baudin. *A Socialist Empire: The Incas of Perú (L'Empire socialiste des Inka,* Paris: Travaux et mémoires de l'Institut d'Ethnologie, vol. V, 1928). Transl. Katherine Woods, ed. Arthur Goddard. Princeton: D. Van Nostrand, 1961, p. 24.

[8] Joaquín F. Pacheco y Francisco Cárdenas, eds. *Colección de documentos ineditos relativos al descubrimiento, conquista y colonización de las posesiones españolas en América y Oceania.* Madrid: Imprenta de Quiros, 1864, vol. I, p. 367.

AN OUTLINE OF ANDEAN EPIDEMIC HISTORY TO 1720   495

the Indians who had survived until then.[9] Father Bartolomé de las Casas[10] doubted that 1,000 Indians survived. The disease spread to Puerto Rico early in 1519.[11] The following year it was introduced into the Mexican Indian population during the conquest.[12] Smallpox played an important role in breaking imperial Aztec military resistance to the Spaniards.[13] It killed Emperor Moctezuma's successor Cuitlahuac only four months after his succession,[14] thus weakening Aztec leadership. The disease also seriously weakened the Tarascan kingdom.[15] Once introduced to the continental Indian population, smallpox rapidly assumed epidemic proportions,[16] causing a mortality reckoned at half the population of some provinces,[17] and spread widely through the hemispheric populace.

Starting out at Vera Cruz in 1520, the smallpox epidemic reached Guatemala the following year[18] or slightly later.[19] It carried off half the

[9] *Ibid.*, p. 370.

[10] Bartolomé de las Casas. *Historia de las Indias.* Mexico: Fondo de la Cultura Económica, 1951, p. 270.

[11] Juan B. Lastres. *La salud pública y la prevención de la viruela en el Perú.* Lima: Imprenta del Ministerio de Hacienda y Comercio, 1957, p. 20; Ramiro Guerra y Sanchez. *Historia de la nación cubana.* Vol. I: *Culturas primitivas, descubrimiento, conquista y colonización.* La Habana: Editorial Historia de la Nación Cubana, 1952, p. 230; Pacheco y Cárdenas, *op. cit.,* vol. I, p. 368.

[12] Bernal Díaz del Castillo. *The Discovery and Conquest of Mexico, 1517-1521.* New York: Grove Press, 1956, p. 293; Francisco Cervantes de Salazar. *Crónica de la Nueva España.* Madrid: Hispanic Society of America, 1914, p. 546; Fernando Ocaranza. *Historia de la Medicina en Mexico.* Mexico: Midy, 1934, p. 83.

[13] Díaz del Castillo, *op. cit.,* p. 328; Wyndham B. Blanton, "Medical references in Bernal Diaz's account of the discovery and conquest of Mexico," *Ann. M. Hist.,* 1942, 3d s. *4*: 402.

[14] George C. Vaillant. *The Aztecs of Mexico.* New York: Doubleday, Doran, 1944, Baltimore: Penguin Books, 1950, p. 113.

[15] Hubert Howe Bancroft, et al. *The Native Races of the Pacific States.* New York: D. Appleton & Co., 1876, vol. V, p. 525.

[16] George Cheever Shattuck, et al. *A Medical Survey of the Republic of Guatemala.* Carnegie Institution of Washington, Publ. 499, 1938, p. 40; Francisco J. Clavijero. *Historia antigua de México.* Mexico: Editorial Delfin, 1944, vol. II, p. 232; Antonio de Herrera y Tordesillas. *Historia general de los hechos de los castellanos en las islas y tierra-firme en el Mar Oceano,* 1945, vol. III, pp. 374-376; Francis B. Steck. *Motolinia's History of the Indians of New Spain.* Washington: Academy of American Franciscan History, 1951, pp. 87-88.

[17] Gerónimo de Mendieta. *Historia eclesiastica indiana.* Mexico: Editorial Salvador Chavez Hayhoe, 1945, vol. 3, p. 17.

[18] Shattuck. *op. cit.,* p. 41.

[19] F. Webster McBryde, "Influenza in America during the sixteenth century," *Bull. Hist. Med.,* 1940, *8*: 296.

Cakchiquel population, including two rulers,[20] and greatly decreased the formerly thick population in the northern interior of the Yucatecan Pen·insula.[21] The pestilence apparently continued across Central America to reach the Inca Empire in 1524,[22] 1525,[23] or 1526,[24] possibly by sea from Panama. The reigning emperor Huayna Capac caught the disease while campaigning on his northern frontier in modern Ecuador and perished.[25] His death, combined with that of his heir,[26] left the empire split on the question of succession, a dynastic situation which materially aided Spanish conquest.

Details of the mortality caused by this epidemic in the Andes are not abundant in Spanish accounts obtained long after the event from survivors, but such information as does exist suggests that the mortality which occurred was of a scale equal to, or exceeding, that in central Mexico. There was the same recording of the demise of the ruler Huayna Capac,[27] his brother, sister, and uncle, and a number of nobles of lesser rank plus generals and other officers, as well as thousands of common·ers.[28] Certainly among the most crucial deaths were those of Huayna Capac and his legitimate son Ninan Cuyoche during this same epidemic. Designated by the dying Inca as his successor, Ninan Cuyoche died before notification reached him,[29] opening the way for the dynastic struggle still being waged when Spanish adventurers arrived to capitalize upon it. In terms of numbers, one author [30] claimed that " the greater part " of the Indian population perished. Later, the conquered Indians cited

[20] Bancroft, op. cit., vol. V, p. 601.

[21] France V. Scholes and Ralph L. Roys with the assistance of Eleanor B. Adams and Robert S. Chamberlain. *The Maya Chontal Indians of Acalan-Tixchel*. Carnegie Institution of Washington, Publ. 560, 1948, p. 326.

[22] Pedro Sarmiento de Gamboa. *History of the Incas*. Transl. and ed. Clements R. Markham. Cambridge: Hakluyt Society, s. II, vol. 22, 1907, p. 169.

[23] José Toribio Polo, " Apuntes sobre las epidemias en el Perú," *Rev. hist.*, vol. V. Citations to separate—Lima: Imp. Nacional de Federico Barrionuevo, 1913, p. 5.

[24] Pedro Cieza de León. *The Second Part of the Chronicle of Perú*. Transl. and ed. Clements R. Markham. London: Hakluyt Society, No. 68, 1883, p. 220.

[25] Lastres 1951, op. cit., vol. II, pp. 75-76.

[26] Mauro Madero. *Historia de la medicina en la provincia de Guayas*. Guayaquil: Casa de la Cultura Ecuatoriana, 1955, p. 8.

[27] Cieza de León, op. cit., p. 221; Sarmiento de Gamboa, op. cit., p. 167; Bernabé Cobo. *Historia del Nuevo Mundo* (Ed. Marcos Jimenez de la Espada). Sevilla: Sociedad de Bibliófilos Andaluces, 1892-1893, Madrid: Ediciones Atlas, 1956, vol. 2, p. 93.

[28] Lastres 1951, op. cit., vol. II, p. 76; Joan de Santa Cruz Pachacuti Yamqui. *Tres relaciones de antigüedades peruanas*. Ed. Marcos Jimenez de la Espada. Madrid: Ministerio de Fomento, 1879, p. 307; Miguel Cabello Valboa. *Miscelanea antartica*. Lima: Instituto de Etnología, 1951, p. 394.

[29] Sarmiento de Gamboa, op. cit., p. 168; Cobo, op. cit., vol. II, p. 93.

[30] Polo, op. cit., p. 5.

this epidemic " which consumed the greater part of them " as having made possible the Spanish conquest.[31] An Indian author's identification of the illness as " saranpion birguelas " [32] or " measles smallpox " suggests that the epidemic was one of deadly hemorrhagic smallpox.

When smallpox was introduced to the people of Iceland in 1707, " no less than 18,000 out of a population of 50,000 died of the disease " in an epidemic lasting until 1709.[33] Knowledge of the decimating impact of epidemic smallpox on other susceptible populations requires the assumption of a very high mortality among inhabitants of the Inca Empire. As Vellard[34] generalized: " The first contact constitutes the most dangerous moment, frequently causing the total extinction of small groups in a few years," because of " the total lack of immunity in the indigenous American populations to contagious diseases to which civilized men have become resistant through centuries of inheritance," a factor in Cuban history recognized also by Guerra.[35] It is known smallpox mortality in other populations composed entirely of susceptible persons that leads to the supposition that the Andean population may well have been halved during this epidemic.

As Spanish rule was imposed upon the Andean populations, communication with the Old World fostered repeated introductions of smallpox, until it became endemic in the highland population. The depopulation verified during the administration of Viceroy Montesclaros, who arrived in Lima in 1607, " was attributed to the ravages of smallpox, repeated every seven years, and to other frequent epidemics." [36]

First New World Measles Epidemic. The natives of the New World enjoyed a few years of population recovery through natural increase following the smallpox epidemic of 1520-1526, before they were struck by the second major epidemic caused by an Old World disease agent. This epidemic struck the natives of New Spain in 1531 in the guise of measles.[37] The disease was brought to the continent by a Spaniard[38] who

[31] Reginaldo de Lizárraga. *Descripción de las Indias.* Lima: Pequeños Grandes Libros de Historia Americana, 1946, p. 85.

[32] Felipe de Guaman Poma de Ayala. *Nueva corónica y buen gobierno.* Paris: Institut de l'Ethnologie, 1936, p. 114.

[33] E. Wagner and Allan E. Stearn. *The Effect of Smallpox on the Destiny of the Amerindian.* Boston: Bruce Humphries, Inc., 1945, p. 14.

[34] Vellard, *op. cit.,* p. 87.

[35] Guerra y Sanchez, *op. cit.,* vol. I, p. 229.

[36] Jean Nuix. *Reflexiones imparciales sobre la humanidad de los españoles en las Indias.* Madrid: Ibarra, 1782, p. 84, n.

[37] Mendieta, *op. cit.,* vol. 3, p. 174; Ocaranza, *op. cit.,* p. 84.

[38] Steck, *op. cit.,* p. 88.

HENRY F. DOBYNS

very likely acquired the infection in the Caribbean Islands. Perhaps two-thirds of the Indians remaining in Cuba died in an epidemic there in 1529,[39] which may have been the island episode of the measles epidemic. From New Spain the pestilence swept southward. An official of the imperial exchequer who arrived at Leon de Nicaragua on 12 December 1532 reported to the emperor at the end of April of 1533: " The settlers are poor and in debt for lack of gold, which results from there having died from sickness, especially measles which has struck them latterly, so many Indians that some citizens have remained without a one." [40] The Nicaraguan Spaniards were at that early post-conquest period still reliant upon Indian slaves for their economic support.

This same epidemic carried off perhaps half the Indians under Spanish control in Honduras. Robert S. Chamberlain [41] placed this pestilence in 1533, but contemporary documents indicate that the contagion passed through central America in 1531. On February 25, 1532, an imperial representative at Panama wrote to the empress: " This land is very depressed . . . many Indians have died, and very little gold is recovered." Consequently, no one wished to stay at Panama; all wished to press on elsewhere.[42] A group of citizens wrote their emperor from Panama on 4 September 1531 that: " There used to be very few Indians here, and there are now many fewer after the pestilence." [43]

The Panamanian episode of the measles epidemic evidently began fairly early during 1531, indicating an early beginning in New Spain, if that was in fact the point of origin of continental infection. At any rate, the contagion reached Panama by sea rather than overland. Writing the emperor on 24 May 1531, de la Gama reported that the mines which had been discovered only a year before had given out, and even if there were gold, " there is no one who would recover it because a ship which came from Nicaragua carried a pestilence to this land." This episode of the epidemic was so fierce that " although it has not ended, two-thirds of all the people who used to exist in this land have died, including the Indians native to it, as well as slaves and even some Christians," i. e., Spaniards.[44]

[39] Guerra y Sanchez, op. cit., vol. I, p. 230.

[40] Raúl Porras Barranechea. Cartas del Perú (1524-1543), Colección de documentos ineditos para la historia del Perú, vol. III. Lima: Sociedad de Bibliófilos Peruanos, 1959, p. 46.

[41] Robert S. Chamberlain. The Conquest and Colonization of Honduras, 1502-1550. Carnegie Institution of Washington, Publ. 598, 1953, p. 28.

[42] Porras Barranechea, op. cit., p. 26.

[43] Ibid., p. 24.   [44] Ibid., p. 22.

It cannot be established at present writing whether or not the measles epidemic of 1531 swept on south into the Andean populations. Chances seem excellent that it did so. The mortality recorded among the Indians and slaves of Panama indicates that the disease agent was virulent and quite capable of making its own way through the entire susceptible population to which it could be carried. Measles is much like smallpox in its infectiousness. Introduced in April of 1846 to a Faeroe Island population not exposed to it since 1781, measles infected 6,000 of the 7,782 inhabitants. In 1951 measles infected 4,221 persons of the 4,458 living in the Julianahaab district of Greenland.[45] The critical question is just what the lines of communication were in 1531 between Panama and the Andean peoples. Presumably, if measles made the short overland jump from Panama to the Chibchas in Colombia, it continued south through the subjects of the Inca, for the constant movement of messengers, troops, and colonists among civilized Andean peoples created fairly ideal conditions for transmission of infectious diseases.

Nor was that the only possibility for transmitting measles to the Andean peoples. It should be remembered that a number of Dominican and Franciscan friars had gone from Nicaragua to Peru in the early stages of the Pizarro conquest, returning to Panama about 10 February 1532.[46] If their timing was right, they may well have carried measles directly from infected Nicaragua to the Andean coastal hinterland.

The 1546 Epidemic. The Andean peoples may not have suffered all the epidemics which struck the northern viceroyalty after 1531, but they did feel the ravages of at least some of the later epidemics which greatly reduced the population of New Spain.

In 1546 an epidemic "spread over all the land, of which people without number died," [47] possibly the Andean episode of the epidemic which had devastated New Spain the previous year. The Cuzco city annals note that the llamas and sheep in all Peru suffered from an epizootic which began in 1546.[48]

Known in New Spain as *matlazahuatl*,[49] the disease is difficult to identify. The Nahuatl name implies that one of its major symptoms was a

[45] Jacques M. May. *The Ecology of Human Disease.* New York: M D Publications, 1958, p. 267.

[46] Porras Barranechea, *op. cit.*, p. 26.

[47] Herrera y Tordesillas, *op. cit.*, vol. IV, p. 385.

[48] Polo, *op. cit.*, p. 9.

[49] Hubert Howe Bancroft, *et al. History of Mexico.* Vol. III: *1600-1803.* San Francisco: Bancroft Co., 1883, p. 756.

500   HENRY F. DOBYNS

rash similar to, but distinguishable from, those caused by smallpox or measles. Since Spanish writers at times referred to it as *peste*,[50] it could have been plague, although *peste* connotes both " plague " in a specific sense and " epidemic " in a general sense. Since it involved fever and bleeding from the nostrils,[51] it could have been caused by a number of disease agents. Hans Zinsser [52] thought that it might have been typhus, since he felt that only typhus or plague would have been likely to cause the high mortality.

The 1558-1559 Influenza Pandemic. A general epidemic of " smallpox and measles "—probably hemorrhagic smallpox—struck Peru in 1558.[53] At least one religious society for the care of the indigent ill in Lima was founded in response to the " acute sickness which had the nature of a pestilence from which many died." [54] Many years later, an early Lima newspaper stated that: " there was in this capital an epidemic which wrought cruel ravages among its inhabitants and those of its environs." [55] The disease was not identified. In the area of modern Ecuador it was smallpox " complicated by severe catarrhs." [56] This same contagion seems to have struck Guatemala in the same year.[57] The influenza component originated in Europe, where it ravaged Sicily in July and Spain in October of 1557. It felled so many harvest hands in England in 1558 that much grain remained in the fields.[58] The governor of the Isle of Wright estimated that half the population of Southampton, Portsmouth, and the Isle were affected in early September of 1558.[59] In 1557, influenza in " truly pandemic form " [60] spread from Sicily to Padua, Lombardy, Dalmatia, and Switzerland during August; to Poitiers, Montpellier and Nismes in France during September; to Harderwyk and Alk-

---

[50] Bancroft 1875, *op. cit.,* vol. I, pp. 638-639.

[51] Hans Zinsser. *Rats, Lice and History.* New York: Blue Ribbon Books, 1934, p. 256; Ocaranza, *op. cit.,* p. 84; Mendieta, *op. cit.,* vol. 3, p. 174.

[52] Zinsser, *op. cit.,* p. 256.

[53] Lastres 1957, *op. cit.,* p. 22.

[54] Cobo, *op. cit.,* vol. II, p. 447.

[55] Polo, *op. cit.,* p. 11; Manuel de Mendiburu. *Diccionario historico-biográfico del Perú.* Lima: J. Francisco Solis, 1885, vol. V, p. 48.

[56] Madero, *op. cit.,* p. 65.

[57] Shattuck, *op. cit.,* p. 41.

[58] McBryde, *op. cit.,* p. 287; Charles Creighton. *A History of Epidemics in Britain from A.D. 664 to the Extinction of Plague.* Cambridge: University Press, 1891, vol. I, p. 401.

[59] *Ibid.,* p. 403.

[60] August Hirsch. *Handbook of Geographical and Historical Pathology.* Vol. I: Acute Infective Diseases. Transl. Charles Creighton. London: New Sydenham Society, 1883, p. 18.

maar in the Netherlands, as well as to Spain, during October.[61] Presumably Spanish ships carried this influenza to Spain's colonial empire in the Western Hemisphere, where it must have caused considerable mortality in combination with epidemic smallpox there.

The Epidemic Period of 1585 to 1591. The Andean peoples either suffered recurrent episodes of a major epidemic from 1585 to 1591, or more likely, two distinct epidemics moving in opposite directions.

The Peruvian medical historian Juan B. Lastres [62] considered the 1585-1598 period one of a single recurrent smallpox epidemic which started at Cuzco in April of 1585, spreading rapidly to Huamanga [63] and later to Lima, Quito, and Santa Fe de Bogota, as thousands died. Indians suffered from this disease much more than non-Indians.[64]

That the residents of Cuzco suffered from an epidemic episode in 1585 cannot be doubted. The principal source [65] identified the disease as "smallpox and measles." The fact that the Huamanga city council cut its road to Cuzco [66] showed that the contagion was moving from east to west. The Cuzco annalist [67] identified the disease as "high fevers with mumps" or goiter, suggesting a fever-producing infection affecting facial glands. Another source [68] said that this infection "ruined thousands of inhabitants" of Cuzco.

This epidemic flared up again in 1586,[69] and mortality in Lima alone was nearly 3,000 persons.[70] Since the capital city's population reached only 14,262 fifteen years afterwards in 1600,[71] such a mortality may well have represented twenty or more per cent of the total population. Yet Lima had more medical facilities and a higher proportion of resident Europeans than any other Peruvian settlement. Those who died in Lima

[61] *Ibid.,* p. 8.

[62] Lastres 1957, *op. cit.,* p. 22.

[63] Rubén Vargas Ugarte. *Historia del Perú, virreynato (1551-1590).* Lima, 1942, vol. I, p. 279.

[64] Lastres 1957, *op. cit.,* p. 23; Vargas Ugarte, *op. cit.,* p. 279.

[65] Montesinos, cited in Polo, *op. cit.,* p. 11; Lastres 1951, *op. cit.,* vol. II, p. 76; Lastres 1957, *op. cit.,* p. 22; Vargas Ugarte, *op. cit.,* p. 279.

[66] Polo, *op. cit.,* p. 11; Vargas Ugarte, *op. cit.,* p. 279.

[67] Father Esquivel, cited by Vargas, *op. cit.,* p. 279. Anónimo. *Anales del Cuzco.* Lima: Imp. "El Estado," 1902, p. 231.

[68] José María Blanco, "Diario de la marcha que hizo el Presidente Orbegoso," *Rev d. Inst. Am. de arte,* 1957, no. 8: 99.

[69] Vargas Ugarte, *op. cit.,* p. 279.

[70] Lastres 1957, *op. cit.,* p. 23.

[71] Cosme Bueno. *Geografía del Peru virreinal (Siglo XVIII).* Lima: Daniel Valcarcel, 1951, p. 132.

were " for the most part Indians," [72] yet many Negroes also died there. Since " catarrh and cough," which came on as the skin rash dried up, are mentioned by one colonial writer as leaving few youngsters or old-sters alive,[73] there was perhaps an influenza outbreak which raised the mortality, or else severe bronchial complications followed after the period of acute prime infection identified as measles,[74] and smallpox. "The Indians were cruelly assaulted by this smallpox "[75] and " an innumerable quantity of Indians died." [76] More concretely, six priests died out of sixty in a Jesuit convent in Lima, a mortality of ten per cent even among a probably nearly all European sub-population. The Santa Ana hospital for Indians reportedly had a daily death rate of fourteen to sixteen patients for two whole months,[77] apparently during 1586.[78] Statements such as these clearly indicate that mortality in the Andean peoples dur-ing this period was on a scale comparable to that in major sixteenth century epidemics in New Spain.

An episode of epidemic "high fevers, smallpox and measles" assaulted the population of Quito (modern Ecuador).[79] Nearly 4,000 people, espe-cially children, died in Quito during three months.[80] This mortality reportedly included more men than women, but no Spaniards.[81]

Just when Ecuador suffered this catastrophe is not easily determined. Historians differ markedly. José T. Polo [82] claimed that Marcos Jimenez de la Espada dated the Quito episode from July 1587 to March 1588. Juan B. Lastres [83] wrote: " Jimenez de la Espada thinks that the epi-demic began in Quito in 1588 and lasted until the end of 1589." An ecclesiastical historian placed [84] this peak mortality in 1586. At the other extreme, Velasco asserted that an episode dated at the end of December of 1589 was the first epidemic there.[85] He also claimed a mortality of 30,000 persons in Quito alone.[86] This confusion over dates may arise

[72] Vargas Ugarte, op. cit., p. 280.
[73] Polo, op. cit., p. 16.
[74] By Lizárraga, op. cit., p. 85, although assignment of his remarks to this date is Polo's.
[75] Lastres 1951, op. cit., vol. II, p. 77.
[76] Anónimo. Historia general de la Compañia de Jesús en la provincia del Perú. Mad-rid: Concejo Superior de Investigaciones Científicas, 1944, vol. I, p. 343.
[77] Polo, op. cit., p. 14.
[78] Lastres 1951, op. cit., vol. II, p. 77; Lastres 1957, op. cit., p. 23; Vargas Ugarte, op. cit., p. 279.
[79] Polo, op. cit., p. 16.   [83] Lastres 1957, op. cit., p. 24.
[80] Madero, op. cit., p. 66.   [84] Vargas Ugarte, op. cit., p. 280.
[81] Polo, op. cit., p. 15.   [85] Polo, op. cit., p. 15.
[82] Ibid., p. 16.   [86] Madero, op. cit., p. 66.

from *two* epidemics having reached Ecuador from opposite directions at nearly the same time. Up to this point, the present narrative has traced the course of an epidemic moving east and then north from Cuzco. Now it is necessary to follow an epidemic traveling south from the Caribbean. A Jesuit historian called it " this universal plague similar to measles and smallpox." He thought it came from Mexico, Brazil, and Panama, began in the New Kingdom, and reached Quito and then Lima, " wreaking great havoc, principally among the Indians and the Spaniards born here." [87] In his annual report to the General of his order in 1590, Father Pablo José de Arriaga of the Peruvian Province described the course of this epidemic. " It first appeared in Cartagena . . . later passed to Quito and neighboring places as I have related in my previous letter. Later it spread not only to Lima, but also to Cuzco, Potosi and to all the southern part of the Kingdom of Peru." [88] Summarizing the available sources, José T. Polo,[59] in 1913, wrote that in 1588 and 1589 " There was a great epidemic of smallpox in Peru, Quito and Popayan, which propagated itself from the Kingdom of Santa Fe."

An epidemic smallpox episode in Santa Fe de Bogota occurred during 1587 and " killed up to 90 per 100 of the native race, sadly privileged to be preferred by the cruel illness." [90] The contagion was widespread through the New Kingdom.[91] It was quite possibly an episode of this epidemic which carried off most of the Teques Indians of Venezuela and turned them into refugees.[92]

Mauro Madero, medical historian of Ecuador,[93] traced like Polo a southward moving epidemic. " It passed to this kingdom from Mexico and Panama; it reached the New Kingdom, Quito, Lima, Cuzco and Chile." An historian of the city of Arequipa attributed this pandemic, which reached there in 1589, to a seaborne introduction from the Cape Verde Islands. " Some parties of Negroes brought from the Cape Verdes had come to Panama, and some of them already infected with the epidemic." The Spaniards of the time were so anxious to secure household

[87] Anónimo 1944, *op. cit.*, p. 45.
[88] Printed in Polo, *op. cit.*, p. 55.
[89] *Ibid.*, p. 15.
[90] Pedro M. Ibañez. *Crónicas de Bogotá*. Bogotá: Imprenta Nacional, Biblioteca de Historia Nacional, vol. X, 1923, p. 61.
[91] *Ibid.*, p. 82.
[92] José de Oviedo y Baños. *Historia de la conquista y población de la provincia de Venezuela*. New York: Paul Adams facsimile edition, 1940 (1824), p. 533.
[93] Madero, *op. cit.*, p. 66.

slaves that the Negroes were rapidly distributed to the ports on the west coast of South America, thus reportedly spreading the infection.[94]

There is contemporary and independent corroboration of a Cape Verde Island origin for at least some portion of the South American epidemic. Sir Francis Drake sailed from England with 2,300 men in twenty-five ships.[95] Clearing Plymouth on 14 September 1585, Drake landed a thousand men on the island of Santiago on 16 November, quartering them in town for ten days to two weeks. Re-embarking on 26 November, Drake reached Dominica in eighteen days. Seven or eight days out from the Cape Verde islands, disaster struck. Epidemic disease contracted during the brief occupation of the island capital killed from two to three hundred of Drake's men.[96] Some, though not all, of those who perished had broken out in " small spots which are often found upon those that be infected with the plague " after suffering with extreme hot burning and "continual agues." Drake's force carried the city of Santo Domingo by assault, even though " Deaths continued to occur, from the same disease as at first, both among officers and men, and so continued for many weeks." Most of the few who survived the disease suffered " great alteration and decay of their wits and strength for a long time after." Yet Cartagena was also captured, and Drake's amphibious forces remained there for six weeks from mid-January to late February of 1586.[97] The expedition was then so weakened by the epidemic that Drake and his officers decided to return to England. Capturing St. Augustine, Florida, on their way home, they lost approximately 750 men on the voyage, about one-fourth of the original force, three-fourths of them to the disease contracted in the Cape Verde Islands.[98]

The Spanish attribution of the epidemic to Negro slaves brought from the Cape Verde Islands via Panama, plus Drake's disastrous encounter with epidemic disease in those islands, provide strong evidence that the South American epidemic spreading southward from Cartagena was in fact introduced there by one or both means.

If the disease which decimated the Drake expedition was in fact the same one which swept down the west coast of the continent, it evidently was neither smallpox nor measles, despite Spanish identification of it as such. Either measles or smallpox, because of their modes of transmission, would have infected rapidly all susceptible members of Drake's forces cooped up in the confines of small ships. A disease spread by a

---

[94] Polo, *op. cit.*, p. 17; Lastres 1957, *op. cit.*, p. 25.
[95] Creighton, *op. cit.*, p. 585.   [97] *Ibid.*, p. 587.
[96] *Ibid.*, p. 586.   [98] *Ibid.*, p. 588.

vector is strongly indicated by the long-continued mortality in Drake's forces. Malaria seems to be ruled out by the spots on some of the dead. Bubonic plague is probably ruled out by the English description of the rash as plague-like, since Englishmen of that period should have been quite capable of recognizing the " black death."

Typhus is left as the most likely culprit, although other diseases should not be eliminated entirely from consideration. If epidemic smallpox moving west from Cuzco in 1585 spread north to the Caribbean coast, to be followed by southward-moving typhus introduced by Drake's force at Cartagena and infected Negro slaves at Panama and ports of the west coast of South America, the high mortality in the later stages of the epidemic may be more easily comprehended.

The southward movement of the epidemic was reported to the King of Spain by his viceroy in Peru at the time. Writing on 19 April 1589, the Count of Villar referred to a previous letter in which he had reported that " smallpox and measles " had begun to cause casualties in the province of Quito. The pestilence had " destroyed and killed a great sum of Indians," who suffered most from its rigors. Then the Viceroy reported the news—since his previous letter, the epidemic had spread to the Provinces of Cuenca, the southern part of modern Ecuador, and Paita and Trujillo, in northern Peru.[99]

That was not all the news about epidemic disease in the Andes in 1589, however, for the Viceroy had bad news from the upper provinces of Bolivia. " There were days when more than 10,000 Indians and some Spaniards sickened in Potosí" from "another illness of cough and catarrh with fever," almost at the same time as the other epidemic spread south of Quito. The Viceroy remarked that up until the time of his report, the highland epidemic had not caused " notable harm" and had not reached either Cuzco or Huancavelica.[100] Clearly an influenza epidemic had started in the Bolivian highlands.

By 11 May the Viceroy was claiming that the severity of the epidemic had abated in northern Peru, although " many people continued to die." Yet he then had to apologize to the King for not forwarding all his correspondence, " because everyone is ill and those who are well are very busy curing them." The northern contagion had continued " spreading to other parts with less harm " and reached Lima a few days prior to his

[99] Roberto Levillier (Compiler). Gobernantes del Perú. Cartas y papeles siglo XVI. Vol. XI: El Virrey Conde del Villar, IIa Parte. 1588-1591. Madrid: Colección de Publicaciones Históricas de la Biblioteca del Congreso Argentino, 1925, p. 207.

[100] Ibid., p. 208.

report. The Viceroy reported few deaths in Lima, " and of those mostly Negroes and Indians, but the illness is so general that there is scarcely a person in the place who is not touched with it." [101]

A month later the Count of Villar had changed his tune. Writing to the King again on 13 June, he reported that since his earlier letter the " catarrhal smallpox and measles " epidemic had grown much worse in Lima. " There have died and die daily many people among the natives and Negroes and mulatos and Spaniards of those born here, and now it has spread to those from Spain." The sickness continued, moreover, to spread to new areas.[102] Three days later on 16 June, the Viceroy reported that after the earlier mitigation of epidemic conditions in the Trujillo region, they "turned with greater fury" so that many Indians and even Creoles and Spaniards died, apparently from " catarrh and stitches in the side." [103] The influenza epidemic evidently moved north from Lima to the northern provinces of Peru, causing high mortality among people already weakened by the rash-producing disease agent. The Viceroy also noted that mortality was rising in Lima, where the rash-producing disease seems to have followed the influenza, which infected nearly everyone.

On 28 June the Viceroy ordered an inspector to the towns of Surco, Lati and Lurigancho, where "nearly all " those infected of the many Indians who lived there died. The inspector was to provide hospitalization, bedding, and medicines to the value of 400 pesos in each town.[104] On the twelfth of July, the Count of Villar appointed a surgeon to spend six months treating those laid low by the epidemic in San Juan de Matocana, San Geronimo de Surco and San Mateo de Guanchor.[105] The location of these settlements east of Lima upstream on the Rimac River clearly marks one path by which the rash-producing disease moved up into the central Peruvian Andes.

This " general epidemic " occurred only two generations after Spanish conquest, and in 1589 some Indians still followed the preconquest practice of bleeding themselves by cutting with sharp stone knives.[106] Perhaps as a result of such therapy the disease caused such " great mortality of Indians." [107] There is considerable testimony, as a matter of

[101] *Ibid.*, p. 221.
[102] *Ibid.*, p. 284.
[103] *Ibid.*, p. 285.
[104] Polo, *op. cit.*, pp. 58-59.
[105] *Ibid.*, pp. 60-62.
[106] Cobo, *op. cit.*, vol. IV, p. 200.
[107] Manuel de Mendiburu. *Diccionario historico-biográfico del Perú*. Lima: Imp. Bolognesi, 1878, vol. VIII, p. 101.

fact, that European-born colonists suffered much less mortality than Indians and American-born Spaniards.[108]

The 1589 episode was the most virulent one to strike the city of Arequipa.[109] In the memory of survivors writing after the event, the influenza and rash-producing disease episodes are probably jumbled together. Judging from the viceregal reports of 1589, however, the influenza epidemic should have moved westward through Arequipa to Lima before the rash-producing disease arrived from the north. An historian of Arequipa thought the contagion was " at the same time smallpox, scarlet fever and measles with such a revolution of the bile that they were complicated by furious fevers." The onset of the disease brought severe headaches and kidney pains. A few days later, patients became stupified, then delirious, and ran naked through the streets shouting. Patients who broke out in a rash had a good chance to recover, reportedly, while those who did not break out seemed to have little chance. Ulcerated throat killed many patients. Fetuses died in the uterus. Even patients who broke out in a rash might lose chunks of flesh by too-sudden movement. " It was the usual thing to lose the skin of the face, and remain without lips or nose, just the bone-work." In extreme cases, even the bone ulcerated.[110] No count of victims was possible in Arequipa, where they had to be interred in open ditches in the public squares during the three month long episode.[111]

Another contemporary witness, the Jesuit Provincial in Lima, reported: " Virulent pustules broke out on the entire body that deformed the miserable sick persons to the point that they could not be recognized except by name." The pustules obstructed nasal passages and throats, impeding respiration and food ingestion, occasioning some deaths from these complications. Many survivors lost one or both eyes.[112]

An infinite number of Indians and Creoles reportedly died, more in the city of Cuzco than elsewhere. Montesinos dated the Cuzco episode in 1590, but José T. Polo[113] attributed his comment to 1589. José M. Blanco[114] placed the Cuzco episode in 1590, on the other hand, and noted that the Cuzco city council's 1589 measure of cutting the bridge over the Apurimac River proved an ineffective defense. The infection reached Cuzco around the middle of September, despite the viceregal prohibition on importation of new wine and the many church rituals held during

---

[108] Levillier, op. cit., pp. 208, 284.
[109] Vargas Ugarte, op. cit., p. 280.
[110] Polo, op. cit., pp. 17-18.
[111] Ibid., p. 19.

[112] Ibid., p. 56.
[113] Ibid., p. 20.
[114] Blanco, op. cit., p. 99.

July and August to ward off the contagion. The annalist in Cuzco mentioned cases of lips so ulcerated and breathing so obstructed that patients could hardly speak. Like observers in Lima and Arequipa, the Cuzco annalist noted the ill effects of this epidemic disease agent on the lips and internal throat of those infected. Some of them required artificial aid even to swallow liquids. He, too, noted that the eyes ulcerated. The "tumors, callous excrescences or itchy scabs or very nasty pustules" which released, when they broke, such irritating matter that sufferers could not resist scratching, resulted in a "monstrous ugliness in faces and bodies." The annalist also noted that the disease produced acute depression.[115]

Local episodes of this epidemic continued into 1591, when many people died in the Ica curacy[116] on the Peruvian coast south of Lima. The Jesuit Provincial reported on 20 May 1590 that, according to recent reports there, the epidemic had already reached Chile.[117] Somewhat later the Chilean episode of this epidemic wrought havoc among both the Spaniards and hostile Araucanian Indians of Chile. At least one writer placed "smallpox" mortality among these Indians during this epidemic episode at three-quarters of their population.[118]

The six year-long siege of epidemic mortality in the Andean area certainly indicates that no sooner had one disease swept through the susceptible population than another infection of quite a different nature and even greater virulence, and to which the earlier one had conferred no immunity, appeared and produced even greater mortality.

The Cuzco Diphtheria Epidemic in 1614. The great epidemics which swept the Andean peoples during the sixteenth century clearly reduced the native population, probably by a very large proportion. A relative scarcity of information about similar epidemics affecting the Andean population during the seventeenth century suggests a reduction of population such as to make geographic isolation a more effective barrier against epidemics.

Still, there were some urban concentrations of population in the Andes sufficient to provide a large number of persons susceptible to epidemic infection. These cities were also the residences of literate administrators or others interested in recording such events, so they are known to

---

[115] Polo, *op. cit.*, pp. 16-17.
[116] *Ibid.*, p. 20.
[117] *Ibid.*, p. 55.
[118] Claudio Gay. *Historia físcia y política de Chile. Historia.* Paris: Author, 1845, vol. II, pp. 183-184.

posterity. The Peruvian city of Cuzco suffered an assault of diphtheria during the summer of 1614—" one's throat swelled and one strangled." It was such a severe epidemic that victims were too numerous to be interred in the many churches. As a result, a cemetery was begun in a canyon west of the city on the Ayacucho road.[119] This epidemic lasted from May to the beginning of September and was said to have affected every household in the city, killing without regard to race, class, or age. It called forth a great burst of Catholic ritual activity aimed at propitiating saintly intercessors so as to end the threat.[120] Juan B. Lastres [121] suspected that scarlatina contributed to the mortality.

An epidemic that occurred in the Bolivian mining center of Potosí in 1615 was probably an episode of the Cuzco contagion.[122]

The Measles Epidemic of 1618-1619. Epidemic measles struck Peru in 1618, and the Viceroy took vigorous counter-measures, including publication of a medical tract on the subject, which were acknowledged by the King. The following year, the population of Copacabana, Bolivia, was decimated by measles.[123]

In the spring of 1619 epidemic smallpox broke out in Chile, causing a toll in the neighborhood of 50,000. This contagion reappeared in the autumn of 1620.[124]

These three episodes were ascribed to *sarampión, alfombrilla,* both Spanish terms for measles, and *viruelas,* or smallpox, respectively. It seems possible, however, in view of an apparent tendency of Spaniards in colonial America to confuse rash-producing diseases, that all three were simply episodes of a single epidemic.

Recurrent Measles Epidemics. Several measles epidemics seem to have followed one another at relatively short intervals in Peru during the first half of the seventeenth century. After the 1618-19 epidemic, measles struck again in 1628 and in 1634-35.[125] Then, in 1630, the Indians in the Jesuit missions of Paraguay were struck by a painful disease that in places caused a mortality over twenty per cent. "The whole body was covered with a rash that some called measles and others smallpox, and no one knew what it was."[126] This may well have been another episode in an epidemic which passed through the Andes a year earlier. The mid-

---

[119] Blanco, *op. cit.,* p. 100.
[120] Anónimo, 1901, *op. cit.,* p. 21,
[121] Lastres 1951, *op. cit.,* vol. II, p. 179.
[122] Polo, *op. cit.,* p. 21.
[123] *Ibid.,* p. 22
[124] *Ibid.,* p. 23.
[125] *Ibid.*
[126] Pablo Hernández. *Organización social de las doctrinas guaranies de la Compañia de Jesús.* Bk. II: *Valor de la obra.* Barcelona, 1912, p. 11.

1630's epidemic also spread east of the Andes. Córdoba in modern Argentina suffered from "measles" and fevers between 1634 and 1636.[127]

Recurrent Smallpox Epidemics. Smallpox was reported in Huánuco (Peru) in 1632, but then not again until 1660 in Ecuador.[128] Jesuit missionaries in Chile baptized 700 Araucanians—an unusually large number—in 1654, because of Araucanian desperation during a smallpox epidemic.[129] Some 20,000 Indians reportedly perished during a smallpox epidemic in the Mainas missions in 1669.[130] This epidemic recurred among the jungle Indians along the Ucayali River in 1670.[131]

Modern Eucador, then known as the Kingdom of Quito, suffered from epidemic smallpox in 1680, when more than 60,000 persons died from the disease in that administrative jurisdiction. By 1681 the contagion had spread to settlements along the Huallaga River on the Amazonian side of the Peruvian Andes.

The Measles Epidemic of 1692-1694. Toward the end of the seventeenth century, perhaps coincident with population increase and rising population density, the historical record began to chronicle real epidemic disease again raging through the Andean peoples.

A measles epidemic commenced at the city of Quito in 1692 and spread all through the territory of modern Ecuador.[132] The infection advanced to Lima, Huamanga, Arequipa and on to the Bolivian province,[133] including the mine center at Potosí. It caused great mortality.[134] Cuzco did not, of course, escape this epidemic, which reached the former imperial Indian capital in 1693.[135] The contagion was so widespread in the Andean area as to call forth viceregal measures to limit its further extension.[136] The viceroy's physician published a *Discourse* on the subject.[137]

[127] Ricardo Piccirilli, Francisco L. Romay y Leoncio Gianello. *Diccionario historico argentino,* vol. III. Buenos Aires: Ediciones Historicas Argentinas, 1954, p. 377.

[128] Polo, *op. cit.,* p. 26.

[129] Gay 1847, *op. cit.,* vol. III, pp. 201-202.

[130] Polo, *op. cit.,* p. 26.

[131] Lastres 1957, *op. cit.,* p. 28.

[132] Madero, *op. cit.,* p. 73.

[133] Lastres 1957, *op. cit.,* p. 28.

[134] Polo, *op. cit.,* p. 26; Lastres 1951, *op. cit.,* vol. II, p. 180; Hipólito Unanue. *Observaciones sobre el clima de Lima y su influencia en los seres organizados, en especial el hombre.* Lima: Comisión Nacional Peruana de Cooperación Intelectual, 1940, p. 60.

[135] Anónimo 1901, *op. cit.,* p. 280.

[136] Rubén Vargas Ugarte. *Historia de la iglesia en el Perú.* Vol. III: *1640-1699.* Burgos: Aldecoa, 1960, p. 401.

[137] Polo, *op. cit.,* p. 27.

This was an epidemic which spread through the Andean region as no other appears, in terms of the available records, to have done for some years. Those writing close in time to the two events seem much more impressed by the scale of mortality caused a generation later (1718-1720), so this measles epidemic of 1692-1694 may have been merely the first to affect a recovering Andean population. Another generation of population increase may well have provided enough susceptible individuals to permit the later epidemic a really impressive number of victims.

The Guayaquil Smallpox Epidemic in 1708. In 1708 the Ecuadorian port of Guayaquil was struck by epidemic smallpox. Guayaquil at that time numbered less than 4,000 inhabitants, yet the disease caused a mortality that peaked at twelve persons daily.[138] *i.e.,* a daily mortality rate in excess of three per thousand population. Fortunately, the epidemic did not last long, suggesting a relatively small proportion of susceptibles in the coastal port population. Lima also suffered from an unidentified epidemic serious enough for the ecclesiastical council to order a procession on 22 November.[139] It may have been an episode of the epidemic that affected the population of Guayaquil.

The Epidemic of 1718-1720. Even George Kubler[140] had to recognize that Peru suffered great population losses during 1720. In fact, the Andean region went through a much wider-spread epidemic lasting over one year, with probably more than a single disease agent involved.

There is some possibility that one of the disease agents responsible started its epidemic career in the Andean region itself. At any rate, one ecclesiastical historian noted that "a general epidemic assaulted a great part of the capital and province" of Huánuco from 1714 to 1718. The disease left "bodies in the fields which were food for birds and dogs."[141]

Certainly the year 1718 saw the wide spread of epidemic disease through South America. A modern commentator on population trends remarked on the 1718-1719 epidemic in Spanish Peru "extending through all the vice-royalty, as far as the Paraguayan missions,"[142] and it decimated tribal peoples such as the Mocobi east of the Andes.[143]

---

[138] Madero, *op. cit.,* p. 81.

[139] Polo, *op. cit.,* p. 27.

[140] Kubler, *op. cit.,* vol. II, p. 334.

[141] Bernardino Izaguirre. *Historia de las misiones franciscanos.* Lima: Talleres Tipográficos de la Penitenciaria, 1922, vol. I, p. 79.

[142] Angel Rosenblat. *La población indígena y el mestizaje en América.* Buenos Aires: Editorial Nova, Biblioteca Americanista, 1954, vol. I, p. 73.

[143] Vellard, *op. cit.,* p. 88.

Smallpox was the 1718 disease agent in Socabaya,[144] and Argentina in 1720,[145] but elsewhere the epidemic was one of catarrh—influenza in all probability—which caused weakness, severe bodily pain, bloody saliva, difficult respiration, but little fever, according to the Peruvian physician Unanue. Mortality reportedly reached 72,800 in the Archdiocese of Lima alone.[146] In response to questioning as to mortality during this epidemic, which Unanue [147] termed " the most terrible plague that Peru has suffered," survivors in one Indian group simply tossed a fistful of sand into the air.

Arequipa suffered during July, August, and September (the southern hemisphere winter) of 1718 from very hot, fetid south winds which were thought to have caused an epidemic which left hardly a person in the city or its environs unaffected by the end of September.[148] Aside from a feeling of great weight, faintness of the senses, and shooting pains all over the body, sneezing caused an " effusion of blood through the mouth and nostrils." A third of the Spaniards and two-thirds of the Indians of Arequipa were said to have perished.[149] Although he attributed it to an eclipse, the great Peruvian physician Unanue [150] identified this epidemic as influenza, "a catarrh of an evil type."

The Indian converts in the Jesuit missions of Paraguay also suffered considerable mortality. Where there were 122,084 souls in 1717, there remained only 101,444 in 1720,[151] and the missionaries had then had two years following the epidemic to recruit replacements from previously unconverted populations.

In 1719, " there began in the frontier provinces of Peru an epidemic" which lasted three years and killed "innumerable Indians." [152] This epidemic began in the city of Cuzco in April of that year, and the annalist there reported that this " epidemic fever" began in Buenos Aires at the beginning of 1719 and spread westward beyond the city of Huamanga. The Cuzco chronicler recorded objectively that this epidemic could not have been caused by an eclipse on 15 August, since the sickness preceded the celestial phenomenon. On the other hand, a letter from Cadiz had brought news that the Moors on the coast of Morocco were suffering from the illness at the same time.[153]

[144] Lastres 1957, op. cit., p. 29.
[145] Piccirilli, Romay y Gianello, op. cit., vol. III, p. 378.
[146] Polo, op. cit., p. 28.
[147] Unanue, op. cit., p. 13.
[148] Lastres 1957, op. cit., p. 30.
[149] Polo, op. cit., p. 30.
[150] Unanue, op. cit., p. 59.
[151] Hernández, op. cit., vol. II, p. 13.
[152] According to Bueno, op. cit., p. 137.
[153] Anónimo 1901, op. cit., p. 246.

The Spanish term *tabardillo*, applied to the disease by the Cuzco annalist, was used historically for such a variety of diseases as to permit no
sure identification. A modern Peruvian physician-historian [154] diagnosed
exanthematic typhus from the recorded symptoms and the term. The
Cuzco annalist's description runs: "An intense fever with immense stomach pains and headaches." Symptoms were, however, "so diverse and
contrary that it was impossible to form an exact idea, thus making a cure
impossible." Some of those infected were seized by a frenzy; others
vomited blood. Some died from dysentery after apparently recovering
from the fever. Few pregnant women recovered. The infection was ex-
extremely contagious, as attested by high mortality among the barbers
who treated infected patients, those who buried the bodies, and even the
llamas which packed the bodies of the dead to the churches for burial.[155]
This last fact is, perhaps, a key to diagnosis, and raises some doubts
about Lastres' diagnosis of typhus, which requires a louse vector. The
mortality among llamas suggests two possibilities. One is that the disease
was plague, which can be transmitted by a flea vector. Llamas are cam-
eloid animals, and recent experiments in the U.S.S.R. have shown that
camels are susceptible to plague. They had been thought for some time
to transmit plague to humans in the Near East.[156] Fleas on rapidly cooling cadavers of plague victims would have wasted no time abandoning
them for the thick warm fur of cargo llamas when bodies were tied on
to be carried to cemeteries in the over 10,000 foot altitude of Cuzco. Yet,
had the epidemic been bubonic plague or even typhus, it would seem that
the typical rash would have been described among the symptoms. So the
second possible diagnosis seems to be pneumonic plague, or simply a
recurrence of the severe influenza which was clearly the original epidemic
component. Both could be transmitted aerially. Human influenza epidemics are often accompanied or preceded by epizootics with similar
symptoms among domestic horses, dogs, and cats,[157] so there is no
reason to suppose llamas are immune.
The Cuzco episode of this epidemic lasted from March until November and was felt locally to be even worse than that of 1589. Persons of
all ages and both sexes perished, "but those who suffered most were

[154] Lastres 1951, *op. cit.*, vol. II, p. 300.
[155] Anónimo 1901, *op. cit.*, p. 247.
[156] V. N. Lobanov, "The pathological anatomy of experimental plague in camels,"
Ark. Pat. (Moscow) 1959, *21* (7): 37-42 (English summary in *Scient. Inform. Rep.,*
T-35, 4 Dec. 1959, p. 44).
[157] Hirsch, *op. cit.*, vol. I, pp. 38-41.

the miserable Indians, because of their complexion," which suggests that a rash-producing disease agent may have been at work after all. Mortality in Cuzco passed 700 individuals per day on 10 August. The other days with peak mortality were 6 and 15 August and 2 September. So many persons died that they could not be buried in the churches. Consequently large ditches were dug in the cathedral cemetery, and on 12 August the bishop blessed two cemeteries at some distance from the city.[158] The mortality was estimated at approximately 20,000 in the city of Cuzco, plus 40,000 in the rest of the diocese, or 60,000 in all, while some extremists asserted that over 80,000 died there.[159] One writer attributed the pestilence to a ship, *The French Lion*, which visited the Peruvian coast in 1719. He claimed that innumerable Spaniards and Mestizos and " more than 200,000 Indians died." [160] Typhus was available in Europe in epidemic form to be carried by ship to the New World. The summers of 1718 and 1719 were typhus periods in England, beginning in May and reaching a peak in July that lasted through August, with high mortality.[161] Ireland's hungry population also suffered from epidemic typhus from 1718 to 1721,[162] while the disease was widespread in Germany, Austria, and Hungary until 1720.[163]

Conclusion. While this brief outline is far from being an exhaustive study of Andean epidemic history, it seems sufficient to show that the area was in fact subjected to severe epidemic depopulation prior to 1720. The Andean natives shared with those in Mexico and Central America the devastation of the first New World smallpox epidemic, in all likelihood the most severe single loss of aboriginal population that ever occurred. Scant evidence suggests the Andean Indians remained part of a single epidemic region with those in Middle America until after 1546, then escaped the decimation of the 1576 epidemic in New Spain but suffered as much or more in their own epidemic from 1585 to 1591. Depopulation seems to have inhibited epidemic disease during the seventeenth century until the Andean population recovered near the end of the century, preparing the way for high epidemic mortality again in 1718-1720.

The sources utilized in the present analysis suggest that colonial

[158] Anónimo 1901, *op. cit.*, p. 248.
[159] *Ibid.*, p. 249.
[160] Polo, *op. cit.*, p. 28; Lastres 1951, *op. cit.*, vol. II, p. 300.
[161] Charles Creighton. *A History of Epidemics in Britain, from the Extinction of Plague to the Present.* Cambridge: University Press, 1894, vol. II, p. 63.
[162] *Ibid.*, p. 263.
[163] Hirsch, *op. cit.*, vol. I, p. 551.

Spaniards experienced difficulty in distinguishing between rash-producing diseases and tended to label them all smallpox or measles. This makes identification of historic epidemic disease agents more than ordinarily difficult. Yet these same sources indicate that influenza played a significant role in epidemic mortality and portray the more serious colonial epidemics in 1585-1591 and 1718-1720 as at least dual in causation. The materials here summarized point to the feasibility of additional study of Andean population trends as related to epidemic and endemic diseases.[164]

[164] It is not possible to treat, within the compass of a short analysis aimed toward correcting an existing impression of rareness of epidemics causing high native mortality, all diseases present in Andean populations prior to 1720. This article discusses major disease events whose causes are more or less well identified in contemporary documents. Modern medical knowledge indicates that malaria, venereal diseases, jaundice-producing disease agents, verruga and intestinal parasite infestation should have contributed to native mortality in the Andean region prior to 1720, at least as endemic ills sapping resistance.

All English translations from Spanish which appear in the text are by the author, whenever a Spanish edition is cited. Emilio Mendizábal L. assisted the author in compiling references in Lima.

6

Epidemiology and the Slave Trade

Philip D. Curtin

Historians have begun to show a new interest in the
slave trade. Recent developments in historical demography, economic history, and the history of Africa have solved some of the
old problems and posed new ones. The mere passage of time makes
it possible to go beyond the largely humanitarian concerns of the
nineteenth-century writers, concerns that arose out of the great
debate over slavery as a question of policy. We can now accept the
trade as an evil and move on to the problem of why and how it
took place for so many centuries and on such a scale.

The recent trend toward a world-historical perspective and away
from parochial national history also calls for a new approach to
the broad patterns of Atlantic history. Social and economic development on the tropical shores of the Atlantic was a single p.)c-
ess, regardless of the theoretically self-contained empires of mer-
cantilist Europe. From the late sixteenth century to the early nineteenth, the central institution was the plantation, located in tropical America, worked by slave labor from tropical Africa, but
directed by Europeans and producing tropical staples for European
consumption. The broader patterns of society and economy were
much the same in all the plantation colonies, regardless of metropolitan control. These patterns were not only different from those
of Europe; they were also different from those of European settlements in temperate North America, the Indian Ocean trading

posts, and territorial empires in New Spain and Peru. Yet the commercial influence of the plantations stretched far and wide—to the English settlements of North America, to mainland Spanish America, and even beyond the Atlantic world to the textile markets of India. The whole complex of commerce and production was an entity which can be called the South Atlantic System.

I

The slave trade was a key institution in this system, as it was in the history of the United States; but in the broad view North America was only marginal to the system as a whole. The "cotton kingdom" of the nineteenth century was a late flowering of the slave plantation. The thirteen colonies imported very few slaves before the eighteenth century; even then, they received only about twenty per cent of the British slave trade between 1700 and the American Revolution. Through the whole course of the slave trade, the present territory of the United States imported less than five per cent of all slaves brought to the New World.[1] Important as slavery and its aftermath have been for the history of the United States, the fundamental development of plantation slavery in the Americas took place elsewhere—in tropical America.

The first territory to achieve a full-blown model of the South Atlantic System was Brazil in the late sixteenth century. From these beginnings it spread to the Caribbean, where it reached a kind of apogee in the late eighteenth century, just before the Democratic Revolutions. As a pre-industrial economic order, the system had some remarkable features at the very beginning. Nothing in earlier European economic experience could compare with its

---

[1] The most careful and probably the most reliable recent estimates of the British slave trade between 1701 and 1775 are those of K. W. Stetson, "A Quantitative Approach to Britain's American Slave Trade" (unpublished M.S. thesis, University of Wisconsin, 1967). An authoritative estimate of the total slave imports into the United States indicates that total imports were probably less than 400,000 and certainly not more than 500,000. (J. Potter, "The Growth of Population in America, 1700-1860," in D. V. Glass and D. E. Eversley [eds.], *Population in History: Essays in Historical Demography* [Chicago, 1965]). The size of the total Atlantic slave trade is considerably reduced by recent monographic research from the earlier estimates of fifteen or twenty millions, or even more. Until more research is published, however, a round number of ten million seems a reasonable guess.

dependence on long-distance transportation. Not only was virtually all of output of the plantations consumed in Europe; timber, cattle, and even food were often imported from North America or Ireland. Most remarkable of all, the system apparently required a continuous and growing stream of workers from tropical Africa, a trade in human beings that became the most massive intercontinental migration before the industrial era.

A full explanation of the demographic, economic, and social forces that set this trade in motion is not yet available. It is clear, however, that they included both a European demand and an African supply. On the supply side in particular we still know far too little about the sources of slaves within Africa, about the commercial institutions through which they were delivered to the coast, and about the technological and economic conditions that made it possible for African societies to sell slaves on terms of trade that were extremely favorable to European buyers. The demand side is far better documented, but many difficulties remain. One of these is a location problem which has bothered students of the slave trade since the early eighteenth century: given a European demand for tropical staples, why satisfy that demand by placing the plantations several thousand miles away from the principal source of labor?

One form of answer can be found in the chronological sequence through which the South Atlantic System grew out of its Mediterranean origins. Long before the discovery of the Americas, Europeans had created an embryo of the later South Atlantic System. Venetians, Genoese, Catalans, and others had sugar grown in overseas "colonies" like Crete and Cyprus and Sicily. These early plantations were often worked by slave labor supplied through the existing Mediterranean slave trade, some of it from the Mediterranean basin itself and some of it imported from the slave-trade posts of the northern and eastern Black Sea coasts. In the late Middle Ages, sugar planting migrated westward, first to southern Iberia, then to the Atlantic islands like Madeira and the Canaries.[2] With the great sixteenth-century maritime out-

---

[2] For this development see the work of Charles Verlinden, particularly: *Précedents médiévaux de la colonie en Amérique* (Mexico, D. F., 1954); "Les origines coloniales de la civilisation atlantique. Antécédents et types de structure," *Journal of World History*, I (1954), 378-98; "La colonie vénitienne de

burst into the Atlantic, newer and greater opportunities presented themselves.

The Europeans experimented with a number of alternative locations and forms of development between about 1500 and the middle of the seventeenth century. In the early sixteenth century, plantations were established on São Thomé in the Gulf of Guinea, convenient to a source of slave labor in tropical Africa. Another alternative was to offer technical assistance to an African state, which might then produce goods for the European market. This was tried most intensively by the Portuguese in the kingdom of Kongo at the same period.[3] On the American shore, plantations were also established using varying sources of labor. Indian slave labor served the Portuguese in sixteenth-century Brazil and the Spanish in sixteenth-century Hispaniola.[4] European labor, most of it either forced convict labor or contract labor, was used extensively by the French and British in the Lesser Antilles, especially during the middle third of the seventeenth century.[5] But the combination that appeared to work best, and which spread most widely, was the plantation located in tropical America, staffed by European managers, and worked by slaves from Africa. The solution of the early planners was thus empirical; trial and error showed that the expedient of importing labor from Africa to the American plantations succeeded, while other alternatives failed.

II

Though the full explanation must wait for further research into supply and demand conditions on both sides of the Atlantic, one aspect worth exploring is the epidemiology of migration. Europeans discovered at a very early date that they experienced high

Tana, centre de la traite des esclaves au xive et au début du xve siècles," *Studi in onore di Gino Luzzato*, 2 Vols. (Milano, 1950), II, 1-25; *L'esclavage dans l'Europe médiévale. Peninsule Ibérique-France* (Bruges, 1955).

[3] J. Vansina, *Kingdoms of the Savanna* (Madison, 1966), 41-64.

[4] M. Ratekin, "The Early Sugar Industry in Española," *Hispanic American Historical Review*, XXIII (1954), 1-19.

[5] F. W. Pitman, *The Development of the British West Indies* (New Haven, 1917); Léon Vignols, "L'institution des engagés, 1624-1774," *Revue d'histoire économique et sociale*, I (1928), 24-45; G. Devien, *Les engagés pour les Antilles, 1634-1713* (Paris, 1952).

mortality rates overseas. The Portuguese failure in Kongo is largely accountable to the high mortality rate among missionary and agents sent to Africa. On the American side of the ocean, planters soon found that both the local Indians and imported European workers tended to die out, while Africans apparently worked better and lived longer in the "climate" of tropical America.

Their first explanations were overwhelmingly racial. Europeans in tropical America believed that Negroes were peculiarly immune to the effects of a hot climate, just as Europeans seemed peculiarly liable to death in the climate of the West Indies or the "white man's grave" on the Gulf of Guinea.[6] The same racial theories could be used to explain that American Indians were not useful, since they were a "weak race" that died out on contact with "white civilization." The general conclusion, that certain races had inborn qualities of strength and weakness fitting them for specific "climates," became an accepted "fact" and a cornerstone of pseudo-scientific racism.[7]

This racist explanation has, of course, been contradicted long since, not merely by the general fall of pseudo-scientific racism, but also by the genuine fact that people of European descent now live as successfully as anyone else in tropical environments— those of Cuba, Costa Rica, Puerto Rico, and Queensland, among others. Yet we are left with the judgment of generations of planters in the Caribbean and Brazil that Negroes were somehow much better workers than any other group.

This opinion might be written off as a social or race prejudice —no one wants to work in the hot sun if he can find someone else to work for him—but epidemiology suggests another answer.[8] People die from disease, not from climate, and the world contains

[6] See P. D. Curtin, " 'The White Man's Grave': Image and Reality, 1780-1850," *Journal of British Studies*, I (1961), 94-110.

[7] P. D. Curtin, *The Image of Africa* (Madison, 1964), 227-43, 363-87; R. H. Pearce, *The Savages of America* (Baltimore, 1952), 42-49; P. M. Ashburn, *The Ranks of Death* (New York, 1947), *passim*.

[8] The standard general work on epidemiology is Maxcy-Rosenau, *Preventive Medicine and Public Health* (New York, 9th ed., 1965), edited by Philip E. Sartwell. But the most convenient recent and brief summary is Ian Taylor and John Knowleden, *Principles of Epidemiology* (London, 1964). I should like to express my appreciation to Dr. Alfred S. Evans, professor of epidemiology, Yale University, for his kindness in introducing me to this field.

many different disease environments, each with a range of viruses and bacteria that differ in varying degrees from those found elsewhere. Physical environment and climate obviously play a role, but epidemiological differences exist even where physical environment is the same. In the United States, for example, measurable differences in the incidence of disease are found in a single region, even between an urban area and the surrounding countryside.

One cause of this diversity is relative isolation. Diseases themselves change radically over short periods; new strains of virus or bacteria appear, and old strains die out. These changes are not merely random; they are often a response to the immunities of the host population. (A recent and striking example is the appearance within the past two decades of a new strain of the malarial parasite, *Plasmodium falciparum*. This strain is resistant to the chloraquin preparations, which earlier varieties of *P. falciparum* were not, yet the new anti-malarials came into use only at the end of the Second World War.) At the same time, the host population itself develops immunities to the endemic diseases of its environment. Thus, each disease environment has a constantly changing equilibrium between the host population's pattern of immunity and its range of endemic desease. The more isolated a human community, the more specialized and individual its disease environment is likely to become.[9]

In the longer sweep of history over the past two or three millennia, increasing intercommunication has made disease environments more nearly alike, not more diverse; but each breach of previous isolation has brought higher death rates, as unfamiliar diseases attacked populations whose environment provided no source of immunity.[10] The Atlantic basin on the eve of the great European discoveries was especially open to this pattern of high death rates from new diseases. All the shores of the Atlantic were relatively isolated from one another. As men moved across the ocean from one disease environment to another, their death rates rose—the increased mortality of human migration. As diseases

[9] See T. Dublin and B. S. Blumberg, "Inherited Disease Susceptibility," *Public Health Reports*, LXXVI (1961), especially 499, 502.
[10] William H. McNeill, in *The Rise of the West* (Chicago, 1963), has traced this pattern in world history.

moved with them from one previously isolated environment to another, they spread to non-immune host populations, who then experienced the increased mortality of disease migration.[11]

This interchange of diseases and peoples was extremely complex, and the data are far from complete. The historical process will not be fully understood until comparative statistical and medical studies have been made of the many isolated peoples who were brought into contact with the ecumenical range of disease between the sixteenth century and the present. This would include many different American Indian groups, the Maori and other Polynesians, the Australian aborigines, and the Koisan-speaking peoples of southern Africa.

Present medical knowledge, however, can outline certain theoretical limits and some of the conditions to be expected when a nonimmune population meets a range of new diseases. Some theoretical expectations can be based on the process of immunization itself. The most significant immunities are acquired, not inherited. The ordinary procedures for artificial immunization are based on the the fact that people can create antibodies which will oppose specific forms of infection. The individual can be immunized either by giving him antibodies directly, or else by inducing a light infection so that his own organism will produce the required antibodies. Similar immunities are, of course, produced by the attack of a disease, but the form of immunity and its duration will vary greatly. It may last only a few weeks after a common cold, or a lifetime after yellow fever. It may be partial, making recurrent attacks less harmful, or it may be a total immunity to all future infection from that source.

Childhood disease environment is the crucial factor in determining the immunities of a given adult population. Not only will the weakest members of society be removed, leaving a more resistant population of survivors; childhood and infancy are also a period of life when many infections are relatively benign. This is so of yellow fever—a disease of special importance to the tropical Atlantic—which is rarely fatal to children but frequently fatal to adults. In addition, children often experience infection in such a mild form they are not even aware of it, yet they acquire

[11] In spite of its age, August Hirsch, *Handbook of Geographical and Historical Pathology*, 3 Vols. (London, 1883), continues to be the most convenient reference work for historical epidemiology.

an immunity that protects them in later life just as effectively as a severe attack would have done.[12] (Before the widespread use of poliomyelitis vaccines, tests showed that, for every recognized case, one hundred to one thousand persons were infected without being conscious of the fact and developed the characteristic immunity.) In general, then, the individual will be safest if he stays in the disease environment of his childhood; if he migrates, a fully effective set of immunities to match a new disease environment could not be expected to appear in his generation.

But immunities are also inherited. These are less important than the acquired immunities, but they raise special problems. First of all, medical science has so far discovered most of these inherited immunities only by statistical inference. We are, therefore, in an area of uncertainty. Second, the very fact that some immunities are heritable raises again the old and discarded racist hypothesis that Negroes could easily work in the tropical climates, simply because they were Negroes. It is, therefore, important to consider the present state of medical knowledge.

One kind of heritable immunity is universal: all children inherit antibodies transmitted by the mother to the fetus, and these protect the child during the first months of life, before its own ability to generate antibodies is fully developed. People of differing blood groups also appear to have differing degrees of immunity to some diseases. These are nothing like the perfect immunity given by an attack of yellow fever, but they are statistically detectable. Family histories also indicate statistical tendencies of susceptibility (or relative immunity) to particular diseases.

In addition, whole populations exposed to early and constant infection may undergo genetic change. Those individuals whose genetic inheritance predisposes them to serious illness from a particular disease may die in childhood, leaving no descendents. Other individuals, whose genetic tendency allows them to escape with a milder illness from the same cause, are likely to live and reproduce. As a result, the genetic make-up of each succeeding generation will shift slightly toward a tendency to mild infection rather than fatal infection. Genetic changes of this sort, however, do not appear to alter the *incidence* of infection; people will still

[12] Taylor and Knowleden, 162-64.

be attacked by the disease in the same proportion, but more will experience a mild illness and fewer will die. Recent studies indicate that this type of genetic influence is important to the epidemiology of poliomyelitis, rheumatic fever, and tuberculosis.[13]

Malaria is another disease which can be influenced by heredity —and one of considerably greater importance in the tropical Atlantic. The important factor in this instance is an inherited hemoglobin characteristic known as the sickle-cell trait, from the characteristic shape of some blood cells under the microscope. This trait is a balanced polymorphism—the circumstance where a particular organic weakness, which would be expected to disappear through natural selection, recurs generation after generation because it also has balancing "good" qualities. Sickle-cell trait is the best known of all balanced polymorphisms, and it can serve to illustrate the process in general. It is found in certain malarial areas, and particularly in Africa. Where it is present, three types of people can be distinguished—those with normal hemoglobin, those with the inherited sickle-cell trait, and those with both the sickle-cell trait and the anemia that often accompanies it. Since sickle-cell anemia is usually fatal in childhood, many of this third group would be expected to die before reproducing; and known laws of genetics suggest that the sickle-cell trait itself should die out over a period of time. But the sickle-cell has another characteristic which permits it to survive. It provides some protection against *P. falciparum*, the dominant form of malaria in tropical Africa and an important cause of infant mortality. Thus, in that environment, malaria tends to cut off those without the sickle-cell trait, while anemia cuts off those with the trait plus anemia. The two causes of early death balance each other, and the trait persists.[14]

It is important to distinguish between these epidemiological characteristics, which are genetic or heritable, and race, which is also heritable. The crucial distinction is that genetic immunities are a variable independent of physical appearance. In addition, the immunities of great historical significance are relatively short-

[13] *Ibid.*, 159-60, 221-24; personal communication from Professor Alfred S. Evans.

[14] For balanced polymorphisms in general, see Dublin and Blumberg, *passim*.

lived. A balanced polymorphism such as sickle-cell trait, for example, tends to disappear from a population once *falciparum* malaria is no longer present. In addition, it is not a "Negro" trait. Even though it is found in tropical Africa, where many Negroes live, it is also found among some white populations in the Mediterranean basin, and it is absent among certain Negro groups in West Africa. Finally, the scientific interest of the balanced polymorphism to genetic studies can obscure the possible historical role of the sickle-cell trait. Statistical studies of Puerto Rican deaths from malaria by race indicate that, between 1937 and 1944, 4.29 per cent of "white" deaths were from malaria, as against 4.19 per cent of "colored" deaths from the same cause. Whatever the differential immunities of the modern Puerto Ricans' ancestors in Africa and Europe, their twentieth-century differences are quantitatively insignificant.[15]

III

On the shores of the pre-Columbian Atlantic, different immunities to disease were caused by different disease environments. These disease environments fell into three separate groups, each created by different circumstances of physical environment and isolation. Europe and North Africa were in the belt of intense intercommunication stretching from the north Atlantic to China. Most diseases of the temperate Afro-Eurasian land mass were already endemic there, and the Europeans had a wide range of immunities to match. They lacked, however, the diseases and the immunities of the Old World tropics.

In tropical Africa, intercommunication was less intense, and disease environments would have been more diverse than those of Europe. Even though Africa had most of the full range of Old World temperate diseases—and its own assortment of tropical diseases, including *falciparum* malaria, yellow fever, sleeping sickness, yaws, and bilharzia—each African community was relatively isolated from its neighbors. It would, therefore, have been unlikely that any single African people would have an endemic assortment that covered the whole range of diseases and

[15] See W. Zelinsky, "The Historical Geography of the Negro Population of Latin America," *Journal of Negro History*, XXXIV (1949), 203.

strains of disease available in the Sub-Saharan region. As a result, Africans had a wide range of immunities, but travel, even within Africa, would be likely to increase the death rate.

In the Americas, a third set of disease environments had been isolated from the Old World for a very long time. Little is known about them, but the lack of frequent communication between one region and another was even greater than in tropical Africa. Each region would, therefore, be expected to have little protection from the diseases of its neighbors, and virtually none against the strange diseases that were to come from across the Atlantic.

When, in the sixteenth century and later, the Africans and Europeans crossed the ocean, they infected the American Indians. Europeans encountered new diseases from the African tropics, and Africans met new strains of Afro-Eurasian diseases. The possible role of New World diseases is not clear in the medical records of the period. (Even the former belief in a New World origin for syphilis is now in serious doubt.)[16] The basic pattern is nevertheless clear enough: everyone in the Americas, or who came to the Americas, paid a price in increased death rates for his entry into this newly created disease environment.

Even though we lack statistical data for sixteenth-century American populations, the quantitative impact on the Indians is known in outline. Especially in the tropical lowlands, many groups died out as a people before they had an opportunity to build immunities against the joint assault of African and European disease. The mortality was most striking and drastic with the densely settled population of the Greater Antilles where the Spansh first landed—and to which they brought the first Africans. Indians on the South and North American mainlands fared somewhat better, and so did the Caribs of the Lesser Antilles, though they, too, almost disappeared. In this case, isolation seems to have protected them from simultaneous attack by the full range of Old World diseases. With the highland peoples of Middle America, Colombia, and the Andes, a cooler environment prevented the spread of malaria and yellow fever, both of African origin. Thus, though these peoples sustained steep declines of population over the sixteenth and part of the seventeenth century, they were

[16] The most extensive study of the medical records of the sixteenth century Americas is Ashburn; see 176-90, 238-44. See also, Maxcy-Rosenau, 274.

able to maintain themselves and ultimately to recover, once new immunities had been acquired.[17]

Epidemiological factors were thus responsible for depopulating some of the best agricultural land in the tropical world. The most obvious reason for locating the productive centers of the South Atlantic System in the American tropics was simply that land was there for the taking, and it was far better land for intensive agriculture than any available in tropical Africa. But land without people has no economic value. Labor had to come from somewhere else, even though bringing people into this disease environment was bound to exact a price from the increased mortality of human migration.

It is impossible to know precisely the size of this mortality rate in the sixteenth or seventeenth centuries, but some data are available for the late eighteenth and early nineteenth centuries. It is justifiable to accept these as suggestive of earlier mortality rates among migrants to the American tropics. While it is possible, and even probable, that diseases had changed somewhat during three centuries of adjustment to new host populations, it is unlikely that early nineteenty-century mortality rates were higher than those of earlier centuries. Indeed, the growing intensity of communication in the Atlantic over these centuries suggests that they should have been somewhat lower. Improving medical care may also have lowered mortality rates over time; but even the use of chinchona against malaria was irregular, and death rates from the more important diseases could hardly have been altered before about the eighteen-forties.[18]

Statistics on military mortality are the most useful source for the mortality of migration, since they make it possible to isolate groups moving from one disease environment to another. In 1835, the British government became concerned about the death rates of British troops overseas and ordered a series of statistical

[17] Ashburn, passim; S. F. Cook and W. Borah, "The Rate of Population Change in Central Mexico, 1550-1570," Hispanic American Historical Review, XXXVII (1957), 463-70; W. Borah and S. F. Cook, The Aboriginal Population of Mexico on the Eve of the Spanish Conquest (Berkeley, 1963); J. H. Steward (ed.), Handbook of the South American Indians, 5 Vols. (Washington, 1946-49).
[18] Curtin, Image of Africa, 58-87, 177-97, 343-62.

studies by Major Alexander Tulloch.[19] These reports, based on the medical transactions of the British Army (begun in 1816) were carried out with a scientific care that was only then beginning to be applied to statistics. Among other things, they show quantitative levels for the mortality of migration from Britain to either the West Indies or West Africa, and from West Africa to the West Indies. (See Tables 1-3.) Tulloch's data are also useful for comparative purposes, since he took the two decades 1817-36 as a common base period, and his samples normally contained significant bodies of men of common background and subject to a common epidemiological experience. They are by far the best data we now have, or are likely to discover.

To study the movement of British troops, Tulloch began with the expected civilian mortality rate among men of military age in the United Kingdom. Deaths from all causes among this group, calculated from actuarial tables and census data, were at the rate of 11.5 per thousand per annum. Once men from this group were recruited into the army, however, the death rate (based on 1830-36) rose to 15.3 per thousand—a predictable increase from the relatively crowded and unsanitary conditions of barracks life.[20] Movement overseas, however, produced far more substantial changes as the men entered new disease environments. (See Table 1.) Service in the Mediterranean, the temperate climate of South Africa, or North America produced a range of mortality that was not drastically different from that of the United Kingdom itself —between 12 and 20 per thousand per annum. (Two Mediterranean exceptions, Gibraltar and the Ionian Islands, were unusually high because of severe epidemics within the period of the survey.)

The tropical world, however, produced a strikingly different

---

[19] Great Britain, *Parliamentary Papers* (hereafter, *PP*), 1837-38, XL (*Accounts and Papers, V*) [138], "Statistical Account of Sickness, Mortality and Invaliding among Troops in the West Indies"; 1839, XVI (*Reports from Commissioners, III*) [166], "Statistical Report of the Sickness, Mortality and Invaliding among the Troops in the United Kingdom, Mediterranean and British North America"; 1840, XXX (*Accounts and Papers, II*) [228], "Statistical Report of the Sickness, Mortality and Invaliding among Troops in Western Africa, St. Helena, Cape of Good Hope and Mauritius"; 1842, XXVII (*Accounts and Papers, II*) [358], "Statistical Report of the Sickness, Mortality and Invaliding among Her Majesty's Troops Serving in Ceylon, the Tenasserim Provinces, and the Burmese Empire."

[20] *PP*, 1839 [166], 4-7.

TABLE 1

Death rates per thousand mean strength per annum, among
British military personnel recruited in the United Kingdom
and serving overseas, from all causes, 1817-36, unless otherwise
noted.

Eastern Frontier District, South Africa (1818-36)	12.0
Nova Scotia and New Brunswick	14.7
Cape District, South Africa (1818-36)	15.5
Malta	18.7
Canada (Quebec and Ontario)	20.0
Gibraltar (1818-36)	22.0
Ionian Island	28.3
Mauritius (1818-36)	30.5
Tenasserim (1827-36)	44.7
Ceylon	75.0
Windward and Leeward Command, West Indies	85.0
Jamaica Command (1803-17, War Office data)	127.0
Jamaica Command (1817-36)	130.0
Windward and Leeward Command (1803-16, War Office data)	138.0
Sierra Leone Command, deaths from disease only	483.0
Cape Coast Command, Gold Coast (1823-26)	668.3

Sources: *Parliamentary Papers*, 1837-38, XL [138], 5-7, 44-45; 1839, XVI
[166], 4-7, 6a, 15b, 22a, 25b, 39a; 1840, XXX [228], 4b, 7, 19, 19b; 1842,
XXVII [358], 5-7, 44-45.

result, and it can be separated into three broad regions of increasing
mortality. Around the tropical Indian Ocean, mortality rates
ranged from 30 to 75 per thousand. In the American tropics, the
rate rose to a level between 85 and 138 per thousand. Finally,
West Africa showed a disastrous mortality range from 483 to
668 per thousand mean strength per annum. This level is confirmed by the qualitative impressions of early visitors to the African coast, and by a variety of other statistical data for the early
nineteenth century.[21] Even if the Europeans had not had the better
agricultural possibilities of tropical America at their disposal,
their reluctance to locate plantations in tropical Africa would be
explained by these figures. Whatever the possibility of European
residence in West Africa (once the migrants had acquired the
proper immunities), the mortality rate of each entering group

[21] The early nineteenth-century mortality of newly arrived Europeans
varied between about 350 and 800 per thousand. See Curtin, *Image of Africa*,
483-87, for a collection of sample data.

was simply too high to allow more intensive occupation than that of a few thinly-manned posts for the slave trade.

One of the often neglected inefficiencies of the slave trade is, indeed, the loss of life in the African posts and aboard the slave ships. A study of the slave trade of Nantes between 1715 and 1774 shows, for example, that crew mortality from disease alone varied between about 150 and 250 per thousand per voyage, though it was usually higher than 200 per thousand. During the same period, Nantes slave traders lost only 145 slaves per thousand from disease in transit.[22] Another and smaller sample of 116 slave ships sailing from English ports in the seventeen-eighties shows a crew death-rate from disease of 210 per thousand per voyage, and a further loss of 263 per thousand from desertion or discharge overseas.[23] At least in the eighteenth century, the maritime slave trade took proportionately more lives of crewmen than of slaves, in spite of the notoriously bad conditions of the "middle passage."

African migrants to the New World by way of the slave trade also experienced increased mortality rates after their arrival. Tulloch's sample of African soldiers serving in the West Indies was made up of men recruited mainly from among the slaves recaptured at sea by the British Navy as part of its anti-slavery blockade. They were not, therefore, from any particular region, but from the whole of West Africa with a special concentration from western Nigeria and Dahomey and only a few from either the Congo basin or East Africa.[24] This was an excellent sample of the kind of men who were sent to America as slaves—they *were* part of the slave trade before they joined the army.

When these men served as soldiers even in Sierra Leone, they had death rates markedly higher than other non-European troops serving in their respective countries of origin. (See Table 2.) Mortality among African troops in the Sierra Leone Command between 1819 and 1836 was 31.1 per thousand per annum from dis-

[22] Gaston Martin, *L'ère des négriers (1714-1774)* (Paris, 1931), 43, 115.

[23] Thomas Clarkson to Lords of Trade and Plantations, July 27, 1788, in Great Britain, Privy Council, *Report of the Lords of the Committee of Council for ... Trade and Foreign Plantations ... Concerning the Present State of Trade to Africa, and Particularly the Trade in Slaves ...* (London, 1789).

[24] For a statistical study of the origins of Sierra Leone recaptives, see P. D. Curtin and Jan Vansina, "Sources of the Nineteenth Century Atlantic Slave Trade," *Journal of African History*, V (1964), 185-208.

TABLE 2

Mortality per thousand mean strength per annum among non-European British troops serving in their region or country of origin.

Maltese Fencible Corps	9
Hottentot Cape Corps	11
Bengal Native Troops	11
Madras Native Troops	13
Royal African Corps, West Africa	32

Source: *PP*, 1840, XXX [228], 15-16.

ease—double the death rate of British troops serving in England.[25] Tulloch was puzzled by this high figure, but a probable explanation is possible. These men were not, in fact, serving in their country of origin. They had already moved from one African disease environment to another. Even without hard data for a comparable sample of men who were able to stay home, a reasonable estimate would put their mortality from disease alone within the range of 15 to 20 per thousand per annum. The soldiers' mortality rate thus increased by more than 50 per cent, simply as a result of movement *within* tropical Africa—an indication of the price exacted by the diversity of African disease environments.[26]

When men recruited in the same way were moved from Africa to the West Indies, a second increase in mortality would be expected, and it occurred. (See Table 3.) The death rate rose from about 30 per thousand to 40 per thousand. The price of movement to America was thus a further 30 per cent increase in mortality, and the death rate of these new arrivals in the American tropics was markedly higher than that of 25 per thousand per annum, calculated for the Jamaican slave population over three years of age during the period 1803-17.[27]

[25] *PP*, 1840, XXX [228], 15-16.
[26] This level of increased mortality following movement within Africa is relatively low compared with the experience of some drafts of forced labor at railroad building and other projects during the colonial period. It is estimated, for example, that 10-15 per cent of all the workers died in the construction of the Pointe Noire-Brazzaville line in Moyen Congo, and annual mortality rates ran as high as 452 per thousand in 1927 and 172 per thousand in 1929. V. Thompson and R. Adloff, *The Emerging States of French Equatorial Africa* (Stanford, 1960), 142; Lord Hailey, *An African Survey* (London, 1938), 1590.
[27] *PP*, 1837-38, XL [138], 49. See, also, G. W. Roberts, *The Population of Jamaica* (New Haven, 1957), 171-72.

TABLE 3

Death rates from disease, per thousand mean strength per annum among British troops recruited in Africa and serving in the West Indies.

Jamaica Command, 1803-17	49
Bahama Islands, 1817-36	41
Windward and Leeward Command, 1817-36*	40
Jamaica Command, 1817-36	30
Slave population of Jamaica, 3 years of age and over, 1803-17	25

Source: PP, 1827-28, XL [138], 11, 50, 73.

* The statistics for this command can be taken as most trustworthy. Not only is the mortality figure an approximate median; the sample force had an average mean strength of 2,047 over these decades, while the Bahama Islands had a smaller sample of only 355 men and the Jamaica command had only a force of labor troops with a mean strength of 286 men.

High as this rate was, it was lower than that of European troops serving in the same command. Tulloch's sample of European troops in the Windward and Leeward command can be set aside because the usual yellow fever epidemics missed these islands during the survey period. (Table 1.) The other three samples closely bracket their mean at 131 per thousand per annum. The rate of 40 per thousand for African troops in the Windward and Leeward Command is not only the mean of the four samples; that command also had the largest and probably the most representative sample. (In this case, the non-occurrence of yellow fever would not be significant, since fever was not an important cause of death among the African troops.) One finding of Tulloch's survey is that these African migrants to the New World outlived a comparable group of European migrants by a ratio of 3.2 to one. This difference is in line with the expectations of epidemiological theory. Africans, even with a combined background of Old World temperate diseases and Old World tropical diseases, would be expected to die at somewhat increased rates on migration to the New World; but Europeans who lacked the relative immunity to malaria and yellow fever, would be expected to die at still higher rates.

Other data from the eighteenth century confirm this pattern, though they cannot be taken to be as reliable as Tulloch's survey. A sample of white and black troops serving Great Britain in the

West Indies between 1796 and 1807—hence in wartime conditions—showed an annual average mortality of 244 per thousand
effectives per annum among the Europeans and an annual average
of only 59.2 per thousand among those of African descent. These
statistics are weak, partly because it is only probable—not certain
—that these African troops were recruited by purchase in Africa,
rather than by purchase from among the West Indian slaves.
Nevertheless, the ratio of differential mortality was 4.1 to one
in favor of the Africans. Another survey of French troops serving
on Martinique and Guadeloupe between 1802 and 1807 shows an
annual average death rate of 302 per thousand.[28] If these earlier
surveys are at all reliable, Tulloch's rate of 130 per thousand may
well lie at the low side of the range of death rates among European
immigrants.

IV

The planters' belief in the superiority of African labor, therefore,
had a basis in fact. They merely mistook the outward and visible
sign of color for the independent variable of disease envionment.
This error is curiously like their other error of writing about the
horrors of a tropical "climate." As every visitor to the West Indies
will recognize, the climate, measured by any standard of human
comfort, is more pleasant in summer than that of the eastern or
central United States, and the winter climate is one of the greatest
economic assets of the Carribbean. But the planters saw only that
newly arrived Europeans died, and they attached this fact to the
most obvious difference from the environment they had known
in Europe—the tropical climate.

From an economic point of view, the price paid for a slave or
an indentured white worker was a claim to future labor. Assuming
that the cost of maintaining each was about equal, the slave was
preferable at anything up to three times the price of the European.
(The fact that indentures were limited in time, while slavery was
not, would make little difference. A death rate of 130 per thousand per annum would practically use up a draft of seven-year indentures before their time had expired.) On the demand side, at

[28] F. Guerra, "The Influence of Disease on Race, Logistics and Colonization in the Antilles," *Journal of Tropical Medicine and Hygiene*, LXIX (1966),
23-35.

TABLE 4

Principal Causes of Death Among British Troops Recruited In
Britain
(in deaths per thousand mean strength per annum)

Disease	(1) Among Dragoons Serving in Britain 1830-36	(2) White Troops— Windward and Leeward Command 1817-36	(3) White Troops— Jamaica Command 1817-36
Fevers	1.4	36.9	101.9
Diseases of the Lung	7.7	10.4	7.5
Epidemic Cholera	1.2	—	—
Violent Deaths	1.3	—	—
Diseases of the Liver	—	1.8	1.0
Intestinal Diseases	—	20.7	5.1
Diseases of the Brain	—	3.7	1.2
Dropsies	—	2.1	—
Other (with mortality rates less than 1 per 1,000 per annum)	4.2	2.9	2.0
Total	15.8	78.5	121.3

Sources: PP, 1837-38, XL [138], 7, 44; 1839, XVI [166], 4.

least, here was sufficient reason for the slave trade from Africa as
the preferred alternative to labor recruitment in Europe.

Tulloch was also concerned with the cause of death, and this
aspect of his survey throws further light on the epidemiology of
migration. Statistics on the cause of death are obviously weaker
than those for gross mortality. (Even today, it is easier to establish the fact of death than to know its cause.) Nineteenth-century
disease classifications and methods of diagnoses were far from
accurate by modern standards. "Fevers" as a category covered
yellow fever, malaria, typhoid, and a great deal more—not merely
because they were grouped together for purposes of classification,
but also because medical men could not always make valid distinctions between them. "Eruptive fevers" in the same way covered smallpox, syphilis, yaws, typhus, and measles, at the very
least. "Diseases of the lungs" can be taken to mean principally
pneumonia and tuberculosis, but it might include influenza as
well. Intestinal diseases were clearly dysentery, but without
further distinction.

TABLE 5

Principal Cause of Death Among British Troops
Recruited in Africa
(in deaths per thousand mean strength per annum)

Disease	Sierra Leone Command (1819-36)	Windward and Leeward Command (West Indies) (1817-36)	Difference Between Cols. 1 and 2
Fevers	2.4	4.6	+2.2
Eruptive Fevers	6.9	2.5	—4.4
Diseases of the Lungs	6.3	16.5	+10.2
Diseases of the Liver	1.9	.9	—1.0
Intestinal Diseases	5.3	7.4	+2.1
Diseases of the Brain	1.6	2.2	+ .6
Wounds	1.4	—	—1.4
Dropsies	—	2.1	+2.1
Other	6.2	3.8	
Total	32.0	40.0	

Sources: *PP*, 1837-38, XL [138], 11; 1840, XXX [228], 16.

Even so, Tulloch's data made it clear that Europeans died in
the West Indies principally from "fevers." (See Tables 4 and 5.)
These fevers were mainly yellow fever and malaria, both of them
Old World diseases brought by earlier African immigrants.[29]
Diagnostic distinctions between the two major tropical fevers
were notoriously bad at the time, but a rough division is possible.
Yellow fever occurred only in periodic epidemics. In Jamaica, for
example, where "fevers" accounted for more than 100 deaths per
thousand per annum over the whole period of the survey, yellow
fever epidemics occurred in 1819, 1822, 1825, and 1827. "Fever"
mortality thus varied from only 67 per thousand in the best year
to 259 per thousand in the worst. If the figure 67 per thousand
represents a death rate mainly from malaria, then about 60 per
cent of the fever deaths were from this cause, and 40 per cent
from yellow fever.

The pattern in the Windward and Leeward Command was
somewhat different. Barbados, where many of the troops were
stationed, was unusually free of malaria. In addition, the Lesser
Antilles passed through a period without serious yellow fever

[29] For the Afro-Eurasian origin of these diseases, see Ashburn, 102-40.

epidemics during the decades of the survey,[30] an indication that the fever mortality—36.9 per thousand per annum—was mainly malaria. Compared to Jamaica, white troops in the Lesser Antilles died at a higher rate from dysentery, but this difference is probably accountable to differences in water supply.

Among African troops, "diseases of the lungs" accounted for most of the increased deaths, though pneumonia and tuberculosis, the principal killers, were also found in the African homeland.[31] Part of the increased mortality was undoubtedly the result of crowded conditions in barracks or slave quarters, and even more may have come from lack of immunity to certain strains of disease not present in Africa. But it may be that genetic susceptibility played some role. Early epidemiologists believed that Negroes were particularly susceptible to lung disease if they moved from Africa to either Europe or North America.[32] Even today, Negro Americans are slightly more susceptible than white Americans to certain forms of tubercular infection. While the differences today are far less than those suggested by Tulloch's figures, it is likely that African environmental conditions over many generations have produced a genetic susceptibility that is still detectable.

The experience of Tulloch's African sample with "fevers" illustrates the point that immunities from one disease environment are not necessarily valid against all possible strains and varieties of a particular disease encountered in another. The West African "fever" environment was probably the most dangerous in the world to outsiders. Fever death rates of European soldiers were 382.6 per thousand per annum in the Cape Coast Command

[30] Yellow fever epidemics occurred in Grenada, St. Kitts, Barbados, and Antigua in 1816, but these were largely over by February of 1817, the first year of Tulloch's sample. The disease appeared in St. Vincent in 1822, but otherwise only the French islands of Martinique and Guadeloupe among the Lesser Antilles were attacked during the remainder of the period; though a very serious epidemic affecting all the Lesser Antilles reappeared in 1852-53 (Hirsch, I, 322-25).

[31] The death rate from "diseases of the lungs" among African troops in Jamaica, however, was only 7.5 per thousand per annum, a figure reasonably in line with that of African troops in Sierra Leone itself. (PP, 1837-38, XL [138], 50.) The Windward and Leeward Command's figure has been accepted as more reliable, however, largely on account of the larger size of the sample.

[32] Hirsch, III, 151-52, 225-28.

and 410.2 per thousand in Sierra Leone,[33] while African troops in Sierra Leone died from fevers at the rate of only 2.5 per thousand per annum. Once they migrated to America, however, Africans of the same origin sustained nearly twice that rate in the Lesser Antilles, and a rate of 8.2 per thousand per annum in Jamaica.[34] The probable explanation is that the West African pattern of apparent immunity to *falciparum* malaria was not effective against other varieties of malaria, nor against other strains of *P. falciparum*.

Once in America, both Europeans and Africans should have begun to acquire new immunities from the new disease environment. The medical mythology of Europeans involved in the South Atlantic System on either shore of the ocean always included a belief in the "seasoning sickness"—the first attack of tropical disease, which left survivors with the expectation of better health. The planters also thought of slaves as passing through the same seasoning process, and seasoned slaves commanded higher prices than newcomers. Military planning was also occasionally based on the concept of seasoning; European troops were given periods of residence in the West Indies before being sent into combat.

Tulloch was understandably concerned with the quantitative aspects of seasoning. His data were weak, however, since his samples had only two dimensions—place of recruitment and annual mean strength. Some of the soldiers in a particular unit might be twenty-year veterans of the tropics, while others were fresh from England. He therefore took pains to trace the medical history of a series of drafts of European troops sent to Jamaica, and he found that the death rates rose during each successive year of service, rather than falling as the common belief in seasoning would suggest. One sample moved from 77 deaths per thousand per annum in the first year, to 87 in the second and third years, and then to 93 per thousand from the fourth year onward. The same tendency was also found in other data from the Windward and Leeward Command.[35] If the samples were

[33] PP, 1840, XXX [228], 7, 19.
[34] PP, 1837-38, XL [138], 50.
[35] PP, 1837-38, XL [138], 89, 92.

representative, seasoning was a longer process than many believed it to be.

In Africa, however, he discovered another seasoning pattern. By chance, the non-commissioned officers serving with African troops were easily divisible into two groups. In the years 1819-24, the British non-coms were freshly arrived from Europe, and they died at a predictable West African rate of 397 per thousand per annum. After 1830, the main body of British troops was withdrawn, leaving behind a group of non-commissioned officers who were already veterans of the African environment. Between 1830 and 1836, these men died at the rate of 72 per thousand per annum, only 18 per cent of the initial rate.[36] The survivors had clearly been seasoned, though their death rate was still more than double that of the African troops under their command. Tulloch's findings therefore suggest a rather slow seasoning process in the American tropics, as against a rapid and costly one in tropical Africa.

The difference can be partly explained by differing patterns of malaria on the two sides of the ocean. West Africa is a hyperendemic area for *falciparum* malaria; new arrivals could hardly escape infection for as long as a year. Once permanently infested with the parasite, the survivors would experience few clinical symptoms—but only if they were regularly reinfected, as they would have been in West Africa. In addition, Sierra Leone was struck by an especially serious epidemic of yellow fever in 1829. Thus the veteran non-coms in Sierra Leone after 1830 can be counted as having survived the two most dangerous diseases of that region. In the West Indies, on the other hand, *Anopheles gambiae*, the most deadly of the African malarial vectors, was missing. Many American forms of malarial parasite were less deadly than the virtually universal *P. falciparum* of the African coast. A European arriving in the West Indies would almost certainly have malaria sooner or later; but its onset was not likely to be so rapid as in West Africa, nor was death so likely. In addition, yellow fever epidemics were less frequent in the West Indies.[37] An individual island might escape for as long as thirty years at a time, just as the Lesser Antilles did during the survey period.

[36] *PP*, 1840, XXX [228], 7.
[37] Hirsch, I, 328-29, 335.

V

Whatever the seasoning process among the immigrants themselves, a new generation born and raised in the American tropics
should have been relatively immune to the American disease
environment. One would, therefore, expect the early slave trade
and a trickle of European migrants to produce a tropical American
population capable of growth by natural increase—if not immediately, at least within a century or so after the trade began. If
this had happened, the high mortality of migration would have
been limited to the sixteenth and part of the seventeenth century.
In fact, this did not happen. The most striking demographic
peculiarity of the South Atlantic System was its failure to produce
a self-sustaining slave population in tropical America.[38] As a
result, the slave trade was necessary not merely to increase the
American production of tropical staples, but even to maintain
the population level. The final result was an increasing flow of
slaves from Africa to America, far into the nineteenth century.

An overall figure for the excess of deaths over births among
American slave populations cannot be established, but the gener-

[38] Population data concerning the immigration and emigration of white
populations in the West Indies and Brazil are extremely scarce, but it appears
more than likely that the white populations of the South Atlantic plantation
colonies also failed to become self-sustaining during the period of the slave
trade. The sex ratios of white populations in the French and English Caribbean colonies were very heavily overbalanced with men. Estimates for the
French Caribbean about 1700 put the sex ratio at three thousand to four thousand white men per thousand women. (Gaston Martin, *Histoire de l' esclavage
dans les colonies françaises* [Paris, 1948], 26.) This pattern developed from
the fact that most white immigrants were either indented servants or else part
of the group of merchants, officials, or planters who came to the New World
as young men hoping to make their fortunes and return home. Given the fact
of an initial mortality of migration at more than ten times the European mortality rate, as Tulloch's data show, the pattern of short-term immigration must
have exacted a very high price indeed. E. Revert states bluntly for Martinique
that the white population could only be maintained by continuous immigration, at least up to 1848. (*Géographie de la Martinique* [Fort-de-France,
1947], 19.) Yet the European populations of these West Indian colonies grew
throughout the eighteenth century. In other territories, such as Cuba and
Brazil, however, a self-sustaining and even a naturally growing white population may well have emerged at an earlier date. In Cuba, for example, the white
sex ratio in 1827 was 1,185 males per thousand females, as compared with a
white Jamaican sex ratio of 1,432 as late as 1844. (R. Guerra y Sanchez *et al.*
[eds.], *Historia de la nación cubana*, 10 Vols. [Havana, 1952], III, 348;
Roberts, 73.)

al picture for tropical America is clear. Eighteenth-century commentators on the slave trade gave estimates of net natural decrease that varied between about 20 and 50 per thousand per annum for the Caribbean.[39] Similar estimates put the population loss among Brazilian slaves at 50 per thousand per annum for the period 1772-1873 and at 30 to 40 per thousand for the late period of slavery, 1872-85.[40] More recent calculations show a natural decrease in Jamaica from nearly 40 per thousand per annum over the period 1703-34, down to a little less than 20 per thousand per annum in the years 1734-39.[41] Barbados' slave population experienced a natural decrease of 43 per thousand per annum between 1712 and 1762.[42] The fact of natural decrease, if not a solidly established rate, is confirmed for other islands in the Caribbean as well.[43]

One cause, perhaps the chief cause, of this excess of deaths over births is to be found on the supply side of the Atlantic slave trade. Slaves were cheap in Africa, whether measured in terms of their marginal productivity on the plantation, or by the replacement cost of breeding and raising a slave to working age in the tropical Americas. Planters therefore preferred to buy more men than women, and they rarely followed a policy of encour-

[39] For samples of eighteenth-century estimates, see L. Peytraud, *L'esclavage aux Antilles françaises avant 1789* (Paris, 1897).

[40] A. Gomes, "Achegas para a história do tráfico africano no Brasil—Aspectos numericos," *IV Congresso de História Nacional, 21-28 Abril de 1949* (Rio de Janeiro, 1950), 65-66 (volume 5 of *Anais* of the *Instituto Histórico e Geográfico Brasileiro*).

[41] Roberts, 36-37.

[42] D. Lowenthal, "The Population of Barbados," *Social and Economic Studies*, VI (1957), 452.

[43] See Pitman, *passim*; Martin, *Histoire de l'esclavage dans les colonies françaises*, 125; E. V. Goveia, *Slave Society in the British Leeward Islands at the End of the Eighteenth Century* (New Haven, 1965), 234; L. M. Díaz Soler, *Historia de la esclavitud en Puerto Rico, 1493-1890* (Madrid, 1953), 117; Julio J. Brusone, in Guerra y Sanchez *et al.*, IV, 188. The United States, however, was a striking exception to this pattern of natural decrease among the slave population. R. R. Kuczynski pointed out the remarkable contrast between the North American colonies and Jamaica more than thirty years ago, in *Population Movements* (London, 1936), 15-17. Net slave imports into the territory of the later United States were probably no more than 500,000 in all, but Negro population at the time of emancipation was more than 4.5 millions. In Jamaica, by contrast, net imports during the whole period of the slave trade have been estimated at more than 700,000, while the Negro population at the time of emancipation was only 350,000.

aging a high birth rate in order to produce a self-perpetuating slave gang. The preference for male workers in turn reflected on supply, and the slave trade carried a remarkably consistent proportion of about two men for every woman. Other things being equal, this in itself would be expected to produce a birth rate per capita 33 per cent lower than that of a balanced population. In addition, birth rates were low even in proportion to female slaves—a reflection of the planters' common decision not to encourage breeding. The evidence from Jamaica indicates that female slaves themselves avoided having children in the conditions of slavery, and they knew about abortives and techniques for contraception in Africa.[44]

Since newly arrived slaves had very high mortality rates for people in the prime of life, we can assume that morbidity rates were correspondingly high. This had a large (if unmeasurable) influence on per-capita birth rates among migrants. One result was a curious paradox in the relation of the slave trade to demographic patterns in the Americas. Where economic growth was most rapid, and slave imports were greatest, population decrease from an excess of deaths over births tended to be most severe. Since the African-born part of the population was the portion with the marked sexual imbalance, the higher morbidity rates, and the higher mortality rates, it was they who pulled down the growth rate of the population as a whole. On the other hand, colonies without notable economic growth over a few decades began to import fewer slaves. They could then begin to achieve more favorable rates of population growth.

The comparative position of the various British West Indian colonies after the end of the British slave trade in 1808 is an interesting illustration of this demographic peculiarity. Barbados, which had virtually ceased importing slaves before the official abolition of the trade, achieved a self-sustaining population shortly after 1808.[45] Jamaica, however, had substantial slave imports up to the end of the trade. As a result, its slave popula-

[44] For discussions of planters' policies on slave breeding or replacement from Africa, see B. Edwards, *The History, Civil and Commercial of the British Colonies in the West Indies*, 2 Vols. (London, 1794), II, 147-54; R. Pares, *West India Fortune* (London, 1950), 123-24; Roberts, 219-47; G. Debien, *Plantations et esclaves à Saint-Domingue* (Dakar, 1962), 44-51.

[45] Lowenthal, 453.

tion still had an excess of deaths over births at 5 per thousand per annum in the period 1817-29. British Guiana, on the other hand, passed through its period of rapid development just before the ending of the slave trade. As a result, it was left in 1817 with a slave population 65 per cent African-born and a rate of natural decrease at 11 per thousand between 1817 and 1829. As the African-born died in each territory, the population decline stopped, as it did in Jamaica by the early eighteen-forties.[46] Meanwhile, Cuba and Brazil had the most rapidly developing planting economies in tropical America, with continued (if illegal) slave imports to the mid-century and beyond. As a result, the pattern of a naturally decreasing slave population persisted there into the second half of the nineteenth century.[47]

Epidemiological factors by themselves cannot explain the origins and development of the South Atlantic System, but they clearly impinged on the system in extremely important ways. They influenced economic decisions and economic patterns, the demography of tropical America, and the planters' preference for Africans over other workers. Nothing that has been said here, however, should be extended to slavery or the slave trade outside the core area of tropical plantations. North America was certainly different, as was highland South America. The role of epidemiological factors in the core area nevertheless suggests that North American slavery might well be re-examined in the light of comparative studies from tropical America. In the same sense, American Indian history would profit from a broad and comparative look at the history of similarly isolated peoples on other continents. In Africa itself, the relative isolation of many human communities suggests that epidemiological factors *must* have been of great importance throughout the history of the continent —and especially at the moment when isolation was broken in the early colonial period. The role of epidemiological factors in the history of the slave trade is, therefore, only one instance among many where the role of disease in history has not yet been fully explored.

[46] Roberts, 39-41.
[47] Julio J. Brusone, in Guerra y Sanchez et al., IV, 167-81; Gomes, 65-66.

7

The Influence of Disease on Race, Logistics and Colonization in the Antilles

Francisco Guerra

Humboldt once asserted that the history of the Antilles was a narrative of sugar and slaves (1826); these twin factors were indeed so dominant that the study of Caribbean medical history is closely interwoven with economic and racial references. On the other hand the political and military history of the Antilles is chequered by the story of disease, for it was frequently disease alone which proved to be the turning point in many an important historical event.

Medical historians have tended to neglect the Antilles, and no information is readily available on the evolution of medicine in the Caribbean during the colonial period. Many have assumed that medical practice and events in the Caribbean were a mere echo of metropolitan medicine, without any distinguishing factors to consider; yet on the contrary, historical research of the Caribbean is of unique importance for the understanding of the transfer of disease between peoples of differing cultures, the natural selection of races by immunity factors, the analysis of mass migrations under epidemics, and the outcome of military operations in areas with endemic tropical diseases, in addition to the usual aspects of medical history.

Caribbean Geopolitics

Throughout the sixteenth century the Caribbean was, for all practical purposes, a Spanish *mare nostrum,* and the Antilles remained sparsely settled due to Spanish commitments in the colonization of the American continent (Parry and Sherlock 1956). The Alexandrian Bulls giving Spain legal dominion over these territories were not formally challenged until the seventeenth century apart from isolated acts of piracy. The naval tactics of Menendez de Avilés (1519 - 1574), and the convoy system adopted by the Spanish fleet, afforded on the whole, sound protection for Spain's commerce with America. It must be remembered that the early exploits of Hawkins (d.1589), Drake (1540 - 1596) and others, were aimed at securing a share of the slave trade and defying the Spanish monopoly of commerce; these exploits resulted in skirmishes on land or sea, but never in established colonies with lasting effects on

general colonial policies. The outstanding feat of the Dutch Admiral Piet Heyn, who captured in 1628 the whole Spanish treasure fleet north of Cuba, was never repeated and its consequences were obliterated within a matter of years. The continual harassment of the Spanish ports in the Caribbean and the sporadic severance of her maritime links by pirates or privateers did not permit England, France or the Dutch to develop either a commercial outlet or stable political dominion. In 1536 it was possible for a single French privateer to capture Havana and in the course of the same century many other ports fell prey to privateers of different nationalities and were held to ransom, but nothing less than economically sound colonization could lead to truly national policies, for Spain was never to surrender her dominion or her commerce as the result of actions she deemed to be piracy. The geographical position of the Antilles offered natural harbours with hinterlands suitable for the support of both squadrons and troops of European powers other than Spain, as well as the possibility of establishing colonies in which to develop commerce. But again, the colonial strategy of those powers depended on the successful settlement of large numbers of their nationals, capable of fostering an agricultural economy of tropical produce such as sugar, coffee, indigo, and spices, which in turn could open a market for consumer goods of metropolitan manufacture. These settlements could then provide strong backing for garrisons and the vital marine installations.

The first endeavours of settlers such as Belain d'Enambuc (1558 - 1636) in St. Christopher or those of Raleigh (1552 - 1618) in Guiana, petered out for lack of open support either by France or England when faced by the strong political and military opposition of Spain. A much clearer conception of commerce supported by insular dominion in the Antilles was evident in the Dutch States General, following their success of 1592, when control of the East Indies spice trade was gained despite Portuguese hostility (Guerra 1965); this policy became more evident in opposition to Spain after the Antwerp truce of 1609 and took final shape with the institution of the Dutch West Indies Company in 1621. The Dutch made an early start in the Caribbean but their settlements in the lesser Antilles and Guiana never expanded and their major Brazilian colonies were first overrun by the Portuguese in 1625 and then definitively in 1653, mainly because of the limited supply of man power. Thereafter the Spanish dominion in the Antilles, from the middle of the seventeenth century, was threatened by two equally powerful nations, France and England. France initiated a grand design of Caribbean policy in 1626 when Cardinal Richelieu (1585 - 1642) created *La Compagnie des Isles de l'Amerique*, with the object of colonizing St. Christopher and Barbados; in 1633 and 1642 further companies were set up for Guiana (Crouse 1943). However, at that time the naval strength of France was extremely limited and not until the advent of Colbert (1610 - 1683), who multiplied her navy tenfold and vastly improved ports and arsenals, did the reorganized colonial companies manage to flourish (Mims 1912). After the loss of Canada in 1759 - 1763 France's geopolitical balance in America was disrupted and Choiseul (1719 - 1785) had to expand the meagre Guiana settlement and to boost the population of St. Domingue and other islands in the Antilles by re-settling Acadians there together with immigrants of French stock. Similar endeavours were made under Napoleon (1769 - 1821) with the expeditions to St. Domingue and Martinique.

England, possessing a navy unmatched by that of any other power, was in a more favourable position to gain control of the Caribbean. British ships were usually victorious in naval engagements and captured ports and entire colonies, but as the Venetian Ambassador (Burns 1954) commented after Drake's attack on Cadiz in 1596, " the English knew how to conquer, but did not know how to hold on." In the Caribbean that statement was justified as regards the early English settlements in Guiana, Providence Island and St. Christopher. It was under Cromwell (1599 - 1658) that the western design of the Caribbean colonies really began to be systematically pursued by England. The Venables expedition of 1655, though it failed to overcome Santo Domingo, was able to occupy Jamaica despite the tenacious resistance of the small Spanish population. After the Restoration the development of the West Indian plantations was accepted as a factor of British crown policy. The Spanish decline under Bourbon rule brought the interests of England

into conflict with those of France in the Antilles and the political dominion of both nations remained quite fluid in that area during the eighteenth century.

Racial Struggles

Paradoxically enough, though sugar and slaves were characteristic of the Antilles, neither the crop nor the forced labour were indigenous to that area: sugar cane was brought to Santo Domingo from the Canary Isles about 1508 (Guerra 1965), and the slaves needed for the cultivation of the imported crop began to be introduced from Africa from 1510 and systematically after 1518 (Parry and Sherlock 1956). The arrival of Negro labour caused a progressive modification of the Caribbean population, intensified during the seventeenth and eighteenth centuries by the continued decline of the aboriginal Siboneyes, Tainos, Caribs and Arawaks, in addition to the simultaneous immigration of white colonists and soldiers of European stock. By the end of the eighteenth century the Negro had become the dominant racial element, outnumbering the whites by 10 to one. The medical implications of this racial modification cannot be overlooked, for as a primary result the aboriginal Indians of the Antilles were practically exterminated—not by forced labour and ill-treatment, as historians would have us suppose—and not so much as the consequence of war, but because of the devastations caused by diseases imported by the colonizers; smallpox, influenza and measles among others. On the other hand in this tropical zone the white Europeans went through the process of acclimatization to unfamiliar diseases to which the American Indian and the African Negro possessed either a greater resistance or a certain degree of immunity. Whether some virus diseases, such as yellow fever, existed in America before the arrival of Europeans or whether such viruses were imported by the slave trade from Africa, is one of the most controversial points in the history of epidemic diseases (Carter 1931).

During the first two centuries of colonization the Antilles witnessed the struggle of the Indian against the colonist and more than once the Caribs made it impossible for the Spaniards or the French to arrive at a peaceful settlement. But in the first years of the eighteenth century national rivalries among European powers in the Caribbean and the struggle of the Amerindian against the European began to be overshadowed by the appearance of a more complex

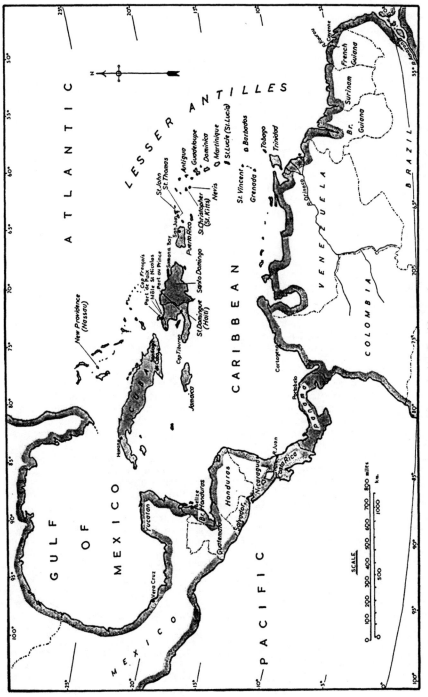

25

Map of the Caribbean Area

racial problem which exploded with unsurpassed violence. On various occasions, when it suited their purpose, French, British, Spanish and Dutch had allied themselves with another race group—Negro or Carib—as mutual dislike divided both these races, and the Caribs had remained numerically important and aggressive in some islands. In 1795 at St. Vincent, for instance (Burns 1954), the French allied with the Caribs against the British and the Negroes, destroying every installation in the Island and killing every inhabitant but for those encircled at Kingstown. After the British recovery the entire Carib population, over 5,000 people, was exiled to Roatan, British Honduras, in 1797.

However, the real menace to the white population in the Antilles was the overwhelming proportion of Negro slaves. Plantation life throughout the colonial period was carried on under the constant fear of a Negro revolt, as the enslaved Africans naturally never relinquished their desire for freedom (Perry and Sherlock 1956). An early taste of things to come occurred at the Danish settlement of St. John in 1733 when all the white residents were murdered with the exception of a handful who escaped to St. Thomas. When fresh troops arrived the Negroes were methodically hunted down and shot (Burns 1954). The Jamaican maroon wars of 1734 and 1795 also reflected the insecure condition of the white planters in the British colonies. The natural right of the Negro to freedom was ratified in the French colonies after the declaration of *les droits de l'homme* during the French Revolution which meant the end, not only of social injustice, but also of the economic system which made possible the cultivation of colonial crops (Godechot 1956). The Negro revolt of 1791 in the northern part of St. Domingue resulted in the murder of 2,000 whites, about 10,000 slaves and the destruction of 180 sugar and 900 coffee and indigo plantations (Edwards 1819). For the Negro slaves of the Antilles the final solution of their problem was to achieve freedom by the extermination of the white man and the destruction of everything symbolized by his rule. Racial hatred, as a result of colonization and slavery, was not confined to Carib against white or Negro against white because it obtained in other shades of colour, and St. Domingue was also the scene of the systematic annihilation of 10,000 Mulattoes who supported Rigaud, by the Negro army under Toussaint l'Ouverture in 1798 (Edwards 1819).

The cruelty unleashed by inter-racial struggles in the Caribbean, ugly as it may appear, was in many ways similar to that demonstrated earlier among the Spanish, Dutch, French and British during encounters between privateers and royal troops. In these campaigns national hates and religious differences fermented violence and the ghastly record of death, mutilation, plunder, and the vicious abuse of prisoners is barely matched by other infamous historical episodes.

The Unpredictable Logistics

Political rivalries and the objectives of colonization policies in the Antilles were necessarily carried into effect by military operations. Notwithstanding the care taken in strategic planning, an unpredictable factor, that of disease, appeared and played havoc among the best trained and equipped forces whenever European navies and troops moved from their traditional battlegrounds and went into action in the Caribbean. Yellow fever began to be repeatedly identified and the unknown nature and conflicting observations of its contagion involved the medical corps in a predicament until the twentieth century (Mosely 1787, Moreau de Jonnès 1816).

Nevertheless, high national policy in the Antilles was seldom satisfactorily resolved by naval or military strategy, but rather by the morbidity of the settlements and the ability of the European either to survive infection or to utilize seasoned troops, either white or negro, which were immune to prevailing disease. Some historians such as Scott (1939), Keevil (1958) and Burns (1954) have given isolated glimpses of certain naval and military operations which were known to have been influenced by epidemics; but the rôle of disease was paramount in every Caribbean engagement and a systematic survey of major events is a gloomy repetition of sanitary disasters. Only on a few occasions were diseases common to continental armies worth recording. Moreau de Saint Méry (1796) mentioned that after the greatest naval engagement in the Caribbean, the battle of *Les Saintes* on 18th April 1782 between the British Navy under Rodney (1719-1792) and the French led by De Grasse (1723-1788), all but two of the 180 wounded died of tetanus. In 1805 after the capture of the ship *Diamant* none of the wounded survived, some dying of tetanus, the rest of gangrene. Yet in the medical history of Caribbean engagements the number of wounded represented only a negligible proportion of the casualties (Moreau de St. Méry 1958); epidemics were to account for a mortality rate of 85 per cent of the troops, and in those cases where yellow fever was complicated by dysentery whole regiments were wiped out. Even during the plague epidemic affecting the Napoleonic troops during the Egyptian and Syrian campaign of 1798 - 1799, Larrey (1766 - 1842) and Desguenettes (1762 - 1837) were able to save up to 60 per cent of their troops (Desguenettes 1802); in the Caribbean the medical corps faced a much more voracious enemy.

In 1585 Sir Francis Drake sailed from England with a fleet of thirty ships to ' impeach ' the Spanish king in the Indies. At the Cape Verde islands the expedition encountered yellow fever and more than 200 men died during the trip to the Antilles. Drake occupied Santo Domingo and afterwards Cartagena, the two most important ports in the Caribbean, but after six weeks of operations with 2,300 men, only 800 were fit for service, 750 having already died of disease and the rest were ill. Drake was censured for not holding the occupied territory, but the deplorable condition of his troops and their progressive debilitation, made it impossible for the British to establish any colony. Shortly after the destruction of the Invincible Armada in 1588, Drake, John Hawkins and Baskerville sailed from England in 1595 to capture the treasure galleon in Puerto Rico; yet their victories were shortlived, as an epidemic, thought to have been dysentery, spread among the sailors in January 1596 and Drake himself died of it on the 27th (Burns 1954). The Earl of Cumberland (1558 - 1605) was more fortunate than Drake in Puerto Rico, as he captured San Juan on 6th June 1598. The harbour and the island seemed promising for colonization but yellow fever broke out among the crews, attacking the leader, and after losing over 400 men in a few weeks the British force was forced to return to England (Burns 1954). The large contingent sent by France to occupy Sainte-Lucie in 1665 was the first of her military expeditions to suffer the full impact of disease. Of the 1,500 men landed, only 89 remained alive a few months later, and though dysentery was rife and they suffered from famine, the mortality rate seems to indicate an epidemic of yellow fever. After the French had captured St. Kitts in 1689, Captain Lawrence Wright sailed from Plymouth in 1690 with eleven warships and a regiment in order to recapture the island. The fleet put into Barbados for two weeks in May of that year and encountered yellow fever; by Spring 1691 the expedition was obliged to return to England having lost most of the crews and troops and having accomplished very little

(Burns 1954). When the attack against the French West Indies was stepped up by royal command during 1692, Keevil (1958) indicated that the expedition of Sir Francis Wheeler with 18 warships included a hospital ship and transports for 1,800 soldiers. Upon arrival in Barbados sickness broke out, although 800 replacements from that island helped to cover the losses. In April 1693 Wheeler landed 2,300 men in Martinique but the attack failed due to illness in the forces, and within a few days 1,300 sailors out of 2,100 and 1,800 soldiers out of 2,400 were wiped out by disease (Keevil 1958).

In 1695 another British expedition under Admiral Robert Wilmot and Colonel Lillingston was sent to the northern coast of St. Domingue against the French, and simultaneously the Spanish troops from Santo Domingo joined forces against the French. The British landed over 900 soldiers at Cap-François on 29th May 1695 while the Spaniards moved about 1,900 seasoned troops in the north. After the capture of Cap-François and Port-de-Paix, the British contingent was forced to re-embark on 27th July 1695 due to extensive sickness among the troops in an area notorious for endemic yellow fever, and the French recovered their lost territory without undue effort. Wilmot died, as did his successor Captain Lance, together with more than 1,000 troops (Moreau de St. Méry 1958).

Rear Admiral Francis Hosier's (1673 - 1727) disaster in 1726 - 1727 affords another well-known page of Caribbean medical history; he was sent to prevent the treasure ships sailing from Porto Bello, Veracruz and Havana. In June 1726 Hosier blockaded Porto Bello, but by December he was forced to fall back to Jamaica, his crews decimated and unable to man the ships. Within the next six months he, his successors St. Lo and Hopson, 10 ships' captains, 50 lieutenants and around 4,000 officers and sailors had died (Keevil 1961). They were not the only ones, as Castelbondo recalls (1755), for the Spanish fleet under Pintado, sent in 1730 to face the British squadron, also lost 2,200 sailors through yellow fever (Castelbondo 1755).

The War of Jenkins's Ear which broke out between England and Spain in 1739 afforded further evidence of the control exercised by yellow fever on any military operation in the Caribbean. Vernon (1648 - 1757), who had served in the West Indies from 1708 to 1712 took command of a fleet and troops with instructions " . . . to destroy the Spanish settlements in the West Indies and to distress their shipping by any method whatever." This was intended to be the end of Spain's dominion in the Antilles by severing her vital commercial links. In November 1739 Vernon captured Porto Bello without much difficulty. France sent the Marquis d'Antin in 1740 to support the Spanish defences but the troops and the crews suffered from epidemics at Martinique and Saint-Domingue and after six months the French fleet was forced to sail for home ports, being in no fit state to go into action. Vernon meanwhile had been reinforced by 58 ships and with a landing force of 18,760 troops, most of them unseasoned, and decided to strike the decisive blow against Cartagena in 1741. It is well known that due to some delays in landing and military operations, yellow fever attacked the British forces and soon over 8,400 of them had died. Of the 3,569 soldiers who re-embarked, the seasoned North American troops accounted for 1,140 (Burns 1954). When Vernon's expedition withdrew from Cartagena the British forces decided to fall upon Santiago de Cuba where half Wentworth's remaining forces, writes Keevil (1958), died of yellow fever before the attack was called off. In July 1741 2,260 men died in three weeks. At the end of the campaign out of 6,000 marines only 2,500 returned fit for duty (Keevil 1961).

In 1795 some 5,000 troops under General Peregrine Hopson, after failing to land in Martinique, were easily able to capture Baseterre in Guadaloupe, the French troops withdrawing to the interior of the island. Within a month more than 2,000 men, General Hopson among them, had either died or fallen ill. The French population finally surrendered, but the British expedition was unable to remain very long in control of the island and was forced to re-embark (Burns 1954). A similar occurrence took place in Havana. The British Navy under Admiral Pocock and 10,000 troops under George Keppel, Earl Albermarle (1724 - 1772) took the Morro castle and Havana after a siege which lasted from 5th June to 14th August 1762. But in 1761 a yellow fever epidemic, re-introduced into Havana by prisoners sent from Veracruz to build the Cabañas fort, had already carried off more than 2,000 inhabitants. One month after landing, the British expedition had lost about 3,000 sailors and 5,000 soldiers, and the remaining forces were eventually unable to retain possession of the port (Burns 1954).

The European soldiers used by France in the Caribbean garrisons were also constantly affected by tropical diseases, mostly dysentery and yellow fever. Moreau de St. Méry (1796) mentions that in 1763 and 1764 the first battalion of the Quercy regiment stationed in Fort-Dauphin, lost a considerable number of soldiers. In 1765 the garrison at Port-au-Prince was affected and 407 soldiers, 47 sailors and only 207 civilians, died. When in 1777 M. Dessources, Captain of the regiment at Port-au-Prince, went to Petit-Goave to furnish a garrison of 100 men, 66 members of the fresh troops fell ill eight days after their arrival. The garrison was relieved after 45 days and by that time only nine soldiers were fit for service and in all no more than 17 survived (Moreau de St. Méry 1958). The records of the British Army surgeon John Weir, published by Lempriere (1799), show that in peacetime under garrison conditions the troops in Jamaica suffered from yellow fever in a similar proportion to the French troops in Saint-Domingue and mortality every year was about 20 per cent of their effectives. The British troops, 20th Light Dragoons and the 62nd Regiment in Spanish Town, suffered very seriously from the fever in 1793, 1794 and 1795. Of the 350 men in the 20th Light Dragoons, 67 died in 1793. Out of the four regiments 473 soldiers died from 1793 to 1796. The situation in the rest of the British West Indies was very much the same. In New Providence, which is now known as Nassau in the Bahamas, the whole 47th Regiment died of yellow fever in 1796 within the space of a few weeks, and with the soldiers died their women and children. In 1802 of 300 men of the 7th Fusiliers 220 died and in 1803, after replacements had covered the losses, 250 more men of the same regiment died (Lempriere 1799).

In 1779 after Spain declared war on England, the settlements in Belize were overrun and the British retaliated by capturing the Omea fort. However they were only able to hold out from 20th October to the end of November, when a fever epidemic decimated the British soldiery. As a result the present territory of British Honduras was free of British settlers from 1779 to 1784. Dancer (1781) has offered a medical account of the expedition sent to Nicaragua from Jamaica in 1780 after these events in Belize. Nelson escorted the troops sent to Nicaragua with orders to capture the San Juan river with the object of gaining control of Lake Nicaragua and reaching the Pacific. The castle at San Juan river was taken at the end of April, but the season being so advanced, in a few days only 380 survived of the 1,800 men who

February 1966

went up the river. Even the garrison left in the castle was decimated and the survivors returned to Jamaica, leaving the whole area to revert to the Spanish (Dancer 1781).

In 1780 the combined Spanish and French fleets assembled at Fort Royal, Martinque, under de Guichen's command. Spain had over 10,000 troops stationed there which, with the French contingent, were expected to attack Jamaica and check any resistance that Rodney's fleet could offer. But being the month of June, the Spanish crews and transports were ravaged by yellow fever and the Spanish fleet and the remaining troops had to fall back on Cuba being in no state to go into action (Burns 1954). Again the records of the Spanish colonies show that, in Fort-Dauphin, St. Domingue, when the Spanish Regiment of León crossed into the French colony from Santo Domingo in 1782, from a complement of 1,440, 17 officers, three cadets and 647 soldiers died within three months (Moreau de St. Méry 1958).

The Caribbean Era of Social Revolution

The social changes brought about in St. Domingue by the declaration of the Rights of Man in 1793 were received with alarm by the British in Jamaica and by the Spaniards in neighbouring Santo Domingo, for the ideas of the French National Assembly could prove far too contagious among their own enslaved labour force. In 1793 England and Spain declared war on the French Republic. The British listened to the royalist offers and sent an expedition under Colonel Whitelocke which was well received by the French inhabitants, and the occupation of Jérémie, Leogane, Môle St. Nicolas and other towns was accomplished without much resistance being encountered. By January 1794 Tiburon was also taken in and in May of that year reinforcements arrived from England, as a fever epidemic had affected the troops, although it was not until 4th June of that year that the full force of yellow fever attacked the British troops, shortly after the capture of Port-au-Prince. Edwards (1819) has given detailed figures of the British losses, a sanitary disaster only surpassed by the Leclerc expedition of a few years later in the same area. Within two months of the fall of the capital of St. Domingue the four Grenadier companies were almost wiped out, and 40 officers and up to 600 soldiers died (Moreau de St. Méry 1958).

In April 1795 the total number of British troops left in all St. Domingue did not exceed 2,200, and half of them were not fit for active service. In view of the recovery of Rigaud's mulatto forces, fresh troops were sent out from England, 9,800 soldiers being immediately followed by a further 7,900 (Edward 1819). Although Burns (1954) mentions that Rigaud's forces were affected by the epidemic it does not seem that yellow fever had such a severe effect on the Negro soldiers under Rigaud or Toussaint l'Ouverture, but in any event, the British soldiers, who had practically obtained full control of the French colony, were progressively decimated. In 1796 in the 82nd Regiment, of 980 men 630 died; of the Hussars 700 out of 1,000 men died. By the 30th September 1796 7,530 men from an expedition of 20,000 were left alive, and of these only 3,000 survived to the end of 1797. The hospital expenditure of this campaign was considerable; 10 shillings were accounted for each soldier at the hospital and as a result the expenses of the British Army in St. Domingue up to May 1797 were £4,383,597 (Edwards 1819).

When General Thomas Maitland withdrew the British expeditionary forces from St. Domingue in April 1798 over 20,000 soldiers and seamen had died of disease alone in the campaign between 1794 and 1798, and only 1,100 men remained alive from the whole of the landing force (Edwards 1819). The British annexation of St. Domingue had failed despite its early success and that part of the island fell once more under the control of the Negro forces.

While the British expedition to St. Domingue was in progress, another was sent on 27th April 1796 under General Abercromby to Ste. Lucie, in the expectation of completing the encirclement of the last French possessions in the Western hemisphere. The attack on the forts accounted for the loss of about 500 men killed and wounded, but after the French capitulation on 24th May, the Republican soldiers and Negro supporters withdrew to the mountains, which enjoyed much better climatic conditions. The British forces who under Sir John Moore were left to garrison the coast, towns and forts, amounted in June 1796 to over 5,000 men, but within only five months less than 1,000 were left fit for service. By 1797, for instance, the 31st Regiment had lost 22 officers and 841 men (Burns 1954).

From 1793 to 1796 the British Army in the Caribbean lost around 80,000 men, over half of them from yellow fever epidemics alone; it has been pointed out that this figure is higher than the total of Wellington's losses in the whole

Peninsular war (Fortescue 1910). Another century was to pass before the medical corps was sufficiently knowledgeable to take proper sanitary measures against yellow fever, and as Fortescue (1899) indicates, at the best of times every British battalion in the West Indies during the 18th and 19th century had to be entirely replaced every two years (Fortescue 1910); chances of success in military engagements could only be ensured if the campaigns were carried out over a very short period of time and during the winter.

The examples of military operations in the Caribbean which were ravaged by yellow fever could be continued until the time of the Spanish American War in Cuba at the turn of the 20th century, but it will suffice to close the story of the old colonial wars in the Antilles with an account of the French expedition to St. Domingue in 1802, which has remained the classic example of medical catastrophe. The narrative by the chief medical officer Gilbert (1803) in the *Histoire médicale de l'Armée française à Saint-Domingue* leaves no doubt that the French expeditionary force was contemplating a quick and easy campaign with plenty of promotions and that the medical corps was totally unaware of the sombre lesson learned by the British, a lesson which they were fated to learn at much higher cost. General Leclerc, brother-in-law of Napoleon (1769 - 1821), with Rochambeau as second in command, left Brest with an élite army of 25,000. A further 2,300 soon joined them from Toulon and, supported by 26 warships, they reached Samaná Bay in Santo Domingo in January 1802. General Kerversau went to Santo Domingo with some frigates, while Rochambeau attacked Fort-Dauphin, Leclerc landed near Cap-François, and Boudet reached Port-au-Prince. The health of the army and the navy was excellent and remained so until the proclamation of 25th April 1802. At Cap-François Leclerc's division soon repaired a hospital of 1,000 beds, as this city was entirely burned before their landing, and by May the French were to all intents and purposes again in control of Saint-Domingue. Reinforcements of about 3,500 fresh troops from France kept coming every month. The news also reached them that the forces of General Richepanse had obtained control of Guadaloupe and had re-established slavery there. Freedom meant everything for the slaves and although Toussaint l'Ouverture had been captured, the Negro generals Dessalines, Christophe and their armies had only to wait

and allow the yellow fever to take its inexorable toll. The end came with fulminating force. By the end of November 1802, that is 10 months from their landing, approximately 40,000 French soldiers had died, including 1,500 officers and 180 physicians, surgeons and apothecaries, most of them from yellow fever (Burns 1954). General Leclerc and many officers had succumbed. By May 1803 British warships had blockaded the colony, cutting off Rochambeau's troops from France. Disease continued to reduce the ranks of the French Army and forced it to evacuate the island except for Santo Domingo, Môle St. Nicolas, and Cap-François. On 30th November Rochambeau surrendered to the British together with the 8,000 men who remained of his entire expeditionary force, and he was taken to Jamaica. On the 3rd December five of the six ships which had escaped from Môle St. Nicolas were also captured (Métral 1825).

It has been said that 60,000 Negroes of the Dessalines and Christophe armies died during the same period, but Dessalines himself does not indicate that these losses were due to disease, but rather to " drowning, suffocation, assassination, hanging and shooting ". By May 1804 Dessalines had effected the massacre of the entire white population of St. Domingue, but for a few members of the medical profession who escaped that fate, Mirambeau, who became chief surgeon of the Negro Haitian Army, and Baillergau who was also appointed State Apothecary, and some priests and magistrates who helped to build the social structure of Haiti, previously St. Domingue, the first all-Negro nation in the western hemisphere (Pressoir 1927).

Colonization and Manpower

A survey of most military campaigns initiated in the Antilles as a result of competitive colonization by European powers, establishes beyond doubt that tropical diseases, yellow fever above all, played the dominant rôle among troops of European stock; these epidemics were well identified at least during the 17th and 18th centuries. The effect of yellow fever on the white man can only be compared with that of two other epidemics which can be dated with accuracy: the introduction of smallpox into America by a Negro boy among the troops of Narvaez which joined Hernán Cortés (1485 - 1547) for the conquest of Mexico in 1520; and the arrival in Canada of the cholera-infected ship from Cork in June 1832.

Both American epidemics contend with yellow fever for having exacted the greatest toll of death (Guerra 1953).

A consideration of the effect of disease upon colonization in the Caribbean shows that the only records for the first century were those of the Spanish settlements. Most of them have been surveyed by Carter (1931) who tended to prove that yellow fever was imported into America from Africa; however most of his sources may be interpreted in two ways and indicate America as an independent place of origin for this tropical disease, as the mortality of the early epidemics among the Spanish conquistadors points repeatedly towards the curve of mortality under yellow fever (Carter 1931). Although there were people of African descent with the conquistadors from the early years of the 16th century, they were household servants and had not been imported through the African slave trade to America which only developed around 1518. By that date there are several reliable records of fever epidemics with a high mortality, even before the arrival of Europeans in the Caribbean. Gomara (1552), Herrera (1601) and several other chroniclers stress that Moctezuma was on several occasions compelled to repopulate the Veracruz coast because of the unhealthiness of the area, which was later recognised as one of the endemic areas of yellow fever. Before the arrival of Negro slaves from Africa the Spanish settlements suffered heavily from disease. The first epidemics in Santo Domingo even affected the expeditions of Columbus in 1492 and 1494. In 1495 several hundred soldiers died on the island and the epidemic struck again in 1496, and according to Herrera (1601) carried off one third of the island's population. Columbus mentions the fever and refers to pains in the thighs, but these symptoms and mortality rates provide evidence too scant to allow of accurate identification. Of more than 2,000 Spaniards who accompanied Columbus, a mere 300 remained alive by 1502, and of the 2,500 who came with Ovando 1,500 were shortly to die of fever. The Ojeda expedition to the northern coast of South America in 1509 lost 260 soldiers out of 300, and in Panama, Nicuesa's losses from fever were 700 out of 800 men within a few months. Jaundice is mentioned in some accounts and both Bishop Las Casas and Herrera give a figure of 40,000 Spanish deaths by disease from 1509 to 1539 in the Panama area alone. Concerning the Mexican coast of the Caribbean, Bishop Marroquin reported to the Emperor in 1537

that there was not a year in which 500 men did not die in Veracruz; and the presence of the *vomito* among the symptoms described in the great Mexican epidemic of 1545 cannot be overlooked, for, according to some writers, this epidemic accounted for 800,000 deaths. Even Carter (1931) accepts that the 1648 epidemic in Yucatan, first described by Lopez de Cogolludo (1688), is a classic outline of the effects of yellow fever upon both Europeans and Amerindians. It should always be borne in mind that all the Spanish-American chronicles referring to the colonization of America present the dread of epidemics in the Caribbean as the greatest deterrent to Spanish immigration, despite all the great opportunities of glory and wealth offered to the conquistadors. The latter have been portrayed bushwhacking through unknown territory, declaiming verse, and grasping a sword in one hand, while the other is constantly swatting mosquitoes.

The Dutch, like the British, began to establish trading posts in Guiana at the close of the 16th century. Leigh plantation, founded on the Opayoc river in 1604 failed in the following year, Leigh himself dying in the epidemic. In 1609 Robert Harcourt used Raleigh's influence among the Arawaks in order to start a colony, but by 1614 the few English and Irish survivors had to join the Dutch, and Harcourt returned to England. The settlements in Guiana were further encouraged by Lord Willoughby, but the Surinam colony was attacked by the Dutch in 1667 and a violent epidemic broke out among the English inhabitants forcing them to surrender (Burns 1954).

British Attempts at Colonization

The western design to settle British colonies in the Caribbean was decided upon by Cromwell after the publication in 1648 of Thomas Gage's account of the Spanish possessions in Central America. The expedition was led by Robert Venables (1612 - 1687) but, in spite of being supported by a considerable force of more than 80 ships and 9,500 men, it failed to conquer Santo Domingo in 1655. The British forces then decided to fall back on Jamaica which was known to be thinly populated—about 1,500 people in all. Jamaica's main port, Spanish Town, fell to the British but the Spaniards, under the leadership of Cristobal de Isasi and aided by Negro maroons, were able to resist until 1670. Yellow fever and dysentery soon disabled the senior officers, troops and planters, and although the British received the experienced support of early Portuguese settlers there, thousands of British troops died of disease in a few weeks. In 1655, with the object of reinforcing the British population of the island, many Royalist prisoners were taken there from England; 1,000 Irish girls and another 1,000 boys in their teens, together with 1,200 men from Ireland and Scotland were deported in 1656, as Cromwell was very well aware that the chances of establishing a strong colony on the island were diminishing in proportion to the decrease of settlers there, but most of these people perished. In 1657 the former Governor of Nevis arrived at Port Morant with a party of 1,600 persons, most of whom died within the year; a similar fate overtook 300 New Englanders and many of the families who came to Jamaica from Barbados and Bermuda. In 1660 other groups arrived from England, some including women from Newgate and Bridewell, but disease disposed of most of the newcomers and the Jamaican British population was not appreciably augmented. In point of fact the island came close to being recaptured by the Spaniards during the 15 years of resistance by Isasi's guerrillas, but for a saving factor— the 1,000 men sent from Cuba in 1658 also fell victims to yellow fever (Burns 1954).

The colonization of Ste. Lucie by the French was destined for an inauspicious beginning because of Carib hostility and disruption among the French themselves. The sale of the island in 1657 to du Parquet and later to a new French company in 1664 complicated the legal rights of Lord Willoughby who " bought " Ste. Lucie direct from the Caribs. A party of over 1,000 from Barbados, together with 600 Caribs from Dominica, landed on the island to join forces with the local Caribs who had agreed to owe allegiance to the King of England. The French surrendered and most of them embarked for Martinique, but disease was so widespread among new settlers that within a few months there remained neither British planters, nor British troops to keep control of Ste. Lucie, and the French returned once more to occupy the island (Burns 1954).

French Colonization

From its origins in the 17th century French colonization in the Caribbean offers many examples of the scourge of epidemic disease. The *Compagnie du Cap de Nord*, first created in 1633 for the settlement of Guiana, failed within a short time because of disease and a second expedition had to be sent under Bontemps in 1643; however, of the 300 settlers who arrived at the island of Cayenne a mere handful remained alive only a year later. At the same time Richelieu despatched another expedition in 1655 under Du Plessis and l'Olive to settle Guadeloupe and Martinique. The 550 colonists and indentured Frenchmen who landed in Guadeloupe suffered a sudden epidemic described by du Tertre (1667) with symptoms of headache, jaundice and pain in the thighs; this is generally supposed to have been yellow fever.

At the end of the 17th century all the French colonies in the Caribbean were affected by another yellow fever epidemic which even reached some ports in France. In December 1690 the infection was brought into Fort-Royal, Martinique, by the ship *Oriflamme*, in convoy from Siam with two other cargo vessels, the *Louré* and the *Saint Nicholas*, the contagion having been taken on board in Pernambuco in Brazil. By the 3rd January 1691 the captain of the ship and over 100 members of the crew had died, and the infection spread not only to the inhabitants of Martinique but also to the crew of another ship, the *Mignon* en route for France with four others, all of which lost half their crews by July 1691. In May of that year three other ships, *Le Solide*, *Cheval-Marin* and the *Emerillon* arrived in Fort-Royal and were infected; they left for St.-Croix, losing 40 sailors between the 2nd and the 7th August and contaminating the latter island. The ships reached Port-de-Paix on the 12th August and the sickness spread throughout St. Domingue. Port-de-Paix was again the port of entry for another yellow fever epidemic brought on the 11th August 1692 by a ship carrying 82 soldiers from the garrison in St. Christopher, which had fallen to the British, and 140 exiles; 128 French colonists arrived two days later, over 200 reached Cap-François on the 20th, 250 on the 28th, and by the end of October almost 1,000 exiles from St. Christopher had arrived in St. Domingue, most of them dying shortly afterwards of yellow fever (Cornilliac 1873, Moreau de St. Méry 1958).

The Kourou expedition of 1764 is an example of mass migration clearly demonstrating the effects of epidemics on colonization. Choiseul, Minister for the Colonies and the Navy under Louis XV, appreciated the strategic value of Guiana, *la France equinoxale*, as a substitute for the loss of Acadia and Canada, *la Nouvelle*

France. In 1763 French Guiana, covering 150,000 square kilometres, was populated by only 1,307 whites, 494 free slaves and 10,478 slaves and Arawaks. After the publication of Prefontaine's work on Guiana (1763) an expedition left France with the purpose of founding a mass settlement of those territories with European settlers. From May 1763 to 1764 a total of 10,446 persons of French and German stock sailed from French ports under Thibault de Chauvalon (1725 - 1783). The ships reached the Kourou river but the establishments met a wave of epidemics and most of the settlers were transferred to the Isles due Salut or Devil's Island, and by April 1765 about 3,000 survivors were left and allowed repatriation or were conveyed to other areas in the Antilles. Chaïa (1958), in an interesting study of the Kourou disaster, estimates that between May 1763 and April 1765 over 6,500 colonists died, though only 900 remained in Cayenne from the original expedition. A study of contemporary sources, Bajon (1777) and Campet (1802), in addition to the evidence offered by Moreau de Jonnès (1820) leaves very little doubt that yellow fever was responsible, even though a ship arrived with cases of typhus on board in 1764. Nevertheless, yellow fever dogged the footsteps of the repatriates wherever they went. In June 1764 a total of 418 Acadians arrived at Môle St. Nicolas in St. Domingue, and almost all of them perished. About 800 Germans and Acadians arrived in Limonade between November and December 1764, and only 171 remained alive a year later; in Dondon only 89 survived out of 242. When the news of the Kourou disaster reached the ports of embarkation some Germans decided to settle in St. Domingue instead of Guiana; 2,470 of them were settled in Bombarde under the care of the botanist Fusée-Aublet, by April 1766 only 776 remained alive, and by March 1770 only 334 survived (Moreau de St. Méry 1958).

In this way an experimental scheme for colonization by mass emigration and settlement was doomed to failure and brought about the collapse of France's grand political design for the Antilles.

Racial Discrimination by Disease

In more than one instance primary sources for the study of Caribbean epidemics contain first-hand observations by unbiased authors which have been either ignored or omitted by the modern epidemiologist. The identification of a certain race group with apparent immunity among a population affected by an epidemic is of considerable importance in fixing the point of origin of the disease in question. This factor may clarify the acquired immunity of the aboriginal inhabitants of that area, or even trace the cross immunity of groups migrating from areas already affected by the same or similar infections, as infection occurring shortly after birth may induce lasting immunity, while antibodies from the mother will still afford sufficient protection against the agent. The disastrous effects of smallpox, measles and influenza upon the Amerindian are well known, as is the susceptibility of the European to yellow fever; nevertheless, the survivors of the latter disease were able to withstand the rigours of subsequent epidemics in the Caribbean whereas otherwise healthy newcomers fell victims to yellow fever. This has always been an axiom among settlers in the Antilles. Therefore the study of titration tests in the geographical distribution of yellow fever antibodies among the aboriginal population both of America and Africa, carries considerable weight when interpreted in the light of the primary sources for historical research.

Lopez de Cogolludo (1688) in his classical description of the yellow fever epidemic in Yucatan during 1648 confirms that the disease attacked the most robust and healthy Spaniards with additional violence and carried them off very quickly, but that the Maya Indians were not affected; this has been interpreted by Carter (1931) to imply that the disease centred principally in the towns and did not spread to outlying villages (Carter 1931). With the disappearance of the Tainos, Siboneyes and Caribs from the Antilles it is difficult to find medical observations referring to them, but Pouppé-Desportes (1770) and Cardanne (1784) both indicate that yellow fever very rarely attacked the Caribs and the Creoles in St. Domingue. The apparent immunity of the Negro to yellow fever in the Antilles has been reported by several historians. Moreau de St. Méry (1784), in referring to Limonade, St. Domingue, observed that mortality from yellow fever among the French soldiers was extremely high, but was practically nil among the Negroes. During the yellow fever epidemic of Philadelphia in 1793, thought to have followed upon infection by the French immigrants from St. Domingue, the general belief was that the Negroes were immune, and some coloured groups played an important rôle in the sanitary measures taken during the epidemic. Lempriere (1799), surveying the public health of Spanish Town,

Jamaica, also noted that slaves and free Negroes enjoyed much better health than did the white population and the permanent residents. Valentin (1803), who was chief physician in the St. Domingue Army and subsequently, after the 1793 débâcle, head of the French hospital in Norfolk, Virginia, found very few Negroes affected by yellow fever. Similar references are frequently encountered in other 19th century medical texts.

The widespread belief in the Negro's immunity to yellow fever and the greater susceptibility of the white man in the face of the same epidemic, carried considerable weight in important colonial decisions years later, despite Negro revolts and fears of massacre. It would be wise to remember that the authorities in French and English colonies in the Antilles not only forbade Negroes to carry any weapon, but prohibited, by detailed legislation, their handling toxic drugs because of the possibility that the slaves might avail themselves of the opportunity to poison their masters and their domestic animals, which in fact frequently happened. The Negro mutiny at St. John in 1733 and the Jamaican maroon war of 1734, made the British colonies apprehend that the rate of loss among European troops would eventually lead to the Negro people controlling the Antilles by virtue of resistance to epidemic disease and sheer numerical force. The *Journals of the Assembly of Jamaica* (1794) carry the record that as early as 1782 a planter, William H. Ricketts, proposed a plan to raise a corps of free coloured people for the internal defence of Jamaica, and thus became the first commander of the Prince of Wales's Corps of free Mulattoes, which was later disbanded when peace was declared. In 1794 Ricketts repeated his proposal for 358 coloured troops under 30 white commissioned officers, including one surgeon and two mates, and this set the pattern for future colonial troops in the Caribbean. In Jamaica coloured Rangers or Black Shots were recruited and in 1795 the British Government finally authorised the raising of the two West India Regiments (Jamaica Assembly 1794). At St. Vincent the Negro slaves who fought with the British against the French and Caribs were enrolled in the St. Vincent Rangers, who were later incorporated with the 2nd West India Regiment. These troops soon proved so valuable where white troops succumbed to sickness that the number of Negro regiments with white officers was increased to twelve. During the second Maroon war of 1795 in Jamaica, the Negro troops were provided with a strange ally, for the British Governor, Lord Balcarres, asked for 40 Spanish dog-handlers from Cuba with 100 mastiffs to hunt down Maroons. This measure was hotly criticized in London, but it produced immediate results and the Maroons surrendered, although until that time they had been murdering whites and plundering plantations (Burns 1954). Quite early on Moreau de Jonnés (1817) appreciated the full implication of the British policy of using Negro troops, even though the French political environment made it impossible to follow suit and in any event it was too late to apply the system in St. Domingue and other colonies already lost. Nevertheless, his tables are worth reproducing, as the mortality figures of white and Negro troops show considerable differences (Moreau de Jonnés 1817).

MORTALITY RATES PER 100 TROOPS AMONG FRENCH AND BRITISH TROOPS IN THE ANTILLES 1796 - 1807.

| | French Antilles | | | British Antilles | |
| | Mar- | Guade- | | Euro- | |
Year	tinque	loupe	Year	peans	African
1802	57	60	1796	40¼	3
1803	44	46	1797	32¼	4
1804	30	29	1798	17½	8
1805	40	49	1799	11¼	7½
1806	8¼	10	1800	15½	6¼
1807	10⅓	15	1801	22¼	6
			1802	22	5

From Moreau de Jonnés 1817

MORTALITY AMONG FRENCH AND BRITISH TROOPS IN THE ANTILLES 1796 - 1807.

French Antilles

| | Martinque | | Guadeloupe | |
Year	Effectives	Dead	Effectives	Dead
1802	884	507	3126	1889
1803	1156	511	3530	1163
1804	1291	389	2131	616
1805	2493	996	2676	1094
1806	2588	214	2514	249
1807	2673	276	2286	346

British Antilles

| | European troops | | African troops | |
Year	Effectives	Dead	Effectives	Dead
1796	15881	6484	2495	75
1797	11503	3766	3080	118
1798	8416	1602	3055	252
1799	7202	876	3354	258
1800	7890	1221	4320	286
1801	10315	2340	4604	276
1802	9038	940	3840	199

From Moreau de Jonnès 1817

Corollary

A survey of Caribbean medical history affords many important lessons. Each of the racial groups in the West Indies was affected by disease in a different way. The principal factor in the extermination of the Amerindian in the Antilles was the spread of virus diseases, such as smallpox, influenza and measles, which were imported by the Europeans. In turn the latter were particularly ravaged by another virus, and epidemics of yellow fever played a dominant part in determining the outcome of military operations initiated by the colonizing powers, and the colonies themselves. By the 18th century the Negroes had become, by reason of sheer numerical force, the most important racial group in the Antilles. Furthermore, by dint of his greater resistance to attacks of yellow fever the Negro provided, paradoxically, the backbone of the colonial army in the British West Indies, and thus set a practicable pattern of military establishment which furnished the means for a continuancy of slavery in the Caribbean, and of colonial dominion by European powers for decades to come.

References

BURNS, SIR ALAN. *History of the British West Indies*. London, G. Allen & Unwin Ltd., 1964. 4°, 821 p. illust.

CARTER, HENRY ROSE. *Yellow Fever. An epidemiological and historical study of its place of origin*. Baltimore, The Williams & Wilkinson Co., 1931. 4°, xii, 312 p. illust.

CHAIA, JEAN. Echec d'une tentative de la colonisation de la Guyane au XVIIIᵉ siecle. Etude médicale de l'expédition du Kourou, 1763 - 1764. *La Biologie médicale*, Paris 47 (4), 1 - 83, 1958.

CORNILLIAC, JEAN JACQUES JULES. *Etudes sur la Fièvre Jaune à la Martinique de 1669 à nos jours*. Fort de France, Imp. du Gouvernement, 1873. 8°, 791, 54 p. tables.

CROUSE, NELLIS M. *The French struggle for the West Indies. 1665 - 1754*. New York, Columbia University Press, 1943. 4° (4) 1. 324 p. plates, map.

DANCER, THOMAS. *A brief history of the late expedition against Fort San Juan*. Kingston, D. Douglass and W. Aikman, 1781. Folio, 63 p.

DESGENETTES, RENE NICOLAS DUFRICHE BARON. *Histoire médicale de l'armée d'Orient*. Paris, Croullebois & Bossange, 1802. 8°, 2 vols.

DU TERTRE, JEAN BAPTISTE. *Histoire générale des Antilles habitées par les Francois*. Paris, T. Jolly, 1667 - 1671, in 4°, 3 vols.

EDWARDS, BRYAN. *The history, civil and commercial, of the West Indies*. 5th edition. London, Whittaker and others, 1819. 4°, 5 vols.

FORTESCUE, SIR JOHN WILLIAM. *A history of the British Army*. London, Macmillan & Co. Ltd., 1899 - 1930. 4°, 13 vols. maps.

GASTELBONDO, JUAN JOSE DE. *Tratado del methodo curativo, experimentado, y aprobado de la enfermedad del Vómito Negro, epidémico, y frequente en los puertos de las Indias Occidentales*. [Madrid], s.n. [1755]. 8° [4] 1. 61 p.

GILBERT, NICOLAS PIERRE. *Histoire médicale de l'armée française à Saint-Domingue en l'an 10, ou memoire sur la Fièvre Jaune, avec un apperçu de la topographie médicale de cette colonie*. Paris, Gabon et Co., an 11 [1803]. 8°, 103 p.

GODECHOT, JACQUES. *La grande nation, l'expansion révolutionaire de la France dans le monde, 1789 - 1799*. Paris, Ed. Montaigne, 956. 4°, 2 vols.

GUERRA, FRANCISCO. *Historiografia de la Medicina Colonial Hispano-Americana*. México, Abastecedora de Impresos, 1953. 4°, 324 p.

GUERRA, FRANCISCO. Drugs from the Indies and the Political Economy of the sixteenth century. *Analecta Medico-Historica*, I, 29 - 54, 1965.

HUMBOLDT, FRIEDRICH H. ALEXANDER, BARON VON. *Essai politique sur l'Ile de Cuba, avec une carte, et un supplément qui renferme des considerations sur la population, la richesse territoriale et le commerce de l'Archipel des Antilles et de Colombia*. Paris, Gide fils, 1826 - 1827. 8°, 2 vols. 818 p. 1 map.

JAMAICA, ASSEMBLY. *Journals of the Assembly of Jamaica, from January the 20th, 1663 - 4* (to 22nd December, 1826). Jamaica, A. Aikman, 1811 - 1829. Folio, 14 vols.

KEEVIL, JOHN J., LLOYD, CHRISTOPHER and COULTER, JACK L. S. *Medicine and the Navy 1200 - 1900*. Edinburgh, E. & S. Livingstone Ltd., 1957 - 1963. 4°, 4 vols.

LEMPRIERE, WILLIAM. *Practical observations on the diseases of the Army in Jamaica, as they occurred between the years 1792 and 1797*. London, T. N. Longman and O. Rees, 1799. 8°, 2 vols.

LEON, RULX. *Les maladies en Haiti*. Port-au-Prince, Imprimerie de l'Etat, 1954. 8°, xxxiv, 345 p.

METRAL, ANTOINE MARIE THERESE. *Histoire de l'expédition des Francais à Saint-Domingue, sous le consulat de Napoléon Bonaparte*. Paris, Fanjat aîné, 1825. 4°, xii, 348 p. port. map.

MIMS, STEWARD L. *Colbert's West India policy*. New Haven, Conn., Yale University Press, 1912. 4°, xviii, 385 p.

MOREAU DE JONNES, ALEXANDRE, Observations pour servir à l'histoire de la Fièvre Jaune des Antilles; suivies de tables de la mortalité des troupes Européennes dans les Indes-Occidentales. *Bulletin de la Societé médicale d'Emulation*. Paris, 6, 237 - 247, 1817.

MOREAU DE JONNES, ALEXANDRE. *Essai sur l'Hygiène militaire des Antilles*. Paris, Impr. de Migueret, 1816. 8°, 83 p.

MOREAU DE SAINT MERY, MEDERIC LOUIS ELIE. *Description topographique, physique, civile, politique et historique de la partie francaise de l'Isle Saint-Domingue*. Paris, Librairie Larose, 1958. 4° xlviii, 1565 p. illus., 3 vols.

MOSELEY, BENJAMIN. *A treatise on tropical diseases; on military operations; and on the climate of the West Indies*. London, T. Cadell, 1787. 8°, xix, 544 p.

PARRY, J. H. and SHERLOCK, P. M. *A short history of the West Indies*. London, Macmillan & Co. Ltd., 1956. 4°, xii, 316 p. illust.

PRESSOIR, CATTS. *La Médicine en Haiti*. Port-au-Prince, Imprimerie Modèle, 1927. 8°, xii, 254 [2] p.

SCOTT, H. HAROLD. *A history of Tropical Medicine*. London, Edward Arnold & Co., 1938. 4°, 2 vols.

8

Fear of Hot Climates in the Anglo-American Colonial Experience

Karen Ordahl Kupperman

ENGLISH people contemplating transplantation to the southern parts of North America and to the West Indies in the sixteenth and seventeenth centuries expressed profound anxiety over the effect hot climates would have on them. Heat and the environment it engendered were expected to be alien and even hostile to men and women from England's temperate climate. This article is a study of the interaction between perception and reality, particularly of the way in which evidence was interpreted to sustain the preconceptions English colonists brought with them. The settlers' health fared badly in both the southern mainland colonies and the West Indies. This fact confirmed their expectations and contributed important evidence that hardened generalized anxieties into medical dogma by the eighteenth century. The link between weather and disease then became axiomatic. In 1598 George Wateson, drawing on his experience as a merchant in Spain, wrote "the first working textbook of tropical diseases," which warned of the diseases engendered by "intemperate Climats."[1] From that time through the colonial period, excessive heat was seen as the major reason for southern sickliness.[2]

Early modern science taught that human beings and their native physical environment normally existed in a state of ecological harmony. That is, the human constitution was responsive to and shaped by climate, air, and diet. It followed that men and women who had been bred in England were unsuited to environments that were radically different, such as those of the

[1] David Beers Quinn, *England and the Discovery of America, 1481-1620* . . . (New York, 1974), 206; George Wateson, *The Cures of the Diseased, in Remote Regions* . . . (London, 1598), sig. B and *passim*.

[2] Gary Puckrein, "Climate, Health and Black Labor in the English Americas," *Journal of American Studies*, XIII (1979), 179-193. For a vivid example of the association of heat and unhealthiness see Sir George Yeardley to Sir Edwin Sandys, June 7, 1620, in Susan Myra Kingsbury, ed., *The Records of the Virginia Company of London*, 4 vols. (Washington, D.C., 1906-1935), III, 298, hereafter cited as *Va. Company Recs*.

southern regions of the New World, with their heats and damps and different dietary regimens. Consequently, those who ventured to such places, stayed there, and ate the indigenous foods risked sickness in the short run and a drastic change in physiology and psychology in the long run as their bodies responded to the new environment.

This line of thought was supported by the medical science of the day based on the Hippocratic theory of the four humors. The four elements, air, fire, earth, and water, were believed to be represented in the human body by the humors blood, yellow bile or choler, phlegm, and black bile or melancholy. Good health resulted from the proper balance of these humors, but each climate created its own characteristic balance. Therefore a move to a radically different climate could cause profound distress while the body tried to adjust. Choler, corresponding to fire, predominated in hot areas: "That Choler abounds between the Tropicks, is but reasonable as well as matter of fact; for the inflaming Sun must needs kindle its like in its neerest Subjects." The body, by its various discharges or excretions, would rid itself of an excess of one or more humors: thus the "bloody flux" that afflicted so many colonists indicated an attempt to achieve the proper amount of blood.[3]

The royalist Richard Ligon fled England in 1647 and spent three years in Barbados where he was a keen and witty observer of the scene. Ligon described his first encounter with the heat of the West Indies, saying that it was hardly to be believed that one from a cold climate could "indure such scorching without being suffocated." He and his companions felt as if they were being "fricased" and experienced "great failing in the vigour, and sprightliness we have in colder Climates." Conversely, Richard Hakluyt marveled that "borne naturalles" of Japan and the Philippines could live in England.[4] Sir William Vaughan, author of several medical

---

[3] Thomas Trapham, *A Discourse of the State of Health in the Island of Jamaica* (London, 1679), 84; William Vaughan, *Approved Directions for Health, Both Naturall and Artificiall*, 4th ed. (London, 1612), 84, 120; John Hammond, *Leah and Rachel, or, the Two Fruitfull Sisters Virginia and Maryland* . . . (1656), in Peter Force, comp., *Tracts and Other Papers, Relating Principally to the Origin, Settlement, and Progress of the Colonies in North America* . . . , 4 vols. (Washington, D.C., 1836-1847), III, No. 14, 10; John Lawson, *A New Voyage to Carolina* . . . (London, 1709), 18-19; John Smith, *The Generall Historie of Virginia, New England, and the Summer Isles*, in Edward Arber and A. G. Bradley, eds., *Travels and Works of Captain John Smith* . . . , 2 vols. (Edinburgh, 1910), II, 565; *Va. Company Recs.*, III, 455; Clarence J. Glacken, *Traces on the Rhodian Shore: Nature and Culture in Western Thought from Ancient Times to the End of the Eighteenth Century* (Berkeley, Calif., 1967), 10-12; Lester S. King, *The Growth of Medical Thought* (Chicago, 1963), 30-31; Richard S. Dunn, *Sugar and Slaves: The Rise of the Planter Class in the English West Indies, 1624-1713* (Chapel Hill, N.C., 1972), 309.

[4] Ligon, *A True and Exact History of the Island of Barbados* (London, 1673 [orig. publ. 1657]), 9-10, 27, 45; Hakluyt, "Epistle Dedicatory" to *The Principall Navigations, Voiages and Discoveries of the English Nation* . . . (1589), in E.G.R. Taylor, ed., *The Original Writings and Correspondence of the Two Richard Hakluyts*, 2 vols. (London, 1935), II, 400.

tracts, expressed the prevailing view: "That which is a mans native soyle, and Countries ayre is best. This by the Philosophers is approved in this principle: Every mans naturall place preserveth him, which is placed in it." Vaughan thought a European could not live near the equator for more than five years.[5]

Change in the balance of the humors may have been what was meant by use of the word *seasoning* to describe the acclimatization of an English person, a process commonly lasting about two years and thought necessary even in southern New England.[6] It was generally believed that the adjustment involved paling and thinning of the blood. William Wood, who was in the vanguard of Massachusetts Bay colonists, said that English traders from Virginia whom he saw in New England were very pale, which he attributed to the drying up of their blood. Since incessant sweating was for many the most remarkable feature of life in a southern climate, the term may have been adopted as an analogy to the seasoning or drying out of wood.[7]

The fear of hot climates was exaggerated in the early years of colonization because Europeans did not realize that the climate of eastern North America was quite different from what their knowledge of climates in comparable latitudes in western Europe led them to expect. Since Newfoundland lies south of London, and Virginia is at the latitude of Spain, promoters expected colonists to face extreme heat in almost all plantations. There was little knowledge of the dynamics of climate and of the effects of the movement of the atmosphere from west to east, which makes the weather on the east coasts of continents so different from that on the west.[8]

People considering or promoting emigration feared effects extending beyond the initial period of adjustment, specifically the possibility that in leaving England they might be leaving their Englishness also, running the risk of becoming more like the Spaniard, whom they perceived as choleric and untrustworthy. The English saw themselves as moderate people living in a moderate climate, and they had firm opinions about the character types produced by the extremes. A late sixteenth-century commentary on colonial plans asserted that a cold climate "brings forth a dull inflexible

[5] Vaughan, *Directions for Health*, 4th ed., 2, 8. By the sixth edition in 1626 he had raised his estimate to 15 years. See also his *The Newlanders Cure* (London, 1630), 6, and John Kirtland Wright, *The Geographical Lore of the Time of the Crusades: A Study in the History of Medieval Science and Tradition in Western Europe* (New York, 1925), 180.

[6] William Hubbard, *A General History of New England from the Discovery to 1680*, 2d ed. (Boston, 1848), 324-325.

[7] William Wood, *New Englands Prospect . . .* (London, 1634), 8; Ligon, *History of Barbados*, 27, 67. David Harris Sacks suggested this possible connection of the two uses of "seasoning" to me in April 1980.

[8] These issues are fully discussed and documented in Karen Ordahl Kupperman, "The Puzzle of the American Climate in the Early Colonial Period," *American Historical Review*, LXXXVII (1982), 1262-1289.

people, obstinately affectinge barbarous liberty & Jelous of all aucthority." Edward Johnson of Massachusetts Bay, on the other hand, believed the perpetual summer of the tropics produced liberty run mad to the point of license. Sir Ferdinando Gorges wrote that people in cold climates were duller than the "sharper wits" of hot countries but had stronger physical constitutions and were capable of having more children. Therefore, though "the invention of Arts hath risen from Southern Nations," those nations had been repeatedly invaded by more hardy and numerous northern peoples.[9]

The conventional wisdom about the effect of hot climates on English constitutions is illustrated by the story of Nicholas Leverton and Hope Sherrard. Leverton had been a minister in the West Indies. Finally he was overcome by "a fit of sickness" and his friends in Bermuda "thought adviseable he should return to England and try his native air." He landed at Sandwich and, as he was preparing to ride to London, the ostler said to him, "Mr. ———, you are somewhat like our minister: I believe you have lived in the hot countries as well as he." In this way Leverton was reunited with Sherrard, who had been his colleague in the Puritan colony at Providence Island. This story is striking because Sherrard had been back in England for several years, yet apparently retained some characteristic look of the tropics. When Leverton settled in England, he named his son Gershom, because he, like Moses, could say: "I have been a stranger in a strange land." For the rest of his life, according to his biographer, "he was subject to warm passions, but they were soon over."[10]

The general agreement that English people would be healthiest in the temperate climates they were used to was frequently offered as a reason to concentrate colonization efforts on New England and Newfoundland. Gorges argued that New England was "more suitable to the nature of our people, who neither finde content in the colder Climates, nor health in the hotter; but (as hearbs and plants) affect their native temperature, and prosper kindly no where else." Edward Hayes and Christopher Carleill, Elizabethan "Projectors," argued that the summer heat of all European places below forty degrees of latitude "is unto our boddies offensyve, Which cannot prosper in dry and scalding heates. more naturall to the Spaniard than us."[11] On the basis of such reasoning Lord Baltimore first

[9] David B. Quinn et al., eds., New American World: A Documentary History of North America to 1612, 5 vols. (New York, 1979), III, 173; Edward Johnson, Wonder-Working Providence of Sions Saviour in New-England (Andover, Mass., 1867 [orig. publ. London, 1654]), 171; Ferdinando Gorges, A Briefe Relation of the Discovery and Plantation of New England (1622), in James Phinney Baxter, ed., Sir Ferdinando Gorges and His Province of Maine, 3 vols. (New York, 1967 [orig. publ. 1890]), I, 228-229.

[10] Edmund Calamy, The Nonconformist's Memorial . . . , 2d ed. (London, 1778), I, 290-295. Calamy rendered Sherrard's name as Sherwood.

[11] Gorges, Briefe Relation, in Baxter, ed., Gorges and Province of Maine, I, 228; [Edward Hayes and Christopher Carleill], "A Discourse concerning a Voyage Intended for the Planting of Chrystyan Religion and People in the North West

decided to found his colony at Ferryland in Newfoundland. After he and his family spent "one intolerable wynter" there, he petitioned the king for land farther south. Baltimore was not prepared to go on with the northern experiment despite Sir William Vaughan's allegation that he had chosen the coldest harbor of the island.[12]

From the 1630s on, propagandists for southern colonies began to stress that the places they promoted lay between the extremes of northern cold and southern heat and therefore would have the riches of hot areas without their evils. Such an argument was made for Maryland.[13] Carolina was also said to experience "a moderate equality of heat and cold between the two violent extreams thereof in *Barbadoes* and *New England*."[14]

The sun and its heat figured prominently in early English thinking about colonization, and in a profoundly ambivalent way. Fear of hot climates was balanced by the belief that the sun was the source of riches. Despite the widespread conviction that English people would sicken and possibly die in hot climates, the majority of those interested in America went or were sent to the southern regions instead of New England or Newfoundland. Early modern science taught that there was a direct trade off between heat and abundance. The sun had a complex relationship with the earth, not only providing warmth but also drawing substances up out of the earth and water. Its purifying power resulted from its attracting poisonous vapors.

Richard Ligon held that the diseases that raged through the Barbadian settlements were partly caused by colonists' faulty reasoning about the sun's role. For example, a pond in which clothes were washed and slaves

---

Regions of America in Places Most Apt for the Constitution of Our Boddies, and the Spedy Advauncement of a State" (1592), in Quinn *et al.*, eds., *New American World*, III, 158-159. Quinn sees "projectors," men who generated speculative schemes of various types, as typical of the Elizabethan period (*Discovery of America*, 232).

[12] George Calvert, Lord Baltimore, to Sir Francis Cottington, Aug. 18, 1629, in Lawrence C. Wroth, "Tobacco or Codfish: Lord Baltimore Makes His Choice," New York Public Library, *Bulletin*, LVIII (1954), 527-534; Baltimore to King Charles I, Aug. 19, 1629, in J. Thomas Scharf, *History of Maryland from the Earliest Period to the Present Day*, 3 vols. (Baltimore, 1879), I, 44-45; Vaughan, *Newlanders Cure*, 68-69.

[13] [Andrew White], "An Account of the Colony of the Lord Baron of Baltimore, 1633," in Clayton Colman Hall, ed., *Narratives of Early Maryland, 1633-1684* (New York, 1910), 7, and "A Briefe Relation of the Voyage unto Maryland, by Father Andrew White, 1634," *ibid.*, 39; Hammond, *Leah and Rachel*, in Force, comp., *Tracts*, III, No. 14, 8, 22; [Beauchamp Plantagenet], *A Description of the Province of New Albion . . .* (1648), *ibid.*, II, No. 7, 6; William Bullock, *Virginia Impartially Examined, and Left to Publick View, to Be Considered by All Judicious and Honest Men* (London, 1649), 4, 32; "Narrative of a Voyage to Maryland, 1705-1706," *AHR*, XII (1907), 329.

[14] E[dward] W[illiams], *Virginia: More Especially the South Part Thereof, Richly and Truly Valued . . .* (1650), in Force, comp., *Tracts*, III, No. 11, 8, 28, 57-58.

bathed after their day's labor was also a source of drinking water. When questioned about the practice, planters explained "that the Sunne with his virtuall heat, drawes up all noysome vapours, and so the waters become rarified, and pure again." Ligon, unconvinced, took his water from a small stream apart. In this case a smattering of scientific knowledge served the colonists badly. Though they had daily and personal experience of the power of the sun, their education caused them to misjudge its efficacy.[15]

The sun's action was also thought to nurture gold, silver, and precious stones within the earth and draw them to the surface: "the influens of the sonne doth norishe and bryng fourth gold, spices, stones and perles." Valuable metals and gems would be found in abundance only in very hot areas.[16] Even where mineral wealth did not materialize, the "Sun with his masculine force" would produce other kinds of riches from the "teeming" feminine earth, for the hottest climate was also the most fruitful.[17] Colonists marveled at how swiftly crops came to fruition, leading to claims of "incredible usurie" in increase as well as multiple harvests every year. From New England to the West Indies, the great heat of the summer was seen as the source of American abundance.[18]

Not only could the plants found in each area be developed, but promoters of early southern colonies argued from fallacious reasoning about the relationship of climate and latitude that plants from many different regions should be introduced and would surely grow in the southern mainland as well as the West Indies. Early Virginia pamphlets promised that the colony would produce oranges and lemons, sugarcane, almonds, rice, and anise, all of which grew in areas where "the sunne is so neerer a neighbour." This reasoning was supported by Caribbean writers such as Ligon who pointed out that sugar was not natural to Barbados but had become, after its introduction, the "soul of Trade" there. Even after

[15] Ligon, History of Barbados, 25, 28; Vaughan, Directions for Health, 6th ed., 14. More striking is Ligon's report that some people continued to drink the water of a bog into which corpses from an epidemic in Bridgetown had been thrown. Those who did died quickly.

[16] Roger Barlow, A Brief Summe of Geographie (1540-1541), ed. E.G.R. Taylor (London, 1932), 179-180; "Commentary on Hayes-Carleill Project," in Quinn et al., eds., New American World, III, 174; [Richard] Eden, "To the Reader," A Treatyse of the Newe India . . . after the Descripcion of Sebastian Munster . . . (1553), in Edward Arber, ed., The First Three English Books on America (Birmingham, Eng., 1885), 7.

[17] Va. Company Recs., III, 220; Ligon, History of Barbados, 84; George Best, "Experiences and Reasons of the Sphere, to Proove All Partes of the Worlde Habitable . . ." (1578), in Richard Hakluyt, The Principal Navigations, Voyages, Traffiques and Discoveries of the English Nation, 12 vols. (Glasgow, 1903-1905 [orig. publ. London, 1598-1600]), VII, 254-255, 266-267.

[18] [Virginia Company], A True Declaration of the Estate of the Colonie in Virginia . . . (1610), in Force, comp., Tracts, III, No. 1, 12-13, and A Declaration of the State of the Colonie and Affaires in Virginia . . . (1620), ibid., No. 5, 4-5; Hubbard, History of New England, 20-21.

such hopes were dashed in Virginia, promoters of Carolina continued to argue that their colony would produce anything grown in the same latitude anywhere in the world.[19] Reports agreed that in the warm colonies both humans and domesticated animals grew larger and experienced more multiple births than in Europe.[20]

There was another side to this picture of superabundance: the sun was so powerful that the planters had to guard their crops and persons against it. Dr. Thomas Trapham, Jamaica physician and member of the General Assembly, wrote that the land in the Jamaican mountains was fertile because it was shaded from the "fierce Rapes of the fiery Phoebus," but that the land around "St. Jago" was poor even for grazing, "the soyle having so long [lain] open to the sterilating Sun." The cacao planters put plantains among their trees to protect them from "the preying sun." Ligon and William Bullock pointed to similar dangers and strategies in Barbados and Virginia.[21] Nor did the sun discriminate in the kind of vegetation it encouraged. Weeds threatened to choke the crops, and thick tangles of vines could appear overnight. Another reservation about the excessive fruitfulness of the south lay in the conviction that the soil would be much more quickly worn out. It was as though any piece of land had only so

[19] [Va. Company], *True Declaration of Estate*, in Force, comp., *Tracts*, III, No. 1, 22; W[illiams], *Virginia Richly and Truly Valued, ibid.*, No. 11, 7-8, 11, 20-29; *A Perfect Description of Virginia* . . . (1649), *ibid.*, II, No. 8, 6, 12; [Plantagenet], *Description of New Albion, ibid.*, No. 7, 32-33; Thomas Hariot, *A Briefe and True Report of the New Found Land of Virginia* . . . (1588), in David Beers Quinn, ed., *The Roanoke Voyages, 1584-1590*, 2 vols. (London, 1955), I, 325; Samuel Purchas, "Virginian Affaires since the Yeere 1620. till This Present 1624," in his *Hakluytus Posthumus or Purchas His Pilgrimes* . . . , 20 vols. (Glasgow, 1906 [orig. publ. London, 1625]), XIX, 147, hereafter cited as Purchas, *Pilgrimes*, and "Virginias Verger . . . ," *ibid.*, 242-243; Hakluyt, "Epistle Dedicatory," to *Principal Navigations*, in Taylor, ed., *Writings and Correspondence*, II, 456; Edward Waterhouse, *A Declaration of the State of the Colony and Affaires in Virginia* . . . (London, 1622), 3-5, 31-32; Daniel Price, *Sauls Prohibition Staide* . . . (London, 1609), sig. F2; "The Discription of the Now Discovered River and Country of Virginia . . ." (1607), in Philip L. Barbour, ed., *The Jamestown Voyages under the First Charter, 1607-1609*, 2 vols. (Cambridge, 1969), I, 100; Patrick Copland, *Virginia's God Be Thanked* . . . (London, 1622), 12-13; Bullock, *Virginia Impartially Examined*, 31-32; Ligon, *History of Barbados*, 84-85; Lawson, *New Voyage to Carolina*, 79; Samuel Wilson, *An Account of the Province of Carolina* (1682), in Alexander S. Salley, Jr., *Narratives of Early Carolina, 1650-1708* (New York, 1911), 175; Robert Horne (?), *A Brief Description of the Province of Carolina* . . . (1666), *ibid.*, 69.

[20] See, for example, John Pory in *Va. Company Recs.*, III, 221; [Va. Company], *State of the Colonie*, in Force, comp., *Tracts*, III, No. 5, 5; Richard Norwood, "The Description of the Sommer Islands, Once Called the Bermudas," in Wesley Frank Craven and Walter B. Hayward, eds., *The Journal of Richard Norwood, Surveyor of Virginia* (New York, 1945), lxxx-lxxxi; and Lawson, *New Voyage to Carolina*, 80-81.

[21] Trapham, *State of Health in Jamaica*, 19, 24, 35; Ligon, *History of Barbados*, 20; Bullock, *Virginia Impartially Examined*, 3.

much allotted fertility, so that if it was particularly abundant, it would sooner become barren.[22] Finally, the generative power of the sun was seen as producing great corruption and putrefaction as well as great abundance; generation and putrefaction inevitably occurred together.[23]

The sun was thought to be especially dangerous for people not used to laboring in its heat. English writers were preoccupied with the question of how a human body changes when introduced into a hot climate. In fact, the body's physiology does change as it becomes acclimatized. The process greatly lessens the strain on the cardiovascular system caused by exposure to a very hot climate because an acclimatized body sheds heat to the environment much more efficiently, partly by dilatation of the blood vessels at the skin's surface, but mainly by the body's "learning" to sweat more quickly and freely. A person new to a very hot environment may sweat 1.5 liters per hour. Within ten days, the rate of sweating will have doubled, and it will reach two-and-one-half times as much within six weeks. Moreover, as the sweat glands become more efficient, the salt content of the sweat is reduced because of the increased secretion of aldosterone. The amount of salt lost in sweat will fall from a peak of 15 to 20 grams per day to 3.5 grams within six weeks of continuous exposure to a hot environment. The acclimatized person has an increased volume of plasma and may have a lower metabolism. Acclimatization is most dramatic in its effects if accompanied by increased physical fitness through moderate exercise. The process reverses itself within three to four weeks after exposure ends, though people who have spent their entire lives in very warm climates have more sweat glands than those from temperate areas, some of whose sweat glands cease to be active in late childhood.[24]

Seventeenth-century observers recognized some of these physiological changes. Ligon may have been pointing to a rise in plasma volume when he said that colonists' blood was paler and thinner in Barbados than it would have been in England. Scientists and settlers knew that the function of the sweating mechanism is to conduct heat from the interior of the body to the outside, but they worried about the result of the process because they

[22] See Philip Bell, governor of Bermuda, to Sir Nathaniel Rich in Arthur Percival Newton, *The Colonising Activities of the English Puritans: The Last Phase of the Elizabethan Struggle with Spain* (New Haven, Conn., 1914), 31-34, and Gov. Samuel Argall to the Virginia Company, Mar. 10, 1617/18, in *Va. Company Recs.*, III, 92. See also Ligon, *History of Barbados*, 69-72, and Dunn, *Sugar and Slaves*, 223.

[23] Best, "Experiences and Reasons of the Sphere," in Hakluyt, *Principal Navigations*, VII, 265. See *Hamlet*, Act II, sc. 2, line 181, for a remark about the sun breeding maggots in a dead dog.

[24] A. R. Lind, "Human Tolerance to Hot Climates," in Douglas H. K. Lee, ed., *Handbook of Physiology*, Section 9, *Reactions to Environmental Agents* (Bethesda, Md., 1977), 93-109; Vernon B. Mountcastle, ed., *Medical Physiology*, 13th ed. (St. Louis, Mo., 1974), II, 1315, 1338-1340; Arthur C. Guyton, *Textbook of Medical Physiology*, 5th ed. (Philadelphia, 1976), 958-960, 967; Robert G. Stone, "Health in Tropical Climates," in *Climate and Man*, Yearbook of Agriculture (Washington, D.C., 1941), 251, 254-255; Jan O. M. Broek, "Climate and Future Settlement," *ibid.*, 231.

believed that "great sweating" left the "inner parts," particularly the stomach, cold and debilitated. They attributed loss of appetite in hot regions to weakness in the stomach: "how can you expect to find heat, or warmth in your stomack, to digest that meat, when the sunne has exhausted your heat and spirits so, to your outer parts, as you are chill'd and numb'd within?"[25] Finally, the whole body became weak and listless. As a remedy, colonists in the tropics, supported by the best science of the time, turned to drinking "strong spirits" and eating hot peppers to warm their insides. Sir Henry Colt, an East Anglian gentleman who emigrated to St. Christopher's in 1630, spent two weeks in Barbados, where he went from drinking "2. dramms of hott water a meale, to 30." He thought he would have gone to 60 drams if he had stayed.[26]

The Spanish physician Nicholas Monardes wrote one of the earliest treatises on New World plants and their properties. His book, which was translated into English in 1577, became a standard work on American diseases and their cure. Monardes endorsed the medicinal use of chili pepper: "It dooeth comforte muche, it dooeth dissolve windes, it is good for the breaste, and for theim that bee colde of complexion: it dooeth heale and comforte, strengthenyng the principall members."[27] To some extent, the taking of chili peppers and alcohol in small amounts was a good adaptive strategy, but not for the reasons the colonists and their medical advisors thought. Though people feel warm after taking them, both promote a degree of hypothermia by increasing the flow of blood to the skin and promoting sweating. Both stimulate gastric secretions, and peppers also increase gastric muscular activity and can, as Monardes indicated, "facilitate the expulsion of gas." In addition, chili peppers are a particularly rich source of vitamins A, B1, and C, and for that reason are important in cultures that live on a high-cereal diet.[28]

Probably no English colonist ate chili peppers to excess, but too many

[25] Ligon, *History of Barbados*, 27, 102; Vaughan, *Directions for Health*, 4th ed., 129; Wood, *New Englands Prospect*, 8.

[26] "The Voyage of Sr Henrye Colt Knight to the Islands of the Antilleas . . ." (1631), in V. T. Harlow, ed., *Colonising Expeditions to the West Indies and Guiana, 1623-1667* (London, 1925), 66. See also John Josselyn, *An Account of Two Voyages to New England* (1675), Massachusetts Historical Society, *Collections*, 3d Ser., III (Boston, 1833), 242-243, and Vaughan, *Directions for Health*, 4th ed., 50. Vaughan thought strong drink was dangerous in the winter when the stomach was "abounding" with heat (*Newlanders Cure*, 70). Dunn gives a particularly vivid picture of social drinking in the 17th-century West Indies (*Sugar and Slaves*, esp. 276-281).

[27] Nicholas Monardes, *Joyfull Newes Out of the Newe Founde Worlde* (1577), trans. John Frampton, ed. Stephen Gaselee (London, 1925), I, 48, hereafter cited as Monardes, *Joyfull Newes*.

[28] Paul Rozin and Deborah Schiller, "The Nature and Acquisition of a Preference for Chili Pepper by Humans," *Motivation and Emotion*, IV (1980), 94; Paul Rozin, "The Use of Characteristic Flavorings in Human Culinary Practice," in Charles M. Apt, ed., *Flavor: Its Chemical, Behavioral, and Commercial Aspects* (Boulder, Colo., 1977), 111-113. See also Vaughan, *Newlanders Cure*, 30-31, and *Directions for Health*, 4th ed., 27.

did not limit themselves to moderate amounts of alcohol. Because the science of the day taught that "strong drink" (spirits) was essential to the digestion in hot weather, it was taken by all, being allotted even to servants and sometimes to slaves. But Caribbean writers agreed that immoderate consumption was a major cause of high disease and mortality rates there. Ligon said that drinking overheated the body, leading to "Costiveness and Tortions in the bowels; which is a disease very frequent there" and the cause of many deaths. He pointed out that ten times more men than women died in one epidemic; since "the men were the greater deboystes," their deaths were directly linked in his mind to overindulgence in spirits. Though Samuel Purchas held that it was the air of the Indies that produced contentiousness in men, most observers linked fighting to drinking and would have agreed with the anonymous *Briefe Discription of Barbados* that the country would be as temperate and wholesome as it was fertile "if the debaucht lives of the people did not prevent nature." As the Virginia Company put it, "well-governed men" live there healthfully.[29]

Robert Beverley, a native-born Virginia gentleman, wrote that the "Gripes is the Distemper of the *Caribbee* Islands." He may have been referring to the dreaded "dry bellyache" that caused "exquisite pain" and could lead to loss of function in the arms and legs. It may have been induced by drinking rum processed in lead pipes. Trapham very shrewdly compared the symptoms to those of cattle in fields around the lead works in Derby, where, he said, the cattle were poisoned by lead fumes. Despite this recognition, however, he thought that the dry bellyache was caused by "sudden contracting cold," which happens in hot areas and is worst when the moon is full. Beverley wrote that the "Gripes" appeared in Virginia only when people drank "filthy and unclean Drinks"; this apparently was occasioned by impatience to drink cider, perry, and beer before they were ready or by using too much lime juice and "foul Sugar in Punch and Flip."[30]

Sudden exposure to a hot climate was seen as particularly dangerous. Reports of all colonies from New England to the West Indies complained of the difficulty of working in the hot summer sun and of the vulnerability

[29] Ligon, *History of Barbados*, 21, 27, 93; Trapham, *State of Health in Jamaica*, 28; Samuel Purchas, *Purchas His Pilgrimage*, 2d ed. (London, 1614), 760; "A Briefe Discription of the Ilande of Barbados," in Harlow, ed., *Colonising Expeditions*, 43; *Va. Company Recs.*, II, 381. See also [Colt], "Voyage," in Harlow, ed., *Colonising Expeditions*, 65-66, 73, 93; *Memoirs of the First Settlement of the Island of Barbados, and Other the Carribbee Islands* (London, 1743), 33; and Antoine Biet, "Father Antoine Biet's Visit to Barbados in 1654." ed. Jerome S. Handler, in *Journal of the Barbados Museum and Historical Society*, XXXII (1966-1968), 62. "Costiveness" and "Tortions" refer to constipation with wringing, twisting intestinal pain.

[30] Beverley, *The History and Present State of Virginia* (1705), ed. Louis B. Wright (Chapel Hill, N.C., 1947), 306-307; Trapham, *State of Health in Jamaica*, 129-139; Hugh Jones, *The Present State of Virginia . . .* (1724), ed. Richard L. Morton (Chapel Hill, N.C., 1956), 85; Dunn, *Sugar and Slaves*, 217, 306.

of unseasoned English people to sickness or even death as a result of the sudden change of climate. John Winthrop recorded that many newcomers died in the hot summer of 1637, and William Bradford believed that the sun's piercing heat made unseasoned people sick. Many accounts of Virginia linked periods of high mortality to "intemperate" heat, a "Torride sommer," or the scorching rays of the sun. On Barbados one man's punishment of standing in the sun all day was "enough to pierce his braine."[31]

Heat stroke may have been the subject of two curious descriptions in which people were said to have been rendered gravely ill by their body's fat melting within them. In one case, described by George Percy in Nevis, the man died. In the other, in New England, the man recovered after about a week. Heat stroke is associated with failure of the sweating mechanism, the reason for which is not known. Symptoms are hot, dry skin and rising body temperature. Victims may be delirious, experience personality changes, and lose consciousness. They may appear to recover but then die of brain damage a few days later. The sinister image of a man's fat melting within him is an index of how threatening and alien hot climates were to early modern English people.[32]

[31] [John Winthrop], *Winthrop's Journal: History of New England, 1630-1649*, ed. James Kendall Hosmer, 2 vols. (New York, 1908), I, 223; William Bradford, *Of Plymouth Plantation, 1620-1647*, ed. Samuel Eliot Morison (New York, 1952), 28; Thomas Dudley to Lady Bridget, Countess of Lincoln, Mar. 12-28, 1631, in Everett Emerson, ed., *Letters from New England: The Massachusetts Bay Colony, 1629-1638* (Amherst, Mass., 1976), 76; Ligon, *History of Barbados*, 110; [Colt], "Voyage," in Harlow, ed., *Colonising Expeditions*, 75n, 98; *Va. Company Recs.*, I, 310, III, 220, 298; H. R. McIlwaine, ed., *Journals of the House of Burgesses of Virginia, 1619-1658/59* (Richmond, Va., 1915), 30; William Strachey, *The Historie of Travell into Virginia Britania*, ed. Louis B. Wright and Virginia Freund (London, 1953), 37-38; [John] Smith, *A Map of Virginia . . .* (1612), in Barbour, ed., *Jamestown Voyages*, II, 334. See also Andrew White, *A Briefe Relation of the Voyage unto Maryland* (1634), in Hall, ed., *Narratives of Early Maryland*, 35; Ferdinando Gorges the Younger, *America Painted to the Life* (London, 1658-1659), sig. A3; and Walter Raleigh, *The Discoverie of the Large and Bewtiful Empire of Guiana* (1598), ed. Vincent T. Harlow (London, 1928), 40. For modern discussion of the issues involved see Dunn, *Sugar and Slaves*, esp. chaps. 8, 9; Darrett B. Rutman and Anita H. Rutman, "Of Agues and Fevers: Malaria in the Early Chesapeake," *William and Mary Quarterly*, 3d Ser., XXXIII (1976), 31-60; Carville V. Earle, "Environment, Disease, and Mortality in Early Virginia," in Thad W. Tate and David L. Ammerman, eds., *The Chesapeake in the Seventeenth Century: Essays on Anglo-American Society* (Chapel Hill, N.C., 1979), 96-125; Thomas P. Hughes, *Medicine in Virginia, 1607-1699* (Williamsburg, Va., 1957); and Karen Ordahl Kupperman, "Apathy and Death in Early Jamestown," *Journal of American History*, LXVI (1979), 24-40.

[32] Percy, *Observations Gathered Out of a Discourse* (1607), in Purchas, *Pilgrimes*, XVIII, 406-407; Josselyn, *Account of Two Voyages*, Mass. Hist. Soc., *Colls.*, 3d Ser., III, 264. For heat exhaustion and heat stroke see Lind, "Human Tolerance to Hot Climates," in Lee, ed., *Handbook of Physiology*, Sect. 9, 102-104; Mountcastle, ed., *Medical Physiology*, II, 1338-1339.

This environment seemed so fundamentally different that English colonists and promoters believed it required an entire body of new medical knowledge. They had no question that hot climates produced diseases different from those of the moderate environment they were used to. "Pestilent Feavours and Calentures," worms, dry bellyache, dysentery, "Frenzies . . . and other hot cholerike sicknesses" were some that disturbed the colonists most. And familiar diseases such as colds were harder to cure; Ligon attributed this to the exhaustion of their bodies from constant sweating.[33] The diseases of hot countries were thought to be bred by the "intemperate and pestilent" air. The air was worst in the tropics, but even in Virginia it had the reputation of being "too hot and aguish."[34] Humidity, combined with heat, was particularly unwholesome. Fogs and dews as well as the moisture-laden night air were considered especially bad, and mariners fled or avoided those places with "infectious *serenas* or dewes."[35]

Only the trade winds made the tropics habitable. William Hubbard reminded his readers that the ancients had not known about these winds when they said that the tropics were unable to sustain life. He thought the heat of the New England summer was sometimes harder to bear than that of the tropics because of the lack of such winds. Only the cold winter saved New Englanders, for "the salubriousness of the air in this country depends much upon the winter's frost."[36]

Some promoters argued that Carolina would be healthier than Virginia because it was closer to the cooling trade winds of the Caribbean or would have more constant weather, less liable to extremes. On the other hand, sharp winter temperatures were thought to protect colonists from the detrimental effects of "continual Summer."[37] And Thomas Trapham

[33] Trapham, *State of Health in Jamaica*, 101-103; Ligon, *History of Barbados*, 45, 67; [Colt], "Voyage," in Harlow, ed., *Colonising Expeditions*, 99; Vaughan, *Directions for Health*, 4th ed., 87-88, 126, and *Newlanders Cure*, 60-62.

[34] Vaughan, *Directions for Health*, 4th ed., 3, 8, 6th ed., 12; [Plantagenet], *Description of New Albion*, in Force, comp., *Tracts*, II, No. 7, 6, 20.

[35] "Robert Dudley's Voyage to the West Indies, 1594-1595," in George F. Warner, ed., *The Voyage of Robert Dudley . . . to the West Indies, 1594-1595* (London, 1899), 69-70.

[36] Hubbard, *History of New England*, 20-21. See also [Colt], "Voyage," in Harlow, ed., *Colonising Expeditions*, 99, and W[illiams], *Virginia Richly and Truly Valued*, in Force, comp., *Tracts*, III, No. 11, 59-60.

[37] William Hilton, *A Relation of a Discovery Lately Made on the Coast of Florida* (1664), in Force, comp., *Tracts*, IV, No. 2, 16, 45; Wilson, *Account of Carolina*, in Salley, ed., *Narratives of Carolina*, 166-169; Horne (?), *Brief Description of Carolina, ibid.*, 66; Thomas Ashe, *Carolina, Or a Description of the Present State of That Country* (1682), *ibid.*, 141; John Archdale, *A New Description of That Fertile and Pleasant Province of Carolina* (1707), *ibid.*, 288; "Francis Yeardley's Narrative of Excursions into Carolina, 1654," *ibid.*, 25; Edward Randolph to the Lords of Trade, Mar. 16, 1698/9, *ibid.*, 208; John Oldmixon, *The History of the British Empire in America* (1708), *ibid.*, 360, 370; Edward Bland *et al.*, *The Discovery of New Brittaine* (London, 1651), 13; Lawson, *New Voyage to Carolina*, 2, 5, 80, 141, 166; John Lederer, *The Discoveries of John Lederer . . .*, trans. William Talbot (London, 1672), sig. A-Av.

believed that colonists of Jamaica escaped many of the Old World's diseases because the constantly moving air had purifying salts, particularly nitre, dissolved in it. To this, and not to the abundance of fresh fruits and vegetables, he attributed the absence of the scurvy that plagued other colonies in their early years.[38]

Some people believed that the extreme swings typical of America's climate rendered it especially unhealthy. These could be felt in a variety of ways. Newcomers to the West Indies were confronted by the most immediate contrast to their accustomed environment. Mainland settlers were struck by the difference between the great heat of summer and the winter's cold. In all colonies, going to bed sweating with the heat and waking up cold in the night was thought to be the source of many "epidemical distempers."[39]

Trapham believed that all processes of nature were more rapid and brisk in hot climates and that a new set of regimes was therefore necessary. Since the body was struggling to create a new balance of the humors, the traditional approaches of bleeding and purging were still recommended. These had to be used with care, however, especially when natural processes were speeded up. Sir William Vaughan reminded his readers that purging and bleeding worked on the beneficial humors as well as the corrupt and therefore could constitute "treacherous wasting of the Oyle of Life." Sir Henry Colt gave detailed medical advice to his son, who was intending to emigrate to the Caribbean. After warning of the dangers of the tropics, he said that a headache could be eased by bleeding but stressed that it was essential to keep the stomach warm at all times by wearing a stomacher, reflecting the belief that sweating renders the body's interior cold and numb.[40]

Colonists sought cures among the products of their new homes. From colony after colony came pleas for physicians to experiment with the herbs and chemicals the settlers were finding. Such requests had also come from the earlier Spanish colonies. For example, Peter de Osma wrote from Peru to thank Nicholas Monardes, the Seville physician who experimented with New World plants and published a medical treatise about them. He said

---

[38] Trapham, *State of Health in Jamaica*, 5-7, 14-15, 17, 81.

[39] Hubbard, *History of New England*, 20; Benjamin Church, *Diary of King Philip's War, 1675-76*, ed. Alan and Mary Simpson (Chester, Conn., 1975), 148; Michael G. Kammen, ed., "Maryland in 1699: A Letter from the Reverend Hugh Jones," *Journal of Southern History*, XXIX (1963), 369; "From the Journal of George Fox, 1672, 1673," in Hall, ed., *Narratives of Early Maryland*, 401; George Alsop, *A Character of the Province of Maryland* (1666), *ibid.*, 366; T. H. Breen, "George Donne's 'Virginia Reviewed': A 1638 Plan to Reform Colonial Society," *WMQ*, 3d Ser., XXX (1973), 455; Virginia Company, *A True and Sincere Declaration of the Purpose and End of the Plantation Begun in Virginia* (London, 1610), 13; Beverley, *History of Virginia*, ed. Wright, 305; [Henry] Norwood, "A Voyage to Virginia," in Force, comp., *Tracts*, III, No. 10, 21; Trapham, *State of Health in Jamaica*, 10-11, 19, 47-48; Ligon, *History of Barbados*, 44-45, 93; *Memoirs of First Settlement of Barbados*, 43.

[40] Trapham, *State of Health in Jamaica*, 67; Vaughan, *Newlanders Cure*, 67, 80-81; [Colt], "Voyage," in Harlow, ed., *Colonising Expeditions*, 99-100.

the doctors in Peru were "nothyng curious." William Strachey similarly complained that doctors in Virginia did not understand the ills of the country. Early English colonists on Tobago attributed sickness to lack of knowledge of the medicinal and nutritional qualities of plants native to the island. Hot areas were seen as sharing the same problems and opportunities; Thomas Hariot took a copy of Monardes with him as a guide to the plants of Roanoke, and the Virginia Company sent its colonists Sir Walter Ralegh's work on Guiana.[41] Science taught that the cure for any disease would be found near the disease's source. Richard Ligon put the point well when calling for "able and skilfull Physitians" to come to Barbados, "for certainely every Climate produces Simples more proper to cure the diseases that are bred there, than those that are transported from any other part of the world: such care the great Physitian to mankind takes for our convenience."[42]

Another way of coping was to learn from the Indians and from inhabitants of other hot countries. Colonists acknowledged a large debt to Indian medical practice, emphasizing that to use the products of America without Indian guidance was very risky. As Richard Hakluyt wrote in a marginal note to a story of the Roanoke colonists being poisoned by a fruit in the West Indies, "Circumspection to be used in strange places." Indian remedies were traded from colony to colony. Trapham and Vaughan also suggested looking at the bathing habits of natives of the East Indies and the Near East. Daily bathing in hot weather, of at least parts of the body, would keep the pores open by removing "relicts of obstructing sweat" so that the corrupted humors could be eliminated. Trapham attributed many of the diseases of hot countries to "constipation of the skin."[43]

Progress was made, even in these early years, in understanding the products of the new environments. This came partly through the activities of experimenters such as Monardes, who encouraged the importation of

[41] Monardes, *Joyfull Newes*, 135; Strachey, *Historie of Travell*, 38; [John Scott], "The Discription of Tobago," in Harlow, ed., *Colonising Expeditions*, 114-115; "For *Master* Rauleys Viage," 1584-1585, in Quinn, ed., *Roanoke Voyages*, I, 135; Hariot, *Briefe and True Report*, *ibid.*, 329, 366; Richard Hakluyt the Elder, *Inducements to the Liking of the Voyage Intended towards Virginia . . .* (1585), in Taylor, ed., *Writings and Correspondence*, II, 337; *Va. Company Recs.*, I, 310, 421, 431, 516, III, 240, 402, 485.

[42] Ligon, *History of Barbados*, 118. On the methods and training of physicians in the colonies see Wyndham B. Blanton, *Medicine in Virginia in the Eighteenth Century* (Richmond, Va., 1931), and Joseph Ioor Waring, *A History of Medicine in South Carolina, 1670-1825* (Columbia, S.C., 1964).

[43] Quinn, ed., *Roanoke Voyages*, II, 518n; Hariot, *Briefe and True Report*, *ibid.*, I, 328-333; Trapham, *State of Health in Jamaica*, 86-87, 95-96, 125-126, 139-142; Vaughan, *Newlanders Cure*, 77-78, and *Directions for Health*, 4th ed., 131-135. See also Henry Spelman, *Relation of Virginea* (1613), in Arber and Bradley, eds., *Travels and Works of Smith*, I, cix-cx; Samuel Argall, "A Letter of Sir Samuell Argoll Touching His Voyage to Virginia," in Purchas, *Pilgrimes*, XVIII, 92; and *A Relation of Maryland* (1635), ed. Francis L. Hawks (New York, 1865), 21.

American plants. Members of the Tradescant family of England made many voyages to America and other warm climates and brought back "curiosities" native to them for study and display.[44] The colonists themselves also experimented; many asked for or were sent herbals and advice on what to look for and how to proceed, and some believed they had found valuable drugs.[45] They preferred to use indigenous agents even for traditional practices such as purging or vomiting, because they were convinced that each environment produced specific relationships between disease and cure. Robert Beverley reported that the fevers and agues of Virginia could be successfully treated with indigenous roots. John Smith gave a long list of previously unknown plants of Bermuda, noting their qualities as purgatives, costives, and vomits.[46] These had to be used with great care, however, because they were thought to be too powerful and rapid in their action in the exhausted and speeded-up bodies of transplanted Europeans. Ligon reported his experience with the so-called "physick nut," which contained a poison so powerful that cattle even avoided the shade of its tree. If administered in a controlled way, Ligon wrote, the poison paradoxically produced good health. Many of these cures were not exportable. Trapham thought that "coker nut" milk was good for "hectick Heat" but dangerous for a cool stomach, and that China root, used in Jamaica to make the patient sweat, would not work at all in a colder climate.[47]

Ligon hoped that survival in the tropics might be assisted by liberal consumption of sugar, a course he personally followed. He reasoned that as sugar preserves plants "from corruption and putrifaction," why should it not also preserve human life? He quoted Dr. William Butler, "one of the most learned and famous Physitians that this Nation, or the world ever bred: 'If sugar can preserve both Peares and Plumbs,/Why can it not preserve as well our Lungs?' "[48]

Hot climates, then, were perceived as dangerous, especially for people used to England's moderation. Emigrating to the southern parts of America meant taking great risks, in fact gambling one's health against the possibility of amassing riches. This gamble took place on the national as well as the personal level. A high proportion of those who went or were

[44] Monardes, *Joyfull Newes*; Mea Allen, *The Tradescants: Their Plants, Garden, and Museum, 1570-1662* (London, 1964), 163-171.

[45] Hariot, *Briefe and True Report*, in Quinn, ed., *Roanoke Voyages*, I, 328-334; Ralph Lane to Richard Hakluyt the Elder, and Master H—— of the Middle Temple, Sept. 3, 1585, *ibid.*, 207-208; McIlwaine, ed., *Journals of House of Burgesses, 1619-1658/59*, 38; *Va. Company Recs.*, III, 238, 447, 476; Thomas Newe to his father, May 29, 1682, in Salley, ed., *Narratives of Carolina*, 185.

[46] Beverley, *History of Virginia*, ed. Wright, 306; Smith, *Generall Historie*, in Arber and Bradley, eds., *Travels and Works of Smith*, II, 628.

[47] Ligon, *History of Barbados*, 66-68; Trapham, *State of Health in Jamaica*, 49, 92, 122-123.

[48] Ligon, *History of Barbados*, 96; *Dictionary of National Biography*, s.v. "Butler, William."

sent by entrepreneurs lost the wager, but high death rates, because they were seen as a necessary result of transplantation, did not diminish enthusiasm for an English presence in the Caribbean and the southern mainland of North America. We cannot know how many colonists lived for the day when they could return to their own native climate.

Heat and high humidity were seen as necessary concomitants. As Beverley wrote of Virginia, "The Natural Temperature of the Inhabited part of the Country, is hot and moist." This heavy, hot climate was not only dangerous but also unpleasant because the immigrants had to jettison much that was familiar and comfortable in order to accommodate to new ways and new forms of nature. Beyond the fear of death and debility was a distaste for an environment so different from their own—a distaste strongly conveyed by their reports of repellent rodents, reptiles, insects, and uncontrollable strange vegetation. The English saw this alienating milieu as the product of intemperate heat. Prospective colonists were warned to give up their expectations about normal types of food, housing, clothing, and pastimes, and were told not to come if these meant too much to them. Ligon wrote of the "deprest" spirits of the Barbadian planters and the "declining and yielding condition" they had been brought to. What others called "slothfulness or sluggishnesse in them" he attributed to "a decay of their spirits" that led to apathy. Only the hope of one day returning to England kept them going.[49]

Familiar foods and drink had to be foregone in some hot places. The Virginia Company encouraged settlers by affirming that salted meat did not putrefy there as in the West Indies. Ligon told his readers not to bring butter, cheese, or candles in the spring and summer, as they would melt and stink. He wrote that the favorite drink on Barbados was "mobbie," a beverage made from boiled potatoes. It could be kept for only four or five days and tasted like "Rhenish wine in the Must." He thought it an unwholesome drink that produced "Hydropicke humours" because potatoes have a moist quality, and he cited the governor's amazement that people could drink it regularly and live.[50]

Virginia colonists reported difficulty in making beer and wine, the former because barley was too expensive and the climate was too hot to make malt, and the latter because of cost, hot weather, and lack of skill. This was particularly serious because, as they said, people need to drink a

---

[49] Beverley, *History of Virginia*, ed. Wright, 296; Ligon, *History of Barbados*, 40-41, 117-118. See also Kupperman, "Apathy and Death," *JAH*, LXVI (1979), 24-40. David Galenson has found evidence that, partly because of working conditions there, servants' contracts to the West Indies were for shorter periods than for the mainland (*White Servitude in Colonial America: An Economic Analysis* [Cambridge, 1981], 110).

[50] [Va. Company], *True Declaration of Estate*, in Force, comp., *Tracts*, III, No. 1, 14; Ligon, *History of Barbados*, 30-32; [Colt], "Voyage," in Harlow, ed., *Colonising Expeditions*, 100; "Voyage to Maryland," *AHR*, XII (1907), 328.

lot in hot weather, and they found a sudden switch to water caused alteration in their bodies. As sack and aquavitae were thought to preserve health, so water weakened the body. Later colonists reported success in making beverages from Indian corn and especially in growing orchards for cider, perry, and brandy. These had to be handled with care, however. Cider was thought to be good for those whose blood was hot, because it cut gross humors. Perry, because it was sweeter and was thought more nourishing, was good for those with cold stomachs but had to be mixed with water for those whose stomachs were hot or very humid.[51]

Native foods were deemed unsatisfying or even dangerous. English settlers in the West Indies learned to eat strange foods: iguana, turtle, and even rats. Cassava bread, considered dry and tasteless, replaced more familiar English grains.[52] Virginia colonists also learned to eat "strange beasts," which some liked better than others. The chief corn on the mainland was maize, which Edward Winslow of Plymouth said was especially suited to hot areas. While many were enthusiastic about Indian corn, everyone looked forward to a time when English seeds would grow there, and some agreed with John Gerard's *Herball* that maize was not nourishing.[53] Moreover, there were poisonous plants, some of which aped edible ones in appearance. Hariot wrote of berries like capers that, after being boiled for eight or nine hours, were "very good meat and holesome." If eaten uncooked, "they will make a man for the time franticke or extremely sicke." Differentiating the good from the bad was especially tricky because colonists believed that plants, like human beings, could change their characteristics when moved from one environment to another. Thus Monardes quoted Peter de Osma as saying that while cassava grown on the islands was poisonous, that from the mainland was benign.[54]

---

[51] *Va. Company Recs.*, III, 365-367, 447, IV, 59; McIlwaine, ed., *Journals of House of Burgesses, 1619-1658/59,* 39; Hariot, *Briefe and True Report*, in Quinn, ed., *Roanoke Voyages*, I, 384; [John] Smith, *A True Relation of Such Occurrences and Accidents of Noate as Hath Hapned in Virginia* ... (1608), in Barbour, ed., *Jamestown Voyages*, I, 173; Lawson, *New Voyage to Carolina*, 51; Hammond, *Leah and Rachel*, in Force, comp., *Tracts*, III, No. 14, 9-10, 13-14; Newe to his father, in Salley, ed., *Narratives of Carolina*, 181; Beverley, *History of Virginia*, ed. Wright, 314; Kammen, ed., "Maryland in 1699," *Jour. So. Hist.*, XXIX (1963), 370; Vaughan, *Directions for Health*, 4th ed., 31-32.

[52] [Colt], "Voyage," in Harlow, ed., *Colonising Expeditions*, 91, 93; Ligon, *History of Barbados*, 27-28; Trapham, *State of Health in Jamaica*, 61-64.

[53] Winslow, *Good Newes from New-England* ... (London, 1624), 62-63; McIlwaine, ed., *Journals of House of Burgesses, 1619-1658/59,* 21, 28; Lawson, *New Voyage to Carolina*, 75; "Voyage to Maryland," *AHR*, XII (1907), 335; Gerard, *The Herball; or Generall Historie of Plantes*, enlarged and amended by Thomas Johnson (London, 1636), 82.

[54] Hariot, *Briefe and True Report*, in Quinn, ed., *Roanoke Voyages*, I, 350, 352-353; Monardes, *Joyfull Newes*, I, 143, II, 4, 35.

Though some considered American pork delicious, others believed it acted quite differently on the body in hot climates than in England. Thomas Gage wrote of his many years in Mexico that no matter how much meat he ate at a meal, he was always hungry again in two or three hours, despite the extra rations of chocolate, conserve, and biscuits he was issued. Since the meat seemed "as fat and hearty" as in England, he could not understand why he became hungry so soon until a "Doctor of Physick" explained that though the meat looked good, it lacked "substance and nourishment." The climate had the effect of producing a fair show but "little matter or substance," an impression that reflected English suspicion of the rapid growth engendered by heat. Fruits were fair and beautiful, sweet and luscious, but had not half the nourishment of an "English Kentish Pippin." This nutritional defect indicated something much more serious. Where meat and fruit exhibited such "inward and hidden deceit," the people were the same. Gage remembered a story that Queen Elizabeth, when shown the fruits of America, remarked that "surely where those fruits grew, the women were light, and all the people hollow and false hearted." Whatever the cause, Gage's experience taught him that all the abundance and variety of food offered "little substance and virtue" and that people's stomachs were always "gaping and crying, Feed, feed."[55]

Ligon was concerned to warn off people who might take the deprivation of familiar pleasures too hard. No coursing, hunting, or hawking was possible, nor was horse racing in the heat. One might shoot or bowl, though in imperfect conditions. Indoor sports were all right if not too "laborious." Not only were sports strictly limited in the West Indies, but, Ligon reported, human senses were poorly served there as well. Perfumes and pastilles lost their scent and taste, drawn forth, as he explained, by the heat and moisture of the air. Flowers growing there were less fragrant and varied than in England, and many English flowers could not stand the heat. The sense of touch was also badly served. Everyone recoiled from another's touch: "take it in the highest, and most active way it can be applyed, which is upon the skins of women, and they are so sweaty and clammy, as the hand cannot passe over, without being glued and cemented in the passage or motion; and by that means, little pleasure is given to, or received by the agent or the patient."[56]

Everything brought to the West Indies was subject to corruption and

[55] Thomas Gage, The English-American, His Travail by Sea and Land . . . (London, 1648), 43, 200. Gage offered descriptions of some Mexican fruits and their taste (pp. 60-61). See also Ligon, History of Barbados, 27; [Colt], "Voyage," in Harlow, ed., Colonising Expeditions, 92; and Vaughan, Newlanders Cure, 56.

[56] Ligon, History of Barbados, 104-107. The satirist Edward Ward wrote of Jamaica that "kissing here grew out of Fashion; there's no joyning of Lips, but your Noses would drop Sweat into your Mouths" (A Trip to Jamaica: With a True Character of the People and Island, 7th ed. [London, 1700], 12). On the beauty of native plants see Ligon, History of Barbados, 74, 84, and Beverley, History of Virginia, ed. Wright, 298-299.

putrefaction. Sir Henry Colt told his son not to bring clothing made of leather because it would rot or mold so quickly. Similarly, Ligon cautioned would-be adventurers that slaves would need a new pair of shoes each month. Everything made of metal rusted. The stones from which Barbadians made their houses sweated moisture that rotted the timbers. They were forced to cover the timber ends with boards soaked in pitch. The living fences Ligon praised on Barbados were especially necessary because all other kinds of fences rotted "by extream moisture, and violent heat."[57]

Other things were vulnerable to the creatures that thrived in the hot, humid environment. Ligon wrote that the hangings in planters' houses were spoiled by ants and eaten by the cockroaches and rats. He described a great variety of insects, lizards, land crabs, and such that inhabited the houses, of which the chiggers (Chegoes) were the worst. The slaves' skins looked, he wrote, as if they had been raked with a currycomb because they were so badly bitten by cockroaches while they slept. No place indoors was safe from the ingenuity of the ants, and the snakes could climb walls six feet high. Trapham attributed the incidence of intestinal worms in Jamaica to the fact that the pond water colonists drank was infested with mosquito eggs. His cure was to eat bitter things or take mercury. Colt wrote that body lice were unknown in the tropics but head lice were unavoidable.[58] Even in New England, John Josselyn noted that the heat brought out many snakes. Sir William Vaughan believed in general that venomous creatures were bred of putrefaction, and John Lawson agreed that vermin were more frequent in warm climates than in those farther from the sun. Robert Beverley said the worst aspects of Virginia were the heat, thunder, and the vermin, in which he included frogs, snakes, and mosquitoes. Mosquitoes and poisonous snakes appear on many such lists.[59] We can sense the intensity of feeling about the alien environment engendered by heat and creatures native to it in a passage in a late work by Capt. John Smith, where he wrote of the "terrible creatures" to be found in Africa, that meet at the watering places and "in regard of the heat of the Country, and their extremities of Nature, make strange copulations, and so ingender those extraordinary monsters."[60]

---

[57] [Colt], "Voyage," in Harlow, ed., *Colonising Expeditions*, 100-101; Trapham, *State of Health in Jamaica*, 14-15; Ligon, *History of Barbados*, 42, 66-67, 113-115.

[58] Ligon, *History of Barbados*, 42, 61-67; [Colt], "Voyage," in Harlow, ed., *Colonising Expeditions*, 65, 73, 83; Trapham, *State of Health in Jamaica*, 103-110; Gage, *English-American*, 27, 163, 166.

[59] Josselyn, *Account of Two Voyages*, Mass. Hist. Soc., *Colls.*, 3d Ser., III, 227; Vaughan, *Directions for Health*, 6th ed., 7; Lawson, *New Voyage to Carolina*, 16; Beverley, *History of Virginia*, ed. Wright, 299-303; *Virginia Richly Valued, by the Description of the Main Land of Florida, Her Next Neighbour* . . . (1609), in Force, comp., *Tracts*, IV, No. 1, 123.

[60] [John Smith], *The True Travels, Adventures, and Observations* . . . (1630), in Arber and Bradley, eds., *Travels and Works of Smith*, II, 877.

Despite all the dangers and the alien environment, however, English people went to the rich southern mainland of North America and the West Indies in overwhelmingly larger numbers in the seventeenth century than to northern regions that were considered to be more like England. For promoters, planters, and medical men in the colonies, adaptation and survival therefore became major concerns, especially the problem of easing newcomers through the seasoning. Experience demonstrated that the young and strong weathered the traumas of adaptation better than those who were sickly on arrival: some writers blamed high death rates in the southern colonies partly on the poor physical condition of immigrants.[61] Regulation of the rhythm of work and emigration also helped. John Hammond said that servants new to Virginia were not required to work much during their first summer, and he and others claimed that servants never worked during the hottest hours of the summer day. Agricultural work was not distributed evenly throughout the year but was concentrated in the late summer and autumn, the time of highest mortality. Virginia settlers early perceived that if new colonists were to arrive in the fall, they would have several months to become acclimatized before they had to face the heat and disease that prevailed during the summer months of hard work. They repeatedly urged this strategy on the Virginia Company, which turned a deaf ear. When, later in the century, practice did shift to sending ships in the fall, it was because that was when the tobacco crop was ready, according to William Bullock, the English colonial promoter, not because the fall was a better time to send colonists.[62]

Colonists were urged to change their eating habits because orderly diet would make them resistant to the ill effects of extreme weather. Trapham chided colonists in the West Indies for continuing English ways of living instead of "substituting new Indian ones." He complained that "we transport northern chilly propensities and customs thereon depending, into the southern hot Climes, and most improper and destructive to health, at least long life." Trapham suggested that Jamaicans give up the habit of eating large meals in the middle of the day. He wanted them to break their fast with chocolate and dine lightly in mid-morning on fruits and meat in broth. It was important to eat light and easily digested foods, "as all the works of nature here are and ought to be most speedy, to

[61] McIlwaine, ed., *Journals of House of Burgesses, 1619-1658/59*, 23; *Va. Company Recs.*, III, 455.

[62] Hammond, *Leah and Rachel*, in Force, comp., *Tracts*, III, No. 14, 12, 14; W[illiams], *Virginia Richly and Truly Valued*, *ibid.*, No. 11, 59-61; Alsop, *Character of Maryland*, in Hall, ed., *Narratives of Maryland*, 357; Carville V. Earle, *The Evolution of a Tidewater Settlement: All Hallow's Parish, Maryland, 1650-1783*, University of Chicago Department of Geography Research Paper No. 170 (Chicago, 1975), 161; McIlwaine, ed., *Journals of House of Burgesses, 1619-1658/59*, 23, 30, 36, 38-39; *Va. Company Recs.*, I, 371, III, 298, 301, IV, 582; Bullock, *Virginia Impartially Examined*, 12.

comply with the universal briskness of motions betwixt the Tropics." He urged colonists to remember that flesh is always more "stubborn" than other foods. At four in the afternoon they should take more chocolate. They could drink plenty of water before chocolate but never after. When they took water, they were warned to follow it with candied warm fruits or roots, such as limes, oranges, or ginger, to prevent chilling their stomachs too much. Finally, at seven or eight in the evening they could have a plentiful supper, for which Trapham suggested a huge variety of meats. Even then, Jamaicans should not eat more than to satiety, and ideally chocolate should constitute half of their food. Chocolate was especially good, because it not only cooled and lubricated the body but provided a natural test of health: if your stomach had "too much choler" to stand it, then you needed "evacuation." After sundown, on Trapham's regimen, one could drink wine in moderation, but he felt that only Madeira wines were suited to the West Indies.[63]

Sir Henry Colt advised his son that when he arrived in the tropics, he should eat less meat and increase his consumption of grains and pulses. His meat should be stewed or in broths.[64] Ligon described the diet of servants and slaves as being almost entirely restricted to carbohydrates. They lived on potatoes, loblolly (a thick maize gruel served cold that the slaves hated), some maize, and "Bonavist," a West Indian pulse. During Ligon's time in Barbados the slaves were newly allowed to cut and cook plantains, which they delighted in. He reported the English servants had salt and pickled fish and meats in addition, though advice manuals warned against salt meat in hot weather. Ligon himself loved many of the fruits of his island but thought some of them might be unhealthy. In general, he felt the meat and bread were "not so well relish'd as in England, but flat and insipid."[65]

Though William Hubbard wrote that winter's cold was easier to deal with than extreme heat, southern colonists could do much to control their personal micro-environments through manipulation of housing and clothing. As early as the late sixteenth century, English colonial promoters were aware that house styles could contribute greatly to health and comfort in very hot climates.[66] Ligon observed that mid-seventeenth-century Barbados houses were not built to maximize comfort. Instead of the high-ceilinged, thick-walled houses open to the constant east wind that he expected, he found that dwellings were low and open to the west, which made them resemble stoves. When the late afternoon sun poured in on planters who were full of "kill-devil" (rum) and were smoking tobacco, he wondered why spontaneous combustion did not occur in their oven-like

[63] Trapham, *State of Health in Jamaica*, 50-60, 67. See also Beverley, *History of Virginia*, ed. Wright, 297-298.

[64] [Colt], "Voyage," in Harlow, ed., *Colonising Expeditions*, 99-100.

[65] Ligon, *History of Barbados*, 27-28, 31, 43-44, 80-84, 110, 113.

[66] Hubbard, *History of New England*, 20; "Commentary on Hayes-Carleill Project," in Quinn et al., eds., *New American World*, III, 174.

houses.[67] Mainland colonists learned to choose the highest ground, open to cooling, cleansing breezes, for their residences. Agreeing that high ground was healthier, William Bullock endorsed this practice but warned against placing houses too far from neighbors, "for that's disconsolate."[68]

Eighteenth-century reports make clear that colonists had learned to build their houses to maximize coolness. Beverley said that houses in Virginia were comfortable even in hot weather because they had cool, open, airy rooms. Chesapeake houses were built around a central hall that drew in breezes; sometimes they were raised to allow free movement of air underneath. Kitchens and other rooms devoted to heat-producing functions were separated from the main house in small buildings, and summerhouses made cool retreats. Underground rooms allowed planters to keep butter and other perishables longer. Common planters' houses as well as those of the great landowners were constructed to allow a free flow of air through them. The naturalist Mark Catesby thought that cutting down forests in South Carolina had opened the land up to the winds, making it cooler in summer, though those who could afford to left the coastal area completely during the hottest months. Janet Schaw, a Scottish gentlewoman who traveled to the West Indies in the 1770s, remarked on how cool the houses were on Antigua because they were shaded by tall palmetto trees.[69]

Clothing was the most easily manipulated element of the personal environment. Colonists were quick to adapt the clothing of slaves and lesser servants to warm conditions. Servants' dress on Barbados consisted

[67] Ligon, *History of Barbados*, 25, 40-43, 55-57, 73-75, 78-79, 102-104.

[68] William Strachey, *A True Reportory of the Wracke, and Redemption of Sir Thomas Gates . . .* , in Purchas, *Pilgrimes*, XIX, 58, and *Historie of Travell*, 33-34, 40; Bullock, *Virginia Impartially Examined*, 61; Earle, *Evolution of a Tidewater Settlement*, 140.

[69] Beverley, *History of Virginia*, ed. Wright, 289-290, 299; Jones, *Present State of Virginia*, ed. Morton, 71, 74; Gregory A. Stiverson and Patrick H. Butler, III, "Virginia in 1732: The Travel Journal of William Hugh Grove," *Virginia Magazine of History and Biography*, LXXXV (1977), 22, 24, 28; [Edward Kimber], "Observations in Several Voyages and Travels in America," *WMQ*, 1st Ser., XV (1907), 153; "An Interview with James Freeman, 1712," in Roy H. Merrens, ed., *The Colonial South Carolina Scene: Contemporary Views, 1697-1774* (Columbia, S.C., 1977), 42, 49; Mark Catesby, *The Natural History of Carolina, Florida, and the Bahama Islands* (1731-1743), *ibid.*, 89; Pelatiah Webster, "Journal of a Visit to Charleston, 1765," *ibid.*, 221; "Charleston, S.C., in 1774 as Described by an English Traveller," *ibid.*, 286; Evangeline Walker Andrews and Charles McLean Andrews, eds., *Journal of a Lady of Quality; Being the Narrative of a Journey from Scotland to the West Indies, North Carolina, and Portugal, in the Years 1774 to 1776* (New Haven, Conn., 1923), 83, 95, 101, 103. For general descriptions of adaptation in house styles, clothing, and food in the 18th-century South see Rhys Isaac, *The Transformation of Virginia, 1740-1790* (Chapel Hill, N.C., 1982), 32-36, 43-46; Gloria L. Main, *Tobacco Colony: Life in Early Maryland, 1650-1720* (Princeton, N.J., 1982), 136-137, 143, 148, 167, 192-205; and Hugh T. Lefler and William S. Powell, *Colonial North Carolina: A History* (New York, 1973), 184-186.

of linen shirts and drawers for men and petticoats for women. The linen garments of the slaves were of canvas, and the materials for Europeans were finer depending on status. Carolina promoters said that a major advantage of the climate was that slaves needed few and cheap clothes.[70]

Settlers above the level of servants also adapted, but apparently reluctantly. Robert Beverley complained that newcomers to Virginia refused to dress in accordance with the climate; they went about in thick clothes suitable for northern places and then complained of the heat. At the same time, John Archdale, the Quaker governor, blamed fevers and agues in Carolina partly on carelessness in clothing. Eighteenth-century medical tracts continued to call for intelligent adaptation in styles of dress. Though newcomers were slow to give up heavy northern clothes, long-time residents of the southern colonies learned to dress much more comfortably. They wore light materials in the summer, with fewer layers. Women in Antigua wore masks out of doors to protect their faces from the sun. Men quit wearing wigs in hot weather, except on very special occasions, and replaced them with thin caps. Though they presented an odd, even slovenly, picture to travelers, colonists were clearly adapting to the special conditions of their adopted homeland.[71]

By the eighteenth century, adaptation had made life in the South more comfortable, and the largely native-born composition of the population reduced the role of seasoning as a killer. And yet, inhabitants of the southern mainland and the West Indies continued to think of their regions as less healthy, less apt to produce robust people because of high heat and humidity. The reply of Lt. Gov. John Hart of Maryland to a questionnaire from the Board of Trade in 1720 began: "Maryland is situated in the center of the British Plantations. The climate is unhealthy, especially to strangers, occasion'd by the excessive heat in summer, and extreme cold in winter; the vernal and autumnal quarters are attended with fevers, pleurisies, etc." When Dr. Alexander Hamilton, the Annapolis physician, returned to Maryland from his journey through the northern colonies, he

---

[70] Ligon, *History of Barbados*, 109, 113-115; [Colt], "Voyage," in Harlow, ed., *Colonising Expeditions*, 100-101; Lawson, *New Voyage to Carolina*, 165; Wilson, *Account of Carolina*, in Salley, ed., *Narratives of Carolina*, 172; Randolph to the Lords of Trade, Mar. 16, 1698/9, *ibid.*, 208; Archdale, *New Description of Carolina*, *ibid.*, 291.

[71] Beverley, *History of Virginia*, ed. Wright, 297; Stiverson and Butler, eds., "Virginia in 1732," *VMHB*, LXXXV (1977), 29, 32; [Kimber], "Observations in Several Voyages," *WMQ*, 1st. Ser., XV (1907), 158; Andrews and Andrews, eds., *Journal of a Lady of Quality*, 87, 114-115; Devereux Jarratt, *The Life of the Reverend Devereux Jarratt, Rector of Bath Parish, Dinwiddie County, Virginia, Written by Himself, in a Series of Letters Addressed to the Rev. John Coleman* . . . (New York, 1969 [orig. publ. Baltimore, 1806]), 14, 26. See also Dunn, *Sugar and Slaves*, 263-264, 281-286. Mountcastle has tables of the insulation value of different types of clothing (*Medical Physiology*, II, 1315). See also Lind, "Human Tolerance to Hot Climates," in Lee, *Handbook of Physiology*, Sect. 9, 93, 102, and Guyton, *Textbook of Medical Physiology*, 958.

ended his journal with the observation that the governments of the northern colonies were to be preferred to the "poor, sickly, convulsed state" of Maryland. "Their air and living to the northward is likewise much preferable, and the people of a more gygantick size and make."[72]

As Hart indicated, seasoning continued to affect newcomers, and a general impression of unhealthiness hung over the southern colonies. Gov. James Glen of South Carolina found he could not place a value on the 25,000 people there by 1751 because he could not know how "how many thousands must have died before such a number could have been established, so habituated to the climate, accustomed with our seasons, their sudden changes, and the methods of guarding against them, and in short so qualified in every respect to make and denominate them useful planters and inhabitants."[73] Janet Schaw, despite her praise for the ingenuity with which colonists adapted to the environment, complained of the heat in North Carolina as well as the West Indies. She hated the mosquitoes and other insects that increased as the heat grew more oppressive. While she believed that the adoption of bad habits killed more people than the heat alone, she clearly subscribed to the theory of humoral change when she described an elderly Englishman who returned from Antigua to his native land. Though he spent his time in a greenhouse there, he found he had become "so absolute an exotick" that he could not stay.[74]

Natives by no means saw themselves as immune to the dangerous effects of the southern climate in the eighteenth century. Several writers warned that a rash style of life could be very harmful. Excessive indulgence in strong drink was one obvious trap, but less clearly harmful acts could bring disaster. Devereux Jarratt, the common planter's son who became a minister, believed that moving from one environment to another within his own region as a young man had brought a prolonged bout of sickness on him. The Rev. Hugh Jones, mathematics professor at William and Mary, argued that all Virginians could be well as long as they took precautions to protect themselves against the sudden alterations of heat and cold that were so dangerous there. Beverley particularly warned against overheating oneself with exercise and then attempting to cool off

---

[72] Hart to the Council of Trade and Plantations, Aug. 25, 1720, in *Maryland Historical Magazine*, XXIX (1934), 252; Carl Bridenbaugh, ed., *Gentleman's Progress: The Itinerarium of Dr. Alexander Hamilton, 1744* (Chapel Hill, N.C., 1948), 199.

[73] Glen, "An Attempt towards an Estimate of the Value of South Carolina, 1751," in Merrens, ed., *Colonial South Carolina Scene*, 183; Robert Witherspoon, "Recollections of a Settler, 1780," *ibid.*, 127; James Oglethorpe, *A New and Accurate Account of the Provinces of South-Carolina and Georgia* (1732), in Trevor R. Reese, ed., *The Most Delightful Country of the Universe: Promotional Literature of the Colony of Georgia, 1717-1734* (Savannah, Ga., 1972), 127; Jones, *Present State of Virginia*, ed. Morton, 84-85; Bridenbaugh, ed., *Gentleman's Progress*, xiii.

[74] Andrews and Andrews, eds., *Journal of a Lady of Quality*, 85-86, 93, 105, 116, 122, 153, 182-183.

too rapidly. Finally, a particularly hot summer could upset the delicate balance of the humors that allowed people to live in these climates. When Dr. Alexander Hamilton returned to Maryland, he learned that the summer had been intemperate: "I should have known the time had been unhealthy without his telling me so by only observing the washed countenances of the people standing att their doors and looking out att their windows, for they looked like so many staring ghosts. In short I was sensible I had got into Maryland, for every house was an infirmary, according to ancient custome."[75]

New dangers also appeared in the eighteenth century with the introduction of yellow fever, the great killer of European Americans in the south. Since epidemics of yellow fever, which intensified toward the century's end, always occurred during hot summers, these outbreaks convinced observers, particularly medical practitioners, that heat caused them. The English experience in the southern parts of America was studied by the transatlantic medical establishment, and this study led to the absolute acceptance of medical environmentalism in the eighteenth century. Those who investigated the problem of fevers were in the forefront of the medical thought of their day; they attacked the problem of disease in hot climates empirically, using the most modern equipment available. Additional urgency was imparted to the task by the British government's need to keep its troops alive in the West Indian theater of the great imperial wars where death from disease mowed down the men. What they lacked was the not-yet-developed paradigm of a germ theory of disease; in its absence, their experiments and observation served to reinforce the old beliefs. As long as the humoral paradigm continued to dominate medical thinking, the link between the human body and climate was accepted as dogma.[76]

Eighteenth-century physicians knew that fevers were the leading cause of death in the southern mainland as well as the West Indies, but they saw fevers as the direct product of hot weather, especially when combined with high humidity. Since heat was the source of these diseases, they could appear, in extraordinary circumstances, in Europe. Dr. James Lind, a Scottish naval physician, wrote that tropical fever had appeared in England

---

[75] Jarratt, *Life*, 29; Jones, *Present State of Virginia*, ed. Morton, 84-85, 93; Beverley, *History of Virginia*, ed. Wright, 305; Bridenbaugh, ed., *Gentleman's Progress*, 198.

[76] On yellow fever in the 18th and 19th centuries see Kenneth F. Kiple and Virginia Himmelsteib King, *Another Dimension to the Black Diaspora: Diet, Disease, and Racism* (Cambridge, 1981), Pts. i, ii. On the end of the humoral paradigm see Charles E. Rosenberg, "The Therapeutic Revolution: Medicine, Meaning, and Social Change in Nineteenth-Century America," *Perspectives in Biology and Medicine*, XX (1977), 485-506. On the "death sentence" that assignment to the West Indies meant for soldiers and sailors see Roger Norman Buckley, *Slaves in Red Coats: The British West India Regiments, 1795-1815* (New Haven, Conn., 1979), 3, and Richard Pares, *War and Trade in the West Indies, 1739-1763* (Oxford, 1936), 259.

during heat waves in 1765 and 1766. Nor did it take much in the way of heat by our standards; the figure mentioned for England was eighty-two degrees.[77] American doctors ordered barometers and the newly accurate Fahrenheit thermometers from Europe and began to take systematic readings of weather variations, which they hoped eventually to correlate with mortality patterns. It was a commonplace that the way to cope with the diseases of any place was first to understand its climate because the link between the two was seen as absolute.[78]

Doctors, like laymen, continued to believe that the human body was drastically changed by moving from a cold to a hot climate. The link between heat and disease for these physicians, as for their seventeenth-century counterparts, was changes in bodily humors produced by exposure to "intemperate climes." Prickly heat and the leg ulcers that afflicted many were seen as attempts by the blood to throw off "fiery" and "acrid" elements, and to excrete them through the skin. Therefore, bathing in cold water or any attempt to control the eruptions was thought to cause more harm to the body by forcing the harmful excretions inward again.[79]

[77] James Lind, *An Essay on Diseases Incidental to Europeans, in Hot Climates, with the Method of Preventing Their Fatal Consequences*, 6th ed. (Philadelphia, 1811). So complete was the identification of hot weather as the cause of fever that West Africa, where death rates from yellow fever and malaria were high among Europeans, was commonly thought to be a place of extreme heat and humidity despite travelers' reports that uniformly described the climate as moderate (P. D. Curtin, " 'The White Man's Grave': Image and Reality, 1780-1850," *Journal of British Studies*, I (1961), 97-100. On the conditions promoting yellow fever and malaria in America see Kiple and King, *Another Dimension to the Black Diaspora*, Pts. i, ii; John Duffy, *Epidemics in Colonial America* (Baton Rouge, La., 1953), chaps. 4, 5; and Rutman and Rutman, "Of Agues and Fevers," *WMQ*, 3d Ser., XXXIII (1976), 31-60.

[78] For such records see Lind, *Diseases Incidental to Europeans in Hot Climates;* William Hillary, *Observations on the Changes of the Air, and the Concomitant Epidemical Diseases in the Island of Barbadoes . . .* (Philadelphia, 1811 [orig. publ. London, 1759]); C. Chisholm, *An Essay on the Malignant Pestilential Fever Introduced into the West Indian Islands from Boullam, on the Coast of Guinea, As It Appeared in 1793 and 1794* (Philadelphia, 1799); and John Lining, "Extracts of Two Letters from Dr. John Lining, Physician at Charles-Town in South Carolina to James Jurin, M.D. F.R.S. Giving an Account of Statical Experiments Made Several Times in a Day upon Himself, for One Whole Year, Accompanied with Meteorological Observations; to Which Are Subjoined Six General Tables, Deduced from the Whole Years Course," *Philosophical Transactions*, XLII (1742-1743), 491-509. For modern discussion of 18th-century theories linking weather and disease see Richard Harrison Shryock, *Medicine and Society in America, 1660-1860* (New York, 1960), 62-63; Owsei Temkin, *The Double Face of Janus and Other Essays in the History of Medicine* (Baltimore, 1977), 459; and James H. Cassedy, "Meteorology and Medicine in Colonial America: Beginnings of the Experimental Approach," *Journal of the History of Medicine and Allied Sciences*, XXIV (1969), 193-204.

[79] Hans Sloane, *A Voyage to the Islands Madera, Barbados, Nieves, S. Christophers, and Jamaica . . .* , 2 vols. (London, 1707, 1725), I, xciv-xcv; Hillary, *Changes of Air and Concomitant Epidemical Diseases*, iv-vi, 26-27.

Constant perspiration continued to be seen as a major cause of disease. It led to laxity of the muscle fibers and, because of a sympathetic connection between the skin and the stomach, to weakness in digestion. Dr. John Tennent of Virginia believed that excessive sweating stole fluid from the blood and produced "heavy sizy [viscous, glutinous] blood." In extreme cases complete "Stagnation of the Blood" caused death, which "indeed is too often the Case." Tennent recommended routine bleeding for everyone going to the West Indies in order to bring the volume of blood into equilibrium with the laxity of the muscle fibers.[80]

Dr. William Hillary of South Carolina thought that relaxation of the muscle fibers on entering a hot climate caused the blood to become "lax, loose, and attenuated," even in healthy people and that this condition produced fevers and other diseases. Others thought that muscle relaxation led to corruption of the humors. The cold winter months brought relief to mainland residents, but some doctors thought that this did not render these areas healthier than the more constant West Indies, because the body was forced to make drastic adjustments several times each year, an exhausting process for even the most healthy.[81]

Though these theories were more complicated, a seventeenth-century reader would have been comfortable with them, based as they were on the same assumptions about human beings in relation to the environment that had informed earlier thinking. Medical thinking based on experiential data from the colonies transformed the vague and unformed beliefs of the late sixteenth and early seventeenth centuries into the certainties of the eighteenth. Evidence from the colonies, interpreted through the lens of the physicians' assumptions about the human body, allowed medical environmentalism to become dogma. The apparently empirical bond between heat and fever, proven experimentally by the colonists, cemented the role of climate in disease in eighteenth-century thinking.

Fear of hot climates was accommodated by the eighteenth century. Southern colonists accepted the danger and discomfort, much as some late twentieth-century Americans accept the risks of cigarette smoking. Most were uneasy about the risks of living in an intemperately hot place, and scientists sought to understand and mitigate the worst effects of heat, but routines of life went on in the face of the danger. Dr. Hamilton thought of Maryland as inherently unhealthy, yet he gave up the idea of returning to Britain in the 1740s despite his continued bad health. He wrote of the

[80] John Tennent, *Physical Enquiries: Discovering the Mode of Translation in the Constitutions of Northern Inhabitants, on Going to, and for Some Time after Arriving in Southern Climates* (London, 1742), 3-5, 25.

[81] Hillary, *Changes of Air and Concomitant Epidemical Diseases*, vii-viii; John Lining, "A Description of the American Yellow Fever in a Letter from Dr. John Lining, Physician at Charles-Town in South Carolina, to Dr. Robert Whytt, Professor of Medicine in the University of Edinburgh," in Chisholm, *Essay on the Malignant Pestilential Fever*, 303-304; George Milligen-Johnston, *A Short Description of the Province of South-Carolina, with an Account of the Air, Weather, Diseases, at Charles-Town* (London, 1770), 43-46, 65-66.

summer's sickliness with resignation and acceptance.[82] By contrast, seventeenth-century people such as Nicholas Leverton had believed that nothing short of return to their native air could cure them when they were sick.

The southern part of America no longer seemed alien; with the woods diminished and English houses dotting the landscape, it had a comfortable look. The vast majority of the population, especially on the mainland, were native-born and therefore did not see the flora and fauna as exotic. The colonists were not really colonists; they were Americans by birth: hot and unhealthy though the land might be, it was their home. Unlike earlier settlers, most of whom had made a decision to emigrate and who therefore looked around them with an appraising eye, eighteenth-century residents were settled in their American environment. Only travelers' accounts and reports to imperial authorities provide a picture of conditions in the eighteenth century comparable to that frequently painted by settlers in the seventeenth.

Within their commitment to the southern colonies, residents had learned that they could do much to make themselves more comfortable and even safer. They learned to construct cooler houses and to wear lighter, less formal clothes. They learned what foods were safe and how to keep them fresh in hot weather. Some of them learned to avoid excesses that rendered them more vulnerable to illness. Until the germ theory of disease was proposed in the nineteenth century and the role of the mosquito in spreading yellow fever and malaria became understood, they could not effectively combat the fevers that made some summers so dangerous, but eighteenth-century colonists felt in control of and at home in their environment.

[82] Bridenbaugh, ed., *Gentleman's Progress,* xiii.

9

Of Agues and Fevers:
Malaria in the Early Chesapeake

Darrett B. Rutman and Anita H. Rutman

ON Tuesday, April 25, 1758, Landon Carter of Sabine Hall, Virginia, recorded in his diary the imminent death of his daughter Sukey. "Her face, feet and hands are all cold and her pulse quite gone and reduced to the bones and skin that cover them and dying very hard . . . severe stroke indeed to A Man bereft of a Wife and in the decline of life." Sukey was probably about seven; Carter was forty-seven but thought of himself as old, and he had lost three wives in all.[1]

Carter's diary entry records as personal tragedy what historical demography is presenting more formally: the fragility of life in the early Chesapeake. Lifespans were in the main far shorter than today, shorter even than in seventeenth- and eighteenth-century New England; childhood deaths were commonplace; and women in their childbearing years ran a greater risk of death than did their husbands, the latter often being left widowers.[2] What were the roots of that fragility? How may it have affected the mind and form of Chesapeake society? Answers to these questions may emerge from an understanding of the endemic nature of malaria in the region.

A caveat is immediately in order. Any entry into the medical life of the past must be undertaken cautiously. On the one hand, Carter and his contemporaries referred to disease in archaic terms and in the context of an archaic medical paradigm. On the other, the nature of modern symptoma-

---

[1] Jack P. Greene, ed., *The Diary of Colonel Landon Carter of Sabine Hall, 1752-1778*, I (Charlottesville, Va., 1965), 221.

[2] Lorena S. Walsh and Russell R. Menard, "Death in the Chesapeake: Two Life Tables for Men in Early Colonial Maryland," *Maryland Historical Magazine*, LXIX (1974), 211-227; Darrett B. and Anita H. Rutman, " 'Now-Wives and Sons-

FIGURE I

THE LIFE CYCLE OF THE MALARIA PARASITE

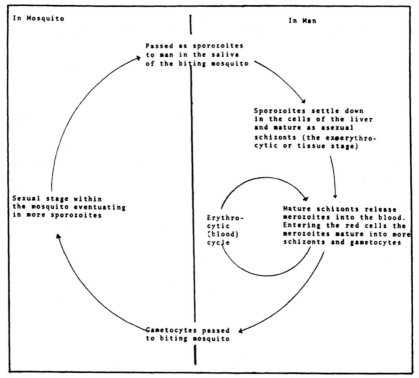

In Mosquito | In Man

Passed as sporozoites
to man in the saliva
of the biting mosquito

Sporozoites settle down
in the cells of the liver
and mature as asexual
schizonts (the exoerythro-
cytic or tissue stage)

Sexual stage within
the mosquito eventuating
in more sporozoites

Erythro-
cytic
(blood)
cycle

Mature schizonts release
merozoites into the blood.
Entering the red cells the
merozoites mature into more
schizonts and gametocytes

Gametocytes passed
to biting mosquito

Source:
    Adapted from G. Robert Coatney *et al.*, *The Primate Malarias* (Bethesda, Md., 1971), 30.

tology can delude the historian, for while the clinical and laboratory manifestations of disease are carefully delineated in modern textbooks, the past
had neither the conceptions nor the means to discern the latter, and the
former seldom appeared in pristine form. "Typicality" is vitiated by the
unique circumstances of the particular patient, by the fact that discrete
diseases can combine in unfamiliar manifestations, and by the fact of treatment itself: in the seventeenth century what effect might phlebotomy
(bleeding) have had on the course of a malarial attack? and in the twentieth
century how many physicians have seen an absolutely untreated case of

in-Law': Parental Death in a Seventeenth-Century Virginia County," in Thad W.
Tate, ed., *The Chesapeake in the Seventeenth Century: Essays on Its Euramerican
Society and Politics* (Chapel Hill, N. C., forthcoming).

malaria through its full course?[3] In brief, the past, with respect to discrete diseases, is indistinct. Literary references to the maladies and ailments of seventeenth-and eighteenth-century Chesapeake colonists abound in surviving letters, diaries, travelers' accounts, scientific works, and the like, but no single reference points unerringly to malaria as it is described today. Hence historians can only build an inferential case for its prevalence, combining the available literary evidence with a contemporary understanding of the disease so that the two are consonant with each other, then test their case against the known attributes of the society—in the present instance, its demographic attributes.

These cautions lead to a first question: malaria—what is it? Put succinctly, malaria is a febrile disease arising as a reaction of the body to invasion by parasites of the genus *Plasmodium*.[4] The life cycle of the *Plasmodium* forms a complex system involving as hosts a female anopheline mosquito and a vertebrate. In anthropomorphic terms, the human host serves as the nursery within which the parasite spends its asexual "childhood"; its sexual "adulthood" is spent in the mosquito. Figure 1 illustrates this complex system in a more "*Plasmodia*-centric," but still simple, form. A highly idealized clinical reaction in the human host is illustrated in Figure 2. From infection by the bite of the female *Anopheles* mosquito through a tissue stage in the liver the reaction is nil. Only as the parasites enter the blood to attack the red cells do the body's defenses rise to do battle and clinical reactions begin. Headache and general malaise are occasional premonitory symptoms, but the internal battle is most marked by fever paroxysms, with the parasite's cycle setting the tempo. Relatively slight paroxysms follow the first entry into the blood; as the cycle proceeds, wave after wave of parasites are rhythmically released, and the host's fever rises and falls in response. Fever "spikes"

[3] The classic caution was entered by Charles Creighton, *A History of Epidemics in Britain*, II (Cambridge, 1894), 1-2. Donald G. Bates, "Thomas Willis and the Epidemic Fever of 1661: A Commentary," *Bulletin of the History of Medicine*, XXXIX (1965), 393-412, is a brilliant modern restatement and elaboration.

[4] The cumulative nature of scientific writing, with its periodic "position papers," has been our key to an understanding of malaria. As basic references and guides to the pre-1972 literature we have used Forest Ray Moulton, ed., *A Symposium on Human Malaria with Special Reference to North America and the Caribbean Region* (Washington, D. C., 1941); Mark F. Boyd, ed., *Malariology: A Comprehensive Survey of All Aspects of This Group of Diseases from a Global Standpoint* (Philadelphia, 1949); G. Robert Coatney *et al.*, *The Primate Malarias* (Bethesda, Md., 1971); and Robert G. Scholtens and José A. Nájera, eds., *Proceedings of the Inter-American Malaria Research Symposium*, printed as a supplement to the *American Journal of Tropical Medicine and Hygiene*, XXI (1972), 604-851, hereafter cited as *Proceedings*. *Cumulated Index Medicus* (Chicago, 1960-   ) provided entry to the most recent studies.

climb progressively higher, frequently accompanied by antecedent chills and postcedent sweatings. Associated with the paroxysms are secondary symptoms. The host may experience headache (sometimes with an accompanying eye pain), loss of appetite, nausea, generalized aches and pains and specific abdominal pain, and occasional respiratory difficulties, weakness, and vertigo. An observer might discern vomiting, skin eruptions, palpable enlargement of the spleen and liver and a generalized swelling of the limbs, nosebleed, diarrhea, jaundice, and pallor, the last indicative of severe anemia. If the body's defenses ultimately prevail, the cycle is broken and at least the parasites in the blood are destroyed. Remission and recovery follow.

From long association with humans, however, *Plasmodium* has evolved its own defenses against theirs. Defeated in the blood, the parasites can remain ensconced in some manner in the liver.[5] Within eight to ten months after the primary attack they will again enter the blood. The cycle begins anew, and the fever returns, calling forth counter defenses on the part of the host. The initial attack starts a process by which an immunity is acquired, and each successive relapse strengthens the immunity until all outward symptoms disappear. The immunity does not last long—only a few years. But the reintroduction of *Plasmodia* by the bite of a female *Anopheles* brings on enough of an internal reaction to reinvigorate the immunity, even though it may not result in an observable reaction in the host.

Thus far our intent has been to sketch quickly and in idealized terms the principal features of malaria, in order to lay ground for a more complicated discussion. First, our reference has been to genus *Plasmodium*, but genus implies species, and indeed there is a multiplicity of species. Four of these infect humans, two of them commonly: *Plasmodium vivax* and *Plasmodium falciparum*.[6] Between these two species there are clear differences in the reaction of the human host. The patterns of fever spikes vary, reflecting different patterns of parasitic development within the body. The intensity of the disease also varies, *vivax* being the more benign, *falciparum* the more virulent; mortality directly associated with untreated *vivax* is estimated at under 5 percent, while mortality associated with untreated *falciparum* can rise as high as 25 percent.[7] The classic relapse pattern is that of *Plasmodium vivax*, there being little or no relapse associated with *falciparum*.

Acquired immunity likewise varies between species. Immunity to *vivax* is

[5] The relapse mechanism of the parasite is not clearly understood. Coatney *et al.*, *Primate Malarias*, 31-37, succinctly reviews the state of knowledge as of 1971.

[6] *P. malariae* and *P. ovale* have been rarities in North America and hence are omitted here.

[7] Emilio Pampana, *A Textbook of Malaria Eradication*, 2d ed. (London, 1969), 19.

AGUES AND FEVERS   35

FIGURE 2

HYPOTHETICAL CLINICAL REACTION TO INVASION
BY MALARIA *Plasmodium (vivax)*
(A PRIMARY ATTACK)

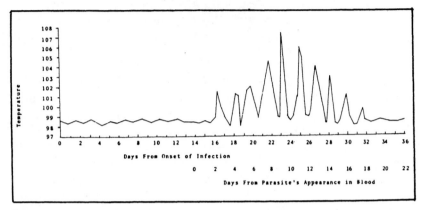

Source:
Following C. Merrill Whorton *et al.*, "The Chesson Strain of *Plasmodium Vivax* Malaria," Pt. III, "Clinical Aspects," *Journal of Infectious Diseases*, LXXX (1947), 237–249.

rapidly acquired and relatively long-lived (approximately three to five years); that to *falciparum* is more solid but shorter-lived and more dependent on regular reinfection for prolongation. And while there is a pronounced innate immunity to *vivax* among blacks, there seems to be no race-specific immunity to *falciparum*. Whites and blacks are clearly susceptible to infection—indeed, a significant portion of modern research on falciparum malaria takes place in black Africa—but blacks seem to tolerate an attack somewhat better than whites. Among both whites and blacks can be found what is termed the "sickle-cell trait," which seems to confer a resistance to infection, although the interdependence of this genetic trait and malaria on the one hand and the long association of blacks with a malarious Africa on the other have made the trait generally more common among blacks than among Caucasians.[8]

[8] Coatney *et al.*, *Primate Malarias*, 283: "There appears to be no racial or innate immunity among Negroes against falciparum malaria as has been observed for vivax malaria. ... However, the Negro does have a tendency to be able to clinically tolerate falciparum malaria infections better than the Caucasians. The presence of genetic traits which inhibit parasite multiplication or survival, such as sickle cell hemoglobin and enzyme deficiencies, have been reported but are not universally accepted." Cf. Peter H. Wood, *Black Majority: Negroes in Colonial South Carolina from 1670 through the Stono Rebellion* (New York, 1974), 88-89.

Within species, moreover, there are strains—an unknown number, of which only a few have been isolated in the laboratory—and there are clear differences in the reaction of the host to particular strains of the same species. Again, the pattern of fever spikes will vary slightly, but more important with reference to both species and strains is the fact that acquired immunities tend to be species- and strain-specific. A person who is infected by *Plasmodium vivax*, St. Elizabeth Strain, for example, tends to develop resistance only to that strain.

Second, we have referred to the mosquito vector as simply the female anopheline, but this masks a complex reality involving a genus *Anopheles* (within the family Culicidae and tribe Anophelini), six subgenera, and a variety of species and subspecies that vary in range, breeding habitat, and biting characteristics, and also as carriers of the parasite. *Anopheles atropos* and *Anopheles bradleyi*, for example, breed in the saltwater pools and marshes of the coast from Texas to Maryland, but *atropos* prefers water with a high salt content, *bradleyi* a low; and while *bradleyi*, in common with most *Anopheles*, tends to confine its biting to dusk, *atropos* will swarm and bite in bright sunlight. *Anopheles crucians* is a species of the southeastern coastal plain, frequenting fresh to slightly brackish swamps and pools and the margins of ponds and lakes. In the early twentieth century it was suspected as the primary vector in tidewater Virginia, because of its high density in the area and its propensity to enter houses to bite.[9] *Anopheles punctipennis* has the greatest range of any North American species, breeding in shaded springs and pools or along the margins of streams from southern Canada to New Mexico and along the Pacific coast. It bites only outdoors, entering houses in late fall only to hibernate. *Anopheles quadrimaculatus* prefers open sunlit waters for breeding, and although it is one of the *anopheles* most highly susceptible to *Plasmodium* (hence most likely to carry the parasite back to human beings), it seems to have a decided preference for the blood of cows and horses. All of the anopheline mosquitoes share certain characteristics. They are creature of short flight, normally ranging no more than one to two miles from their breeding places. They are highly affected by the weather. Optimal conditions for biting include a bright moonlit night, humidity about 85 percent, and a temperature in the low to mid-eighties. In a temperate climate the onset of cold weather brings on a suspension of all anopheline activity.

Species and strains of *Plasmodium* on the one hand; variety of *Anopheles* on the other—yet we have only touched on some of the many variables

[9] James Stevens Simmons, "The Transmission of Malaria by the Anopheles Mosquitoes of North America," in Moulton, ed., *Symposium on Human Malaria*, 114; Stanley B. Freeborn, "Anophelines of the Nearctic Region," in Boyd, ed., *Malariology*, I, 388.

involved in what malariologist Mark F. Boyd has described as the most complex and contradictory of disease systems.[10] A third set of complications relates to the behavior of malaria in communities.

In the malarial system the disease manifestation in humans is only one part. *Anopheles* must be infected by a human host, who, in turn, must be infected by *Anopheles,* with the circular transmission dependent on both. An anopheline mosquito must have access to, and must bite, a person (and not a nearby horse or cow) when the blood of that person is carrying the single form of the parasite that will infect the mosquito—in general, during or shortly after a malarial attack. After enough time has elapsed to allow the completion of the parasitic cycle within the mosquito, the mosquito must bite again, passing on the single form of the parasite that will bring about reinfection. To use technical terms, an *Anopheles* with a sporozoite-clear saliva biting a person free of gametocytes will have no more effect than to provoke a swat and a scratch! Within any given malarial community the degree to which the system is established is clearly dependent on the rate of transmission of the parasite from *Anopheles* to human being and back to mosquito through properly timed bites. At the lowest levels of endemicity few infected mosquitoes are abroad, few in the human population play host to the parasite, and transmission is only occasional. At the very highest levels of endemicity—hyperendemicity—virtually all anopheline mosquitoes are infected, and they are so numerous that no member of the human population can avoid being bitten every night. Human infection is then virtually 100 percent, and transmission is virtually constant. Between these extremes lie an indefinite number of levels of endemicity.

To speak of levels of endemicity is not to speak directly of levels of clinical morbidity—that is, the number of persons in the population displaying observable symptoms. Recall that malarial infection results in the human host in a species- and strain-specific immunity, but one of limited duration that is dependent for prolongation on reinfection (although not necessarily morbidity). In a malarial community the development of individual immunities tends to create a degree of group immunity. How effective that group immunity will be depends on the transmission level, or the level of endemicity. In communities of low endemicity individuals will be infected less often and group immunity will be lower than in areas of high endemicity. Clinical morbidity, group immunity, and endemicity levels interact to force a curvilinear relationship between the first and last, as sketched in Figure 3. If we were to measure the endemic and clinical morbidity levels of a number of communities, we would find that morbidity climbs as endemicity rises, since a

[10] Mark F. Boyd, "Epidemiology of Malaria: Factors Related to the Intermediate Host," in Boyd, ed., *Malariology,* I, 552.

greater percentage of infectious bites by *Anopheles* leads to symptomatic malarial attacks. Yet the rate of morbidity will be balanced at some point by the rate of immunities in the population and then will begin to decline until, in a hyperendemic situation, morbidity is largely limited to children, non-immune newcomers to the community, and pregnant women. Moreover, within any given community the level of endemicity (and consequently clinical morbidity) will tend to stabilize at a fixed figure. The figure may rise or fall as the number of anopheline mosquitoes in the area rises or falls, or as the number of the nonimmune changes, or when the onset of a new strain or species makes prior immunities irrelevant, or even as the spatial organization of the society shifts: a trend toward urban clustering, for example, will tend to decrease the proportionate access of mosquitoes to the population and bring a decline in the endemic level. But although the level of endemicity may change, there will invariably be a tendency toward stasis.[11]

Two other aspects of the malarial system in communities must be sketched before we turn to the subject at hand—malaria in the early Chesapeake region. First, whatever the endemic or morbidity level of a population, there is an areal definition to that population. The point is best made by an example. Consider a village located beside a saltwater swamp in which *Anopheles bradleyi* breed. Given the flight and breeding limitations of *bradleyi*, it is clear that even if our exemplifying village is highly endemic, another, four miles away beside a freshwater pond, need not be. The areal boundaries of the malarious population are thus defined by the mosquito. Presume that the pond by our second village is a breeding area for *Anopheles quadrimaculatus*. What then? It will remain malaria-free only if no one laden with gametocytes travels to it from the first village. In this case the areal boundaries are set by levels of population mobility as well as by the mosquito. The example may seem exaggerated, but the abruptness of areal boundaries was clear even in the 1890s when Walter Reed noted that while malaria was endemic among the soldiers of Washington Barracks, on the low flats bordering the Anacostia and Potomac rivers in the District of Columbia, it was significantly less prevalent "among those who live in the more elevated section of the city" away from the flats.[12]

Second, in a temperate climate such as that of the Chesapeake malaria cannot achieve the hyperendemic level that follows from near-constant transmission. As we have noted, the onset of cold weather inhibits anopheline

[11] A few malariologists, notably Ronald Ross, and statistician Alfred J. Lotka have attempted to reduce the malarial system to a mathematical model. See Mark F. Boyd, "Epidemiology: Factors Related to the Definitive Host," *ibid.*, 683-687.

[12] Hugh R. Gilmore, Jr., "Malaria at Washington Barracks and Fort Myer: A Survey of Walter Reed," *Bull. Hist. Med.*, XXIX (1955), 348.

AGUES AND FEVERS   39

FIGURE 3

HYPOTHETIC RELATIONSHIP OF LEVELS OF
MORBIDITY AND ENDEMICITY AMONG
MALARIAL COMMUNITIES

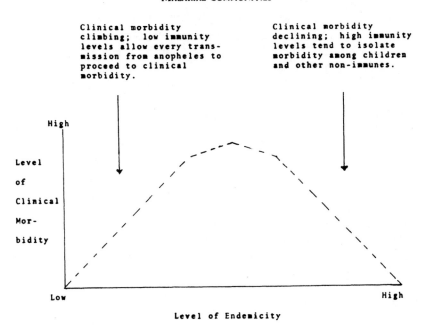

Clinical morbidity
climbing; low immunity
levels allow every trans-
mission from anopheles to
proceed to clinical
morbidity.

Clinical morbidity
declining; high immunity
levels tend to isolate
morbidity among children
and other non-immunes.

High

Level
of
Clinical
Mor-
bidity

Low   High

Level of Endemicity

activity and thus regularly interrupts transmission. In the absence of transmission, morbidity declines, individual immunities diminish, and the non-immune increase; group immunity thus deteriorates, leaving the population vulnerable to what is to come. Latent infections will persist over the winter, and as these bring on a few malarial attacks in the spring, as cases of *vivax* contracted during the previous fall reappear as relapses, and as mosquitoes start biting again, transmission restarts and the malarial system is reinvigorated. The endemic level, having declined during the winter, rises again. Symptomatic morbidity steadily increases through the spring and summer to a peak in the autumn, then abruptly declines with the coming of another winter. Figure 4, a seasonal plot of 614 malaria cases treated at The Johns Hopkins University Hospital in the early 1890s, displays the seasonality of the two major species of malaria then current in the Chesapeake area.

Was there malaria in the early Chesapeake? Historiographically, the question has been asked mainly with reference to Virginia, and the answer has been mixed. Thomas Jefferson Wertenbaker, reflecting a traditional view, wrote in 1914 of the "swarms of mosquitoes" that rose from "the stagnant pools" around Jamestown and attacked the settlers of 1607 "with a sting more deadly than that of the Indian arrow or the Spanish musket ball." In 1930 the tradition was challenged by Wyndham B. Blanton. "No one doubts that there were marshes, mosquitoes and sickness along the James River," but "there is no evidence ... that malaria was responsible for a preponderating part of the great mortalities." Blanton was rebutted by John Duffy in 1953: with malaria in the Carolina lowcountry to the south and among the French and English to the north, "it is highly improbable that the early settlers in Virginia were exempt." In 1957 Blanton replied that there was no natural habitat around Jamestown for *Anopheles quadrimaculatus* (even if true, Blanton ignored the fact that *quadrimaculatus* is but one of many species). He also contended that malaria was not introduced until late in the century—by which time the colonists, by clearing the forests, had created a habitat for mosquitoes—and that it was brought by slaves from the malaria-infested areas of the west African coast.[13] This mini-debate was in reality a non-debate, for the participants had different frames of reference. Blanton's gaze was fixed on the great mortalities of the years to the mid-1620s, from which he extrapolated forward;[14] Duffy, with a broader view of the whole colonial period, inferred from the whole to the part.

All indications are that malaria was imported into the Americas by Europeans. The disease in its milder form (*vivax*) is thought to have been general in Europe in the sixteenth and seventeenth centuries—Oliver Cromwell seems to have been only one of the more prominent sufferers. The more virulent *falciparum* is thought to have been prevalent in large parts of Africa.

---

[13] Thomas J. Wertenbaker, *Virginia Under the Stuarts, 1607-1688* (Princeton, N. J., 1914), 11; Wyndham B. Blanton, *Medicine in Virginia in the Seventeenth Century* (Richmond. Va., 1930), 54; John Duffy, *Epidemics in Colonial America* (Baton Rouge, La., 1953), 207n. Duffy made good use of St. Julien Ravenel Childs, *Malaria and Colonization in the Carolina Low Country, 1526-1696* (Baltimore, 1940), but to that study must be added Wood, *Black Majority*, Chap. 3, and Wyndham B. Blanton, "Epidemics, Real and Imaginary, and Other Factors Influencing Seventeenth Century Virginia's Population," *Bull. Hist. Med.*, XXXI (1957), 454-462. For a malariologist's answer to the general question of the historical development of malaria in North America see Mark F. Boyd, "An Historical Sketch of the Prevalence of Malaria in North America," *American Journal of Tropical Medicine*, XXI (1941), 223-244.

[14] Hence Blanton could make a part of his chain of evidence for the whole 17th century the "happy, intelligent, and vigorous" nature of the Powhatan Indians of 1607, arguing that they would have been otherwise if malaria had been prevalent, for "malaria notoriously destroys happiness, intelligence and vigor." Blanton, "Epidemics," *Bull. Hist. Med.*, XXXI (1957), 457.

AGUES AND FEVERS   41

But the Americas appear to have been free of the disease until the arrival of Europeans.[15] G. Robert Coatney and his colleagues find the evidence of pre-Columbian malaria too scant to be convincing, while to Saul Jarcho the existence of the mosquito in pre-contact America is certain, of *Anopheles* probable, and of malaria improbable although not impossible.[16]

FIGURE 4

SEASONAL DISTRIBUTION OF MALARIA CASES TREATED AT
JOHNS HOPKINS HOSPITAL, BALTIMORE, 1889–1894

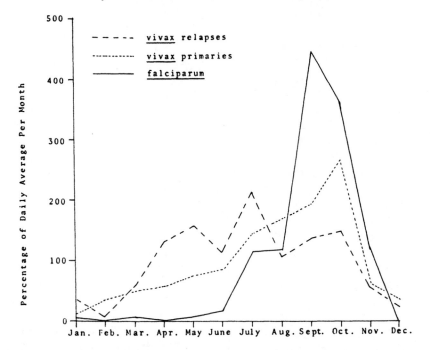

Source and notes:
    Adapted from Mark F. Boyd, ed., *Malariology, A Comprehensive Survey of All Aspects of This Group of Diseases From a Global Standpoint* (Philadelphia, 1949), I, 557. The distribution is expressed as the percentage of daily average per month to allow comparison of different sample sizes and to minimize the effect of months of different lengths. The percentage is arrived at by a series of divisions: $[(E_m \div D_m)/(E_y \div 365.25)] \times 100$ where $E_m =$ the events in a month, $D_m =$ the number of days in a month, $E_y =$ the total events in the sample. Feb. is assigned 28.25 days.

[15] Frederick F. Cartwright and Michael D. Biddiso, *Disease and History* (New York, 1972), 138-140.
    [16] Coatney *et al.*, *Primate Malarias*, 7; Saul Jarcho, "Some Observations on Disease in Prehistoric North America," *Bull. Hist. Med.*, XXXVIII (1964), 9.

If malaria was not indigenous to the Americas, it could only have been introduced by the entry of infected individuals into areas where *Anopheles* breed. When or from where such persons arrived in Virginia—directly from England or by way of the Caribbean—is irrelevant and certainly indeterminable. Although a variety of strains and perhaps even both major species may have been introduced by diverse carriers at a fairly early date, a more probable model, given the flow of immigration and the prevalence of *vivax* in Europe and *falciparum* in Africa, would have strains of the former entering during the first half of the century, followed by the gradual establishment (perhaps spotty) of areas of stable, low-level endemicity. The shattering of this picture would occur as blacks in numbers began arriving from a variety of African areas, bringing with them new strains of *vivax*, and *falciparum*.[17] In this model, symptomatic morbidity—the number of clinical cases—would rise gradually to about 1650, by which time the occasional, seemingly random cases of the early decades would be giving way to seasonal outbreaks. Through the remainder of the century epidemic-like incidents would mark the entry of each new strain or species, the general level of malaria morbidity rising a bit higher in the aftermath of each such outbreak.[18] The model also suggests that a qualitative change occurred sometime in the second half of the century as *falciparum* entered the colony, precipitating more virulent and wracking attacks, a phenomenon also noted by Peter Wood in his study of South Carolina slavery. The evidence from Carolina suggests to Wood that the benign *vivax* was prevalent in the 1670s but was supplanted by the more virulent *falciparum* in the 1680s.[19]

The literary evidence for Virginia supports this model, although in relating the archaic and imprecise terminology of the sources to the modern symptomatology of the disease we enter on the most treacherous ground of medical history. Blanton, for example, keyed his search for malaria on the word "ague" as referring to the combination of chills and fevers so generally associated in the popular mind with the disease. But chills may accompany fevers other than malarial, and malarial fevers are not always accompanied by chills. In a modern study of 201 paroxysms, 137 were found to be

[17] White susceptibility to diseases prevalent among blacks would be the other side of the coin with regard to Philip D. Curtin's thesis of black susceptibility to diseases prevalent among whites. See Curtin, "Epidemiology and the Slave Trade," *Political Science Quarterly*, LXXXIII (1968), 190-216.

[18] This is the picture drawn by a 100-year simulation based on the mathematics in Boyd, "Definitive Host," in Boyd, ed., *Malariology*, I, 683-687. It has been extended to incorporate elementary shifts in the human population and changes in the immunity level to reflect assumptions as to the sequential introduction of species (*vivax* followed by *falciparum*) and the periodic introduction of new strains.

[19] Wood, *Black Majority*, 87.

unaccompanied by chills, leading the investigators to conclude that "the term 'chills and fevers' inadequately described" a malarial attack.[20] Similarly, the words "intermittent" and "remittent," used in the sources as adjectives for "fever," may or may not refer to the characteristic fever spikes of malaria, as may "quotidian," "tertian," and "quartan" used to describe the timing of the spikes. References to chinchona or its synonyms—Peruvian bark, Jesuit bark, or simply "the bark"—may also be indicative of malaria, for chinchona was introduced into Europe as a specific remedy for what is generally considered to have been malaria. Such references are not infallible, for the bark was sometimes utilized for fevers other than malarial, and its efficacy was widely questioned; hence it was not invariably given.[21] Nevertheless, we must have a measure of confidence: even if many of the references to ague, the varieties of fever, and "the bark" are misapplied, the remainder correctly point to malaria. From the sources it seems clear that the "agues and fevers" that were only occasional in the first fifty years in Virginia became both more general and more severe (reflecting the entry of *falciparum?*) in the second fifty and on into the eighteenth century.

There is no need here to review the occasional evidence for seventeenth-century malaria cited by Blanton.[22] Clearly, by the 1680s the "seasoning"— that period of illness which almost inevitably befell a newcomer to the Chesapeake—was associated with what we can take for malaria. Newcomers might assume any sickness that struck them to be a "seasoning," as Robert Beverley noted in his *History of Virginia* and as George Hume did in 1723. To Hume a whole succession of illnesses—from "a severe flux" to a "now and then" bout with "the fever and ague"—added up to "a most severe" seasoning.[23] But the long-time resident of Virginia was more precise. William Fitzhugh wrote of his newly arrived sister in 1687: she has had "two or

---

[20] G. Robert Coatney and Martin D. Young, "A Study of the Paroxysms Resulting from Induced Infections of *Plasmodium vivax*," *American Journal of Hygiene*, XXXV (1942), 141. C. Merrill Whorton *et al.*, "The Chesson Strain of *Plasmodium vivax* Malaria," Pt. III: "Clinical Aspects," *Journal of Infectious Diseases*, LXXX (1947), 241, reported chills in only 46% of 158 primary attacks.

[21] A. W. Haggis, "Fundamental Errors in the Early History of Chinchona," *Bull. Hist. Med.*, X (1941), 417-459, 568-592.

[22] Blanton found 6 references to 1700: *Medicine in the Seventeenth Century*, 52-53; "Epidemics," *Bull. Hist. Med.*, XXXI (1957), 458. A few escaped him, notably John Clayton's. Edmund and Dorothy Smith Berkeley, eds., *The Reverend John Clayton . . . His Scientific Writings and Other Related Papers* (Charlottesville, Va., 1965). To some extent the number of references is a function of the quantity and types of materials extant from the period rather than of the prevalence of the disease.

[23] George Hume to Ninian Hume, June 20, 1723, *Virginia Magazine of History and Biography*, XX (1912), 397-400. Robert Beverley wrote in *The History and Present State of Virginia*, ed. Louis B. Wright (Chapel Hill, N. C., 1947), 306:

three small fits of a feaver and ague, which now has left her, and so consequently her seasoning [is] over." And again, in another letter: "My Sister has had her seasoning . . . two or three fits of a feaver and ague." John Clayton, Virginia's scientific parson, wrote of "Seasonings, which are an intermiting feaver, or rather a continued feaver with quotidian paroxisms," in describing that same year the "distempers" among the English.[24]

By the 1680s sharp geographical differences in levels of health were being noted in the colony. To a French traveler of 1686-1687 the inhabitants of tidewater Gloucester County "looked so sickly that I judged the country to be unhealthy"; those of Stafford and old Rappahannock were obviously healthier, "their complexions clear and lively." The Virginians gave him a reason he considered "quite plausible": "along the seashore and also along the rivers which contain salt, because of the tide, the inhabitants in these places are rarely free from fever during the hot weather; they call this a local sickness; but the salt in the rivers disappears about twenty leagues from the seas, just as one enters the county of Rappahannock, and those who live beyond that point do not suffer from it." Clayton, too, noted the geographic difference, adding a hint of autumnal seasonality: "so far as the Salt Waters reach the Country is deemed less healthy. In the Freshes they more rarely are troubled with Seasonings, and those Endemical Distempers about *September* and *October*."[25] All three phenomena are commensurate with a hypothesis of widespread malaria. As we have seen, autumnal seasonality is inherent in temperate-zone malaria; so too are the susceptibility of newcomers—they must develop immunities to the specific species and strains of *Plasmodia*

"The first sickness that any New-Comer happens to have there, he unfairly calls a Seasoning, be it Fever, Ague, or any thing else, that his own folly, or excesses bring upon him."

[24] William Fitzhugh to Henry Fitzhugh, July 18, 1687, Fitzhugh to Dr. Ralph Smith, July 1, 1687, in Richard Beale Davis, ed., *William Fitzhugh and His Chesapeake World, 1676-1701: The Fitzhugh Letters and Other Documents* (Chapel Hill, N. C., 1963), 229, 230; Dr. Nehemiah Grew to John Clayton, 1687, in Berkeley and Berkeley, eds., *John Clayton*, 26. Richard Harrison Shryock, *Medicine and Society in America, 1660-1860* (New York, 1960), 87, generally associated malaria with the colonial "seasoning"; so did travelers describing the entry of newcomers into the malarious Mississippi Valley of the 19th century. See Michael Owen Jones, "Climate and Disease: The Traveler Describes America," *Bull. Hist. Med.*, XLI (1967), 256.

[25] Gilbert Chinard, ed., *A Huguenot Exile in Virginia, or Voyages of a Frenchman exiled for his Religion with a description of Virginia & Maryland* (New York, 1934), 130, 174; John Clayton to the Royal Society, 1688, in Berkeley and Berkeley, eds., *John Clayton*, 54. Clayton went on to suggest that an investigation of the phenomena might result in "several beneficial Discoveries, not only in relation to those Distempers in *America*, but perhaps take in your *Kentish* Agues." The latter phrase has generally been understood to refer to malaria.

present in an area—and the sharp boundaries between infected and uninfected populations, although in this case the boundaries would seem to have
been only temporary. Time would be required to create in newly settled areas
the conditions necessary to maintain the endemic levels that existed in older
areas.[26]

For the eighteenth century the literary evidence is clearer, and there is no
question among historians as to the prevalence of malaria. John Oldmixon,
who presumably drew some of his information from William Byrd II, wrote
at the turn of the century that "the *Seasoning* here, as in other parts of
America, is a Fever or Ague, which the Change of Climate and Diet
generally throws new Comers into; the Bark is in *Virginia* a Sovereign
Remedy to this Disease." Beverley wrote of the Virginians' "Intermitting
Fevers, as well as their Agues," as "very troublesome" and cited "*Cortex
Peruviana*" as a remedy that "seldom or never fails to remove the Fits." Byrd
dosed with the bark his family, himself, and his fellow commissioners of the
North Carolina boundary survey. In 1735 he referred to the shipment of
"infused" bark to Virginia by England's "Drugsters and Apothecarys"--
that is, bark which had been steeped in water, the water being used in
England and the residual bark shipped to the colonies—as "almost as bad as
Murder." Hugh Jones wrote of a people "subject to feavers and agues, which
is the country distemper, a severe fit of which (called a seasoning) most
expect, some time after their arrival." Chinchona was "a perfect catholicon
for that sickness . . . which being taken and repeated in a right manner,
seldom fails of a cure."[27]

[26] In contrast to descriptions of other parts of Virginia, John Banister's descriptions of the falls area of the James make no mention of illness and disease, implying a
relatively disease-free area during the late 17th century. Joseph and Nesta Ewan,
John Banister and His Natural History of Virginia, 1678-1692 (Urbana, Ill., 1970).
At the end of the 18th century Thomas Jefferson wrote that "Richmond was not well
chosen as the place to shake off a fever and ague in the months of Aug. Sep. and Oct.
till frost. All it's inhabitants who can afford it leave it for the upper country during
that season." Wyndham B. Blanton, *Medicine in Virginia in the Eighteenth Century* (Richmond, Va., 1931), 67. In the 19th and 20th centuries no malarial "fall
line" existed as suggested by the earlier distinction between "the salts" and "the
freshes." See the county morbidity and mortality statistics for 1927-1932 in Frederick
L. Hoffman, *Malaria in Virginia, North Carolina and South Carolina* (Newark,
N. J., 1933).

[27] John Oldmixon, *The British Empire in America,* I (London, 1708), 294;
Beverley, *History of Virginia,* ed. Wright, 306; Louis B. Wright and Marion
Tinling, eds., *The Secret Diary of William Byrd of Westover, 1709-1712* (Richmond,
Va., 1941), 232, 372-373, 386-389, 538, 589; Louis B. Wright, ed., *The Prose Works
of William Byrd of Westover: Narratives of a Colonial Virginian* (Cambridge,
Mass., 1966), 102, 130, 189, 340-342, 348; William Byrd to Mrs. Otway, Oct. 2,

Sources from the latter half of the century contain abundant references to what can be construed as malaria, leading Blanton to conclude that "hardly any section . . . escaped the inevitable 'Ague and Fever.' "[28] Indeed, here and there in the literature are such detailed accounts that one is tempted to diagnose individual cases—Landon Carter's Sukey, for example. Autumnal fevers were pronounced in both 1756 and 1757, Carter writing of the fall of the latter year that it was a "very Aguish Season" when nothing "but the barke" would do, and noting that "it has been more usefull this year than common." During the autumn of 1756 Sukey was among the sixty-odd in his family and labor force to take sick. A year later, in the midst of a still worse fever season, Sukey came down again, falling into a monthly pattern of attacks that extended through the autumn and early winter, subsided during the coldest weather, then reappeared in March 1758. In describing his daughter's illnesses Carter noted time and again the secondary symptoms associated with malaria, from nausea and vomiting to pains and pallor. But most telling is his running account of the course of Sukey's fever. In Figure 5 the description of five days of Sukey's first 1757 fever attack in August is superimposed on a modern fever chart of a quotidian (intermittent-remittent type) clinical attack of *Plasmodium falciparum*. Was Sukey's a case of malaria? Diagnosis from such evidence is impossible: all the historian can hope for is consonance between historical evidence and medical understanding. The literary description of Sukey's illness seems entirely consonant with malaria.[29]

Presuming that, from the literary evidence, a circumstantial case can be made for the presence of malaria in the Chesapeake region, or at least in Virginia, in the seventeenth and eighteenth centuries, what demographic effects might follow? Can we discern these effects and substantiate to an extent the literary case already made? In other words, does the hypothesis of malaria fit, perhaps even explain, the empirical evidence? The question requires consideration of as much as possible of the demographic analysis of early America done to date. It requires, too, the drawing of analogies between early America, for which no direct measurement of malaria or its

---

1735, *VMHB*, XXXVI (1928), 121. Byrd in this letter, as Clayton did in 1687 (n. 22), associated the Virginia "distemper" with "your Kentish Distemper." See also Hugh Jones, *The Present State of Virginia*, ed. Richard L. Morton (Chapel Hill, N. C., 1956), 85.

[28] Blanton, *Medicine in the Eighteenth Century*, 67.

[29] Sukey's illness can be followed in Greene, ed., *Diary of Carter*, I, 127, to her death on pp. 221-222. In the case of prominent men even more positive "diagnosis" is common, for example, the diagnosis of Washington as suffering from "chronic malaria" in Blanton, *Medicine in the Eighteenth Century*, 309.

AGUES AND FEVERS   47

FIGURE 5

EIGHTEENTH-CENTURY FEVER DESCRIPTION SUPERSCRIBED
ON A TWENTIETH-CENTURY FEVER CHART
ARISING FROM AN INFECTION OF *Plasmodium falciparum*

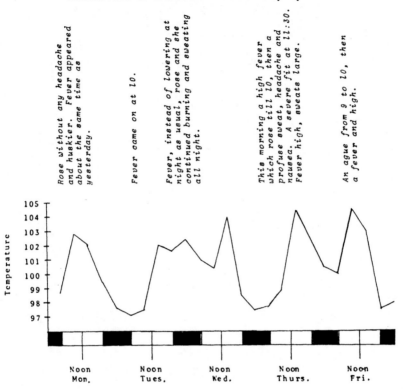

Sources and notes:

Fever description paraphrased from Jack P. Greene, ed., *The Diary of Colonel Landon
Carter of Sabine Hall, 1752-1778* (Charlottesville, Va., 1965), I, 165-167; fever chart adapted
from S. F. Kitchen, "The Infection in the Intermediate Host: Symptomatology, Falciparum
Malaria," in Forest Fay Moulton, ed., *A Symposium on Human Malaria with Special
Reference to North America and the Caribbean Region* (Washington, D. C., 1941), 198, Case
no. 1164. Mon. was the second day of fever.

effects is available, and malarious areas of the world where measurements
have been made during the twentieth century.

Since 1967, when Philip Greven formally introduced early Americanists
to the startling possibilities for research opened by the French demographic
historians, a great deal of sophisticated demographic work has been done on

TABLE I

COMPARATIVE ADULT LIFE EXPECTANCIES: THE CHESAPEAKE REGION AND NEW ENGLAND

Expected Years Yet to Live

Achieved Age[a]	Andover b.1670-1699		Salem d.17th Cent.		Middlesex b.1650-1710		Salem d.18th Cent.		Andover b.1730-1759	
	Male	Female	Male	Female	Male	Female	Male	Female	Male	Female
15	- -	- -	- -	21.4	- -	24.9	- -	- -	- -	- -
20	44.8	42.1	36.1	- -	28.8	19.8	35.5	37.0	41.6	43.1
25	- -	- -	- -	20.0	23.7	16.3	- -	- -	- -	- -
30	38.7	35.9	29.2	- -	19.4	13.6	30.3	32.6	36.3	36.5
35	- -	- -	- -	20.9	15.8	10.7	- -	- -	- -	- -
40	31.4	29.0	24.1	- -	13.0	8.6	25.3	26.3	28.4	30.9
45	- -	- -	- -	14.4	10.0	9.2	- -	- -	- -	- -
50	23.5	22.4	19.1	- -	7.7	9.3	19.6	21.1	24.5	25.0
55	- -	- -	- -	16.2	7.7	7.9	- -	- -	- -	- -
60	15.2	15.9	14.5	- -	5.8	5.0	14.5	16.4	17.2	18.8
65	- -	- -	- -	10.0	5.0	3.7	- -	- -	- -	- -
70	10.2	11.9	10.0	- -	3.6	5.2	10.0	10.0	10.9	12.0
75	- -	- -	- -	- -	2.9	- -	- -	- -	- -	- -
80	6.7	9.5	- -	- -	- -	- -	- -	- -	7.1	8.3
85	- -	- -	- -	- -	- -	- -	- -	- -	- -	- -
90+	5.0	6.2	- -	- -	- -	- -	- -	- -	5.0	5.0

Notes and sources:

[a] Achieved age represents the lower inclusive boundary of a group. In the case of Middlesex: 15-19, 20-24, 25-29, etc.; Andover: 20-29, 30-39, 40-49, etc.; but N. B. Salem: 21-30, 31-40, 41-50, etc., with an estimate of 10 inserted for 71-plus.

For Andover and Salem see Maris A. Vinovskis, "Mortality Rates and Trends in Massachusetts before 1860," *Journal of Economic History*, XXXII (1972), 198-199 (drawing upon the work of Philip J. Greven, Jr., and James K. Somerville respectively). For Middlesex see Darrett B. and Anita H. Rutman, "Now Wives and Sons-in-Law': Parental Death in a Seventeenth-Century Virginia County," in Thad Tate, ed., *The Chesapeake in the Seventeenth Century: Essays on Its Euramerican Society and Politics* (Chapel Hill, N. C., forthcoming). The Middlesex table is based upon data for subjects known to have achieved marriageable age and to have chosen to marry. Both sources discuss at length the populations and procedures underlying the tables.

New England and, recently, on the early Chesapeake region.[30] This work has varied in quality and to some extent in methodology. It has been confined for the most part to explorations of particular locales, and for both regions such local studies are few. Investigation has nonetheless advanced to the point where a few basic phenomena seem to be coming into focus—four in particular with regard to mortality. First, radically different mortality schedules seem to have obtained in New England and the Chesapeake region. Men and women in the northern colonies tended to live considerably longer lives than did their contemporaries to the south. Second, in the Chesapeake and in seventeenth-century Salem, Massachusetts (but not apparently in other New England areas studied so far), women fifteen to forty-five years, the child-bearing years, seem to have run a substantially greater risk of death than did males of the same age. The third finding emerges from the second: even within a particular region and time period mortality rates in general, and sex-specific mortality rates in particular, seem to have varied by locality. Finally, in New England at least, mortality rates shifted over time. In the eighteenth century life expectancies rose from seventeenth-century levels in some areas and for some segments of the population and fell in others, the net effect being a tendency toward convergence—the "washing out" of differences. All four of these phenomena can be seen in Table I, drawn from studies of Andover and Salem, Massachusetts, and Middlesex County, Virginia. But Table I also suggests, in its confusion of sample definitions and age groupings, that such cross-study comparisons furnish grounds for only very broad general statements.

Still, the broad statements are enough to prompt questions. Why a difference in mortality between New England and the Chesapeake? Why a shift in mortality over time within New England? Why, in the seventeenth century, a sex-related difference in mortality during the years between fifteen and forty-five? Piecemeal explanations have been offered with respect to the New England data. Rising mortality rates and falling life expectancies between the seventeenth and eighteenth centuries have been attributed to the rise of population density to the point where infectious diseases could be supported. Although this plausible supposition accounts for some of the data, it does not explain those from Salem where mortality rates tended to fall slightly. Maris Vinovskis has related high death rates among Salem's females in the seventeenth century to maternal mortality—but were the conditions of

[30] Philip J. Greven, Jr., "Historical Demography and Colonial America," *William and Mary Quarterly*, 3d Ser., XXIV (1967), 438-454. Maris A. Vinovskis, "Mortality Rates and Trends in Massachusetts Before 1860," *Journal of Economic History*, XXXII (1972), 184-213, is a good introduction to, and critique of, the New England work, particularly that of Greven, Kenneth A. Lockridge, Susan L. Norton, and Vinovskis's own. The Chesapeake work is cited in n. 2 above.

childbirth so very different between Salem and nearby Ipswich where Susan Norton has found "no significant attrition of the female population during the years when . . . married women would be bearing children"?[31] Did the care of women in childbirth improve so greatly in the eighteenth century as to account for the congruence of male and female life expectancies found by Vinovskis in Salem and reflected in Table I? Most importantly, none of the piecemeal answers applies to the sharp contrast between New England and Chespeake mortality.

Does a consideration of malaria suggest a more general answer? The most obvious impact of malaria is on the general level of public health. Malaria is not notorious as a "killer" disease: the 5 and 25 percent mortality rates cited earlier are extremes. It is rather "the great debilitator"; it lowers the level of general health and the ability to resist other diseases. One modern study estimates that for every death ascribed to malaria in an infected population, five additional deaths are actually due to malaria acting in concert with other diseases.[32] Carter's Sukey is a case in point. Weakened by her bouts with a malarial fever, and undoubtedly anemic, she died in the spring of 1758 from what appeared to be a respiratory infection.

That an inverse relationship exists between the degree of malaria morbidity and the death rate is indicated in modern Guatemala. A malaria eradication program was initiated there in 1957, and the death rate declined 20 percent between 1958 and 1963. In Ceylon, where both eradication and a concerted attempt to expand medical facilities began immediately after World War II, the death rate declined by two-thirds between 1946 and 1953, with roughly 23 percent of the decline attributable to the malaria eradication program.[33] Thus a hypothesis of a malarious Chesapeake and a relatively nonmalarious New England might well explain a considerable part of the disparity between New England and Chesapeake mortality rates.

Note, however, that we refer to New England as "relatively" free of malaria. We mean to imply a difference of degree rather than an absolute difference, for there is evidence of malaria in seventeenth-century New

---

[31] Vinovskis, "Mortality Rates," *Jour. Econ. Hist.*, XXXII (1972), 201; Susan L. Norton, "Population Growth in Colonial America: A Study of Ipswich, Massachusetts," *Population Studies*, XXV (1971), 442.

[32] Peter Newman, *Malaria Eradication and Population Growth: With Special Reference to Ceylon and British Guiana* (Ann Arbor, Mich., 1965), 77.

[33] S. A. Meegama, "Malaria Eradication and its Effect on Mortality Levels," *Pop. Stud.*, XXI (1967), 207-208, 232. The effect of eradication on mortality rates is the subject of an intense debate, one largely fought out in the pages of *Pop. Stud.* We have adjusted Meegama's figures to reflect the latest word offered by R. H. Gray, "The Decline of Mortality in Ceylon and the Demographic Effects of Malaria Control," *ibid.*, XXVIII (1974), 226-227.

England. Duffy describes "attacks of pernicious malaria" in Boston in 1658, western Connecticut in 1668, Salem in 1683, and Boston again in 1690. For some reason, however, the northern boundary of malaria shifted in the eighteenth century, leaving New England entirely free of the disease after roughly the mid-century mark.[34]

The whole question of endemic (as distinct from epidemic) disease is undeveloped in early American historiography in general, and for New England specifically,[35] but one can make a calculated guess that malaria had only a marginal foothold in New England even in the seventeenth century and that levels of endemicity varied among the closed populations of the area. Among some, the disease was virtually nonexistent (but the population, lacking immunity, would be susceptible to sudden, short-lived periods of morbidity); among others, malaria was relatively well established.

This view would be consonant with the findings of modern malariologists who break down national malariometric and morbidity rates into regional and even village rates and find enormous variety. It would also be consonant with the diversity of mortality rates being found by historians of New England and—if we assume that Salem was an area of relatively well-ensconced malaria—with the two peculiarities of Salem's mortality schedule presented by Vinovskis. The first is the suggestion that while in other New England towns that have been studied mortality rose in the eighteenth century, Salem's mortality declined—that there was, in effect, a tendency among the towns for mortality to converge. Such a tendency would be very familiar to students of eradication programs;[36] and what was the disappearance of malaria from eighteenth-century New England but a form of natural eradication? The second is the high death rate for women in their childbearing years, which, although unique to Salem among the seventeenth-

---

[34] Duffy, *Epidemics*, 206-207, 213. Oliver Wendell Holmes's "Dissertation of Intermittent Fever in New England," *Boylston Prize Dissertations* (Boston, 1838), is, from start to finish, a compendium of quotations indicative of malaria in New England.

[35] Richard H. Shryock's complaint in his "Medical Sources and the Social Historian," originally published in the *American Historical Review*, XLI (1935-1936), 458-473, and reprinted in Richard Harrison Shryock, *Medicine in America: Historical Essays* (Baltimore, 1966), is that historians in general, and medical historians specifically, have emphasized the story of medical disasters (epidemics). "It is easier to find records of a sudden 'visitation' than it is to trace obscure, endemic conditions; and once written, the former makes more spectacular reading. Hence the universal attention accorded 'the Black Death.' Hence also the neglect of contemporary endemic diseases, which in the long run were more fatal and perhaps equally significant in their social consequences" (p. 278).

[36] For example, Gray, "Decline of Mortality," *Pop. Stud.*, XXVIII (1974), 226-227.

century New England towns studied, was shared with Middlesex in tidewater Virginia.

Exaggerated maternal mortality can be directly associated with endemic malaria, a relationship intuitively perceived in the malarious South of a half-century ago by country doctors who routinely dosed their pregnant patients with quinine, and more recently demonstrated in a controlled study of 250 pregnant women in urban Nigeria.[37] The nature of the linkage is still undetermined, but the indirect evidence indicates that pregnancy tends to nullify immunities, paving the way for a build-up of parasites, morbidity, and pronounced anemia, with a consequent hazard of abortion, premature labor, and the childbirth death of both mother and infant. Modern medical researchers cannot, of course, measure mortality directly, for of necessity they intervene to stop the course of the disease. Neither can modern medical research duplicate the conditions that exaggerated the hazards in the seventeenth and eighteenth centuries: large households crowded into small houses, exposing anemic, periodically feverish mothers-to-be to contagious ailments; living conditions that can only be described as dirty, with a consequent exposure of the mother to septicemia; and above all, a counterproductive medical practice: the bleeding and stringent dieting that William Byrd imposed on his pregnant and presumably malarious and anemic wife could hardly have been efficacious.[38]

Analogy can, to an extent, supply what the medical research leaves out. Puttalam district, Ceylon, in the late 1930s was an area roughly comparable to Middlesex County, Virginia, in the late seventeenth and early eighteenth centuries. Both were rural; both were devoid of modern medicine; in both, childbirth was managed by traditionally rather than medically oriented midwives; and both (Puttalam district for a certainty and Middlesex for the sake of argument) were malarious. Figure 6 graphs age- and sex-specific death rates for each area. The values are obviously different—for one reason because the figures are based on different statistical populations[39]—but the

[37] Warren K. Stratman-Thomas, "The Infection in the Intermediate Host: Symptomatology, *vivax* Malaria," and S. F. Kitchen, "The Infection in the Intermediate Host: Symptomatology, *falciparum* Malaria," in Moulton, ed., *Symposium on Human Malaria*, 187-188, 203-204; H. M. Gilles *et al.*, "Malaria, Anaemia and Pregnancy," *Annals of Tropical Medicine and Parasitology*, LXIII (1969), 245-263. See also P. Tilly, "Anaemia in Parturient Women, with Special Reference to Malaria Infection of the Placenta," *ibid.*, 109-115; C. A. Gill, "The Influence of Malaria on Natality with Special Reference to Ceylon," *Journal of the Malaria Institute of India*, III (1940), 201-252; and R. Menon, "Pregnancy and Malaria," *Medical Journal of Malaysia*, XXVII (1972), 115-119.

[38] For example, Wright and Tinling, eds., *Secret Diary*, 141-142, 344, 364.

[39] Only a very general comparison can be made because of the different age

similarity of the general configuration of the curves is significant. In both areas females in their fertile years ran an exaggerated risk of death in comparison to males. The link between the two areas may well have been malaria, and for the historian who must work from highly tangential evidence the extent to which female deaths exceed male deaths in a given area may well be a rough measure of the hold of malaria on that area. If the suggestion is sound, Middlesex and whatever part of the Chesapeake region it accurately reflects were highly malarious.

What of the social ramifications of malaria? Although disease is biologically defined, it is also to an extent culturally defined. The sickly appearance of Gloucester County men and women in 1687 and the ghostly pallor of those who lived about the Great Dismal Swamp in 1728 invited comment by

FIGURE 6

AGE SPECIFIC DEATH RATES, PUTTALAM DISTRICT,
CEYLON, 1937–1938; SEVENTEENTH- AND EARLY EIGHTEENTH-CENTURY
MIDDLESEX COUNTY, VIRGINIA

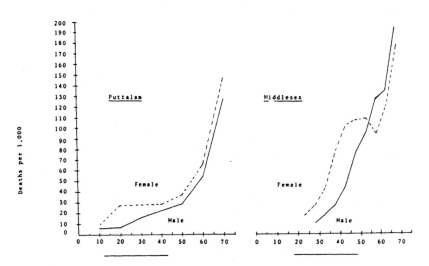

Sources and notes:
    For Puttalam see S. A. Meegama, "Malaria Eradication and Its Effects on Mortality Levels," *Population Studies,* XXI (1967), 225; for Middlesex see Darrett B. and Anita H. Rutman, "'Now-Wives and Sons-in-Law': Parental Death in a Seventeenth-Century Virginia County," in Thad W. Tate, ed., *The Chesapeake in the Seventeenth Century: Essays on Its Euramerican Society and Politics* (Chapel Hill, N. C., forthcoming). High maternity cohorts are underlined. N. B.: The populations at risk varied. See n. 39.

Durand de Dauphine and William Byrd respectively;[40] but did the inhabitants look upon themselves as diseased and sick? Probably not. Even the periodic "agues and fevers" of malaria could be culturally normative rather than culturally exceptional. This is the implication of the almost casual language with which Fitzhugh reported the end of his sister's illness—"and so consequently her seasoning [is] over." Even in Carter's diary most of the seizures are noted in a commonplace way: "Judy's fever left her this day. Lucy her ague and fever at 5 this eve."[41] Only in extreme situations did illness become something more than commonplace, as it did for Carter in the terrible year 1757. "It is necessary that man should be acquainted with affliction," Carter wrote in exasperation toward its end; "and 'tis certainly nothing short of it to be confined a whole year in tending one's sick Children. Mine are now never well."[42] It is, perhaps, this cultural definition of illness that underlies the diverse reactions to endemic and epidemic diseases commented on by Richard Shryock: the former are "taken for granted," the latter provoke hysteria.[43]

That said, however, we propose three ways in which endemic malaria, even if matter-of-factly accepted by its victims, conceivably affected their society. What follows can only be quick, tentative, and suggestive. The subject of the interrelationship of disease and society is only now coming into prominence under such rubrics as "medical anthropology," and potentially useful models from contemporary studies are still few and rudimentary.[44] In addition, we have been able to associate the disease only generally with Virginia through literary evidence, and only with regard to one small

---

groups used (Puttalam has been graphed on the basis of the mid-years of the age groups 5-14, 15-24, 25-34, 35-44, 45-54, 55-64, and age 70 for the cohort 65-plus; Middlesex on the basis of smoothed data for the mid-years of 5-year groups), the different species and strains of *plasmodium* prevalent in the two areas, and, above all, the differences in the populations at risk. In Puttalam the entire population of the district, 1937-1938, was at risk; for Middlesex the population at risk is married and widowed adults, the figures being based on the experience of subjects born over the span of years 1650-1710 who both survived to a marriageable age and chose at some time to marry. If the Puttalam population at risk had been so restricted, the resulting "bulge" of female deaths during the fertile years would undoubtedly have been somewhat greater.

[40] Chinard, ed., *Huguenot Exile;* Wright, ed., *Prose Works,* 202.
[41] Davis, ed., *Fitzhugh Letters;* Greene, ed., *Diary of Carter,* I, 203.
[42] Greene, ed., *Diary of Carter,* I, 194.
[43] Shryock, *Medicine and Society,* 93-95.
[44] For example, V. F. P. M. Van Amelsvoort, *Culture, Stone Age and Modern Medicine* (Assen, The Netherlands, 1964). Burton A. Weisbrod *et al., Disease and Economic Development: The Impact of Parasitic Diseases in St. Lucia* (Madison, Wis., 1973), Chap. 2, is a good overview of this literature, but see also Gerald Gordon *et al., Disease, the Individual, and Society* (New Haven, Conn., 1968), Pt. I.

tidewater area—Middlesex—can we make even a rough statement as to degree. Still, a beginning seems in order.

The most obvious interrelationship between disease and society is that defined by economics. What is the cost to the society of an endemic disease such as malaria? In modern economic scholarship the question has been posed in terms of the economic gain to a society of an eradication program and the answer seems to be coming back as a negative. Robin Barlow has summarized the findings: eradication of malaria brings about a population rise by reducing the death rate and, more important, by raising both the birth rate, as more children are successfully delivered, and the rate of survival through childhood. Moreover, the reduction of mortality, morbidity, and debility increases the quantity and quality of labor output. An immediate economic gain follows, but the society loses in the long run as the added population makes increasing demands on the public sector for services, reduces per capita income, and curtails capital formulation.[45] This econometric approach is cold and impersonal, and it runs counter to the historian's normal prejudice by requiring an "if" proposition—what *if* there had been no malaria in the Chesapeake? But there is some profit in applying it, if only to discount any quick generalization as to malaria and economic backwardness. Without malaria the rate of natural increase in the Chesapeake and the number of people living there would have been greater. This probably would not have resulted in an increased demand for public services, for the concept of public service was weakly defined; yet an increase in a population, dependent on a single cash crop and a finite market, would have resulted in greater production and lower prices—and consequently lower per capita income. Only if receiving lower prices for tobacco had led Virginians to an earlier and more energetic acceptance of economic diversification would the overall economy have improved.[46]

Another approach is perhaps more revealing. The agricultural economy of the Chesapeake region was labor-intensive: in the main a person's economic position depended on the application of labor to land. But disease in

[45] Robin Barlow, "The Economic Effects of Malaria Eradication," *Papers and Proceedings of the Seventy-Ninth Annual Meeting,* in *American Economic Review,* LCII (1967), 130-148. See also Barlow, *The Economic Effects of Malaria Eradication* (Ann Arbor, Mich., 1968); Newman, *Malaria Eradication;* and Gladys N. Conly, "The Impact of Malaria on Economic Development: A Case Study," *Proceedings,* 668-674, a preliminary report on an attempt to measure micro-effects using 300 farm families in eastern Paraguay before and after an eradication program.

[46] John C. Rainbolt, *From Prescription to Persuasion: Manipulation of Seventeenth Century Virginia Economy* (Port Washington, N. Y., 1974), discusses the early and unsuccessful diversification attempts. Avery Odelle Craven, *Soil Exhaustion as a Factor in the Agricultural History of Virginia and Maryland, 1606-1860* (Urbana, Ill., 1926), 69, dates tidewater diversification at about mid-18th century.

general and malaria in particular strike directly at labor.[47] Hence in the Chesapeake one's economic position was constantly jeopardized by disease, as the marquis de Chastellux observed when, with reference to "epidemical disorders" common among the slaves of the Virginians, he reported that "both their property and their revenue" were "extremely precarious."[48] The risk, however, was unevenly spread. The planter who relied on his own labor, with that of his wife and perhaps a single servant or slave, chanced disaster more than did the planter who had built up a labor force of ten or twenty persons. Imagine the small planter struck down by a malaria attack at the moment most appropriate for the transplantation of tobacco seedlings from seedbeds to fields, or when the ripe tobacco leaves had to be cut and housed. A good percentage, perhaps even all, of his year's income might be lost. The intensity of the dependence on labor is illustrated by Peter Mountague of Middlesex County whose one male servant ran away at harvest time in 1701, causing Mountague to complain to the county court in 1702 that he had sustained as a consequence "the whole loss of the last crop."[49] It is true that larger planters could be hard hit. Armistead Churchill of Middlesex lost thirty slaves in one six-month period in 1737.[50] But a large labor force insured against catastrophe. Even at the height of his troubles in 1757 Carter still had laborers in his fields. Moreover, in a society in which working lives were short, the amassment of capital provided defense against the economic effects of death. The short-lived planter, large or small, frequently left orphaned children.[51] But the chances that orphans of the large planter would start their working years with enough capital in the form of labor to protect them from disaster were far greater than those of orphans of the small planter. Generation after generation the latter had to begin their working lives with no

[47] Wood, *Black Majority*, 91, argues that in South Carolina the combination of malaria (together with yellow fever), black resistance to both diseases, and the labor-intensive economy "must have done a great deal to reinforce the expanding rationale behind the enslavement of Africans." Wood attempts to demonstrate that South Carolina's whites, from an early date, *thought* of the blacks as more resistant to disease—this in sharp contrast to Winthrop D. Jordan, *White Over Black: American Attitudes Toward the Negro, 1550-1812* (Chapel Hill, N. C., 1968), 259-265. We have found no evidence in Virginia to substantiate Wood's thesis.

[48] Marquis de Chastellux, *Travels in North-America, in the Years 1780, 1781, and 1782*, 2d ed., II (London, 1787), 297.

[49] Middlesex County, Va., MS Order Book, No. 3, 1694-1705, 483, Virginia State Library, Richmond.

[50] *The Parish Register of Christ Church, Middlesex County, Va., from 1653 to 1812* (Richmond, Va., 1897), 275-276. In this case the loss might well have been to yellow fever, a disease then entering the colony.

[51] Rutman and Rutman, " 'Now-Wives and Sons-in-Law,' " in Tate, ed., *The Chesapeake*.

more, and sometimes less, than their fathers had begun with. These inequalities may well have contributed to economic polarization over time.[52] For the planter who, by virtue of ability, energy, or luck, lived insulated from the economic consequences of disease had a far better chance to improve his economic position and, consequently, still greater insulation.

A consideration of disease and economics has led to one aspect of the structure of Chesapeake society—exaggerated economic polarization. But disease interacts with social structure in other ways as well. Provision must be made for illness. This was in part an individual matter, as it was for Dennis Conyers when he sold one hundred acres on the Piankatank River in Middlesex to Peter Godson on the condition that "the said Peter . . . administer Physick or Physical means to the said Dennis for his own person for the space of one year."[53] For the whole society the provisions for illness take on a more general form. The phenomenon of every planter his own practitioner has long been noted. Equally to the point are the phenomena of every claimant to the title "doctor" being engaged as one and, notwithstanding the aspersions of Byrd, the high esteem accorded physicians in the Chesapeake area.[54] On a still higher level of generalization one can suggest that illness and early death were related to the basic social organization of the Chesapeake. In the continuing study of Middlesex County of which this article is a part, the region is emerging not as an area of isolated plantations and individuals but as a mosaic of close-knit neighborhoods and kinship groups. Few aspects of life reflect this mosaic more clearly than do illness and death. Illness brought visitation, and kin and neighbors clustered about the sickbeds of the county.[55] Death, particularly the death of parents with the consequent orphaning of children, evoked kinship obligations, and

[52] Darrett B. Rutman, "The Social Web: A Prospectus for the Study of the Early American Community," in William L. O'Neill, ed., *Insights and Parallels: Problems and Issues of American Social History* (Minneapolis, 1973), 85, 85n, 112-113, briefly compares polarization in New England and Middlesex.

[53] Lancaster County, Va., MS Deeds, Etc., No. 2, 1654-1702, 116-117, Va. St. Lib.

[54] Philip Alexander Bruce, *Economic History of Virginia in the Seventeenth Century*, II (New York, 1896), 231ff. See Byrd to Sir Hans Sloane, Apr. 20, 1706, *WMQ*, 2d Ser., I (1921), 186: "Here be some men indeed that are call'd Doctors: but they are generally discarded Surgeons of Ships, that know nothing above very common Remedys." Oldmixon, *British Empire*, I, 294, presumably reflecting Byrd, wrote that the Virginians "reckon it among Blessings" that they had few doctors, "fancying the Number of their Diseases would encrease with that of their Physicians." These attitudes are in sharp contrast to the social position accorded physicians in Middlesex society.

[55] The phenomenon can be glimpsed in depositions submitted to the county court in cases involving disputed wills—for example, the probate proceedings surrounding

relations (including such relations as godparents) moved to care for the parentless. The effect was a society of open and mixed households. The home was not an isolated castle but a neighborhood focal point. The typical family was not the neat nuclear one of mother-father-children but a mixed affair of parents, stepparents, guardians, natural children, stepchildren, and wards.[56] It could hardly have been otherwise, given the prevalence of illness, the frequency of early death, and the necessity of caring for the sick and orphaned; and it can be argued that in the Chesapeake region the form and strength of the social bonds were direct corollaries of the fragility of life.

Finally, one can suggest an impact of disease on the culture of the Chesapeake, for while culture to an extent defines disease, the relationship is reciprocal. The associations are so tenuously perceived that questions seem more in order than statements. If there is validity in the ideal *mens sana in corpore sano*, then, conversely, the ill do not think clearly. Might this have been related to the low level of intellectual activity in the early Chesapeake, a level frequently contrasted to that of New England? Dr. John Mitchell's biographers, writing of his years in Urbanna, Middlesex, imply as much. "Continuous bouts of malaria . . . left him with little energy and even less *joie de vivre*"; and most of Mitchell's significant work was done after he removed to England.[57] What would be the attitudes of a population that had a relatively high rate of illness and short life expectancy? Richard S. Dunn's comparison of New England and the English Caribbean is provocative, assuming that the Caribbean and Chesapeake were areas of high malarial morbidity. "The Caribbean and New England planters were polar opposites in social expression. . . . The contrast in life style went far beyond the obvious differences in religion, slavery and climate. The sugar planters 'lived fast, spent recklessly, played desperately, and died young.' . . . Their family life was broken, and since the colonists were predominantly young people without effective guidance, they behaved in a freewheeling, devil-may-care fashion."[58]

---

the will of John Burnham in Middlesex County, Va., MS Deeds, Etc., No. 2, 1679-1694, 22, Va. St. Lib. Here and there, too, it can be seen in literary sources—William Byrd, for example, hovering about the sickbed of John Bowman of Henrico County. Wright and Tinling, eds., *Secret Diary*, 89-94.

[56] A point elaborated upon in Rutman and Rutman, " 'Now-Wives and Sons-in-Law,' " in Tate, ed., *The Chesapeake*.

[57] Edmund and Dorothy Smith Berkeley, *Dr. John Mitchell: The Man Who Made the Map of North America* (Chapel Hill, N. C., 1974), 59.

[58] Richard S. Dunn, "The Social History of Early New England," *American Quarterly*, XXIV (1972), 675; Dunn quotes his own *Sugar and Slaves: The Rise of the Planter Class in the English West Indies, 1624-1713* (Chapel Hill, N. C., 1972). See the latter, pp. 302-303, regarding malaria in the English Caribbean.

Applied to Virginia, Dunn's description probably would be an exaggeration, but Virginia can certainly be described, in comparison with New England, as a present-minded society that was more involved, in Wordsworth's phrase, with "getting and spending" than with abstractions or ideals. Do the Virginians' attitudes toward death reflect the fact of frequent illness and early death? Robinson Jeffers's "patient daemon"[59] was much on the minds of colonials north and south, but while the New Englanders seem to have been both enamored of and terrified by death, the Virginians apparently discerned death more as a matter of fact, of "dissolution"—William Fitzhugh's word—and of business, the willing and disposing of property.[60] The comparison can only be highly tentative for little work has been done on the subject, but two vignettes are suggestive. In September 1658 William Price of Lancaster County told of his last conversation with Roger Radford: "I came into the room where Mr. Radford was sitting upon his bed sick. I asked him how he did. 'Pretty well,' he said. 'You are not, I think, a man for this world. Therefore you had best to make your peace with God and set everything to rights with Mr. Cocke.' He answered: 'No, for he is more engaged to me than I to him.' 'What do you give Polly Cole?' [I asked.] 'I give Polly Cole my land.' "[61] The second vignette was recorded by Philip Fithian toward the end of the eighteenth century. The sudden death of a black child "with the Ague and Fever . . . was the Subject of Conversation in the House." "Mr *Carter* observed, that he thought it the most desirable to die of a Short Illness. If he could have his Wish he would not lie longer than two days; be taken with a Fever, which should . . . gradually increase till it affected a Dissolution—He told us that his affairs are in Such a state that he should be able to dictate a Will which might be written in Five Minutes, and contain the disposal of his estate agreeable to his mind—He mentioned to us the Substance."[62]

[59] Jeffers, "The Bed by the Window" (1931):
> We are safe to finish what we have to
> finish;
> And then it will sound rather like music
> When the patient daemon behind the screen of sea-rock
> and sky
> Thumps with his staff, and calls thrice: "Come, Jeffers."

[60] David E. Stannard, "Death and Dying in Puritan New England," *AHR*, LXXVIII (1973), 1305-1330; W. Fitzhugh to Mrs. Mary Fitzhugh, June 30, 1698, in Davis, ed., *Fitzhugh Letters*, 358.

[61] Lancaster County, MS Deeds, 56-57, Va. St. Lib. The quotation has been modernized.

[62] Hunter Dickinson Parish, ed., *Journal & Letters of Philip Vickers Fithian, 1773-1774: A Plantation Tutor of the Old Dominion,* rev. ed. (Williamsburg, Va., 1957), 182. The deeply religious Fithian continued: "Our School make it [the death]

Economy, social structure, culture—all conceivably bore the imprint of malaria in the early Chesapeake. We do not mean to assert a direct causal association, for the question of the relation of disease to society is far too complex, the variables far too many, and the evidence far too slim. We *do* mean to suggest that malaria was endemic in the early Chesapeake (and relatively absent in New England), and that it is in the nature of societies to adjust to the disease environment in which they exist. These, we argue, should be informing assumptions in early American history, and the processes and consequences of such adjustments, varying by time and place, require the attention of historians.

---

a Subject for continual Speculation; They seem all to be free of any terror at the Prescence of Death; *Harry* in special signified a Wish that his turn may be next." Cf. David E. Stannard, "Death and the Puritan Child," *AQ*, XXVI (1974), 456-476.

10

Smallpox and the Indians
in the American Colonies

John Duffy

Romanticized versions of the conquest of North America—for conquest it was—emphasize the heroic battles and perennial warfare of the frontier. The picture of pioneers in their log cabins warding off Indian attacks, or of small garrisons grimly defending themselves from hordes of savages is a familiar one to all Americans. And certainly such scenes were characteristic of the frontier. Yet the extirpation of the Indians was far more the result of the white man's diseases than his weapons. Once the Europeans gained a foothold, their advance guards of disease bore the brunt of the attack and carried death and devastation on an unprecedented scale far into the Indian territory. Historians of the Indian frontier have long been aware that smallpox and other contagions played a significant role in white-Indian relations in North America, but other than noting the fact, little has been written about it.[1]

Prior to the advent of the whites, North America was little troubled with contagious infections. In contrast to the many complaints of sickness and death which characterized the later seventeenth and eighteenth centuries, early explorers and traders universally commented on the salubrity of the climate and the good health of the Indians. For example, Captain Bartholomew Gosnold, who explored the New England coast in 1602 and named Martha's Vineyard, found "the people of a perfect constitution of body, active, strong healthful, and very witty. . . . For ourselves, we found ourselves rather increased in health and strength than otherwise; for all our toyle, bad dyet and lodging; yet no one of us was touched with any sickness." [2] The absence of diseases was also noticed by the early settlers in New England, one of whom wrote in 1633: " Heare I find three great blessings, peace, plenty and health in a Comfortable measure the place well agreeth with our English bodies that they were never so healthy in their native Contrey generally all heare, as never could

---

[1] William C. Macleod in his *American Indian Frontier* (New York, 1928) briefly mentions smallpox, but devotes much of his attention to venereal disorders. P. M. Ashburn, *The Ranks of Death* (New York, 1947), a first-rate work, deals only cursorily with smallpox. The best short general study of the subject is *The Effect of Smallpox on the Destiny of the Amerindian* (Boston, 1945) by E. W. and Allen E. Stearn which surveys the period from 1492 to the end of the nineteenth century.

[2] P. M. Ashburn, *The Ranks of Death* (New York, 1947), p. 16.

be rid of the head ach, tooth ach, Cough and the like are now better and freer (?) heare and those that were weake are now well long since and I can heare of but two weake in all the plantation Gods name be praised." [3] Little doubt exists that the Indians were relatively free from most of the contagions prevalent in Europe. Smallpox and measles, for example, were certainly absent, and in all likelihood, malaria, yellow fever, typhoid, typhus, and the venereal diseases were among those introduced from the Old World. These infections exacted a heavy toll even among Europeans who had acquired some tolerance to them, but their impact upon the Indians was a major tragedy.

Lest the foregoing present too cheerful a view of health conditions among the early settlers, it must be remembered that in the seventeenth and eighteenth centuries life was short, and sickness and death were omnipresent. Major epidemics swept through Europe with fearful regularity, and endemic disorders steadily winnowed the population. Removal to the New World brought no relief, for contagious sicknesses migrated with the first settlers. And as the wealth and resources of America offered unlimited opportunity for the whites, so their infections found a virgin field in the native population. By way of retribution, the disorders, after ravaging the Indian tribes, occasionally returned with renewed virulence to plague the settlers. However, this danger was relatively minor in relation to the other problems besetting those emigrating to the New World. In the first place, the passage to the colonies, which was made in small overcrowded vessels, ordinarily took from eight to fourteen weeks. Food, on the long voyage, was both scant and dietetically unsound, and sanitation was either neglected or rudimentary. On arrival in the colonies, at least during the first years of colonization, the settlers found a continuation of poor food and inadequate housing. It was small wonder that sickness and disease were a more serious threat to the colonists than the Indians. However, epidemic sicknesses were a familiar evil to Europeans, who looked upon them as the inexplicable instruments of a Divine Providence, whereas for the Indians, they were a new and terrifying experience.

The Spaniards in the sixteenth century were the first to benefit from the services of contagious infections which they, unwittingly, turned loose upon the Indian tribes. Their chroniclers were amazed and, in the case of the Jesuits, shocked at the tremendous casualties which these epidemic diseases inflicted upon the Indians. Certainly such an attitude was justi-

[3] Master Wells to Family, New England, 1633, Sloane MSS (Library of Congress Transcript), vol. 922, no. 90.

fied since the estimates of smallpox deaths alone in Spanish-America during the colonial period run into the millions.   Meanwhile other disorders, too, were exacting a heavy tribute.   The courage and determination of the small bands of Spaniards who pushed on into vast, unknown, and populous lands cannot be gainsaid, but the glorious victories attributed to Spanish arms would not have been possible without the devastation wrought by Spanish diseases.   Spanish arms performed a notable feat; but it was their most potent weapon, sickness, which made the Spanish-American Empire, and later, as an ally of the English and French, was to subdue the Indians in North America.

In contrast to the Spanish missionaries, who worried over the fact that conversion to Christianity so often proved a death warrant to the natives, and that sickness and death were too frequently the result of missionary endeavors, the English in North America during the seventeenth century openly rejoiced when the Lord sent his " Avenging Angels " to destroy the heathen.   The American frontier conception that the only good Indian was a dead one characterized relations between the whites and Indians in British North America from the beginning of colonial times.   Increase Mather records that when the colonists prayed the Lord to destroy the Indians, an answer was prompt in forthcoming, " For it is known that the Indians were distressed with famine, multitudes of them perishing for want of bread; and the Lord sent Sicknesses amongst them, that Travellers have seen many dead Indians up and down in the woods that were by famine and sickness brought unto that untimely end.   Yea the Indians themselves have testified, that more amongst them have been cut off by the sword of the Lord in these respects than by the sword of the English." [4]   A missionary to New York wrote home in 1705, ". . . the English here are a very thriving growing people, and ye Indians quite otherwise, they wast away & have done ever since our first arrival amongst them (as they themselves say) like Snow agt. ye Sun, So that very probably forty years hence there will scarce be an Indian seen in our America, God's Providence in this matter seems very wonderful, & no cause of their Decrease visible unless their drinking Rum, with some new Distempers we have brought amongst them." [5]

[4] Increase Mather, "An Historical Discourse Concerning the Prevalency of Prayer," in *A Relation of the Troubles Which Have Happened in New-England by Reason of the Indians there, from the Year 1614 to the Year 1675, etc.* (Boston, John Foster, 1677), p. 6.

[5] Mr. Moor to the Secretary, New York, November 13, 1705, in the Society for the Propagation of the Gospel in Foreign Parts MSS (Library of Congress Photo.), London Letters, A 2, fpp. 272-78 (hereinafter cited as S. P. G.).

Of the many contagious sicknesses which the Europeans brought to plague the Indians, smallpox was far the most deadly. Although the disease is now largely a thing of the past in the more advanced countries, it was one of the leading causes of death in seventeenth and eighteenth century Europe. For example, the London Bills of Mortality from 1731 to 1765 attribute nine per cent of all fatalities to this infection.[6] In the American colonies, too, smallpox was a major threat, but here it more than compensated for any damages inflicted upon the settlers by its ravages among the Indians. A loathsome and exceedingly fatal sickness, smallpox found in the vulnerable Red Men a fertile field for conquest. Unable to comprehend the nature of this unseen foe, the Indians first died in droves huddled in their camps. Later, when bitter experience had made them wiser, they fled in terror at its approach. The infection menaced both whites and Indians throughout the colonial period; it played a part in all colonial wars, fighting sometimes for the French, sometimes for the British, but in all cases warring against the Indians.

The Pilgrims, who first settled New England, entered that region in the wake of a major epidemic which, some three years earlier, had devastated the New England tribes to such an extent that they were unable to make even a token resistance to white occupation. The disorder which smoothed the path for these settlers was undoubtedly of European origin, but its exact nature is still in dispute among medical historians. Smallpox or bubonic plague are the two most likely suspects, but the evidence is inconclusive.[7] No doubt exists, however, about the smallpox outbreak which occurred in New England in 1633. Increase Mather explains that " the Indians began to be quarrelsome touching the Bounds of the Land which they had sold to the English, but God ended the Controversy by sending the Smallpox amongst the Indians of Saugust who were before that time exceeding numerous. Whole Towns of them were swept away, in some not so much as one soul escaping the Destruction." [8] Another colonial writer declares: " This contagious Disease was so noisome & terrible to these naked Indians, that they in many Places, left their Dead

---

[6] *Gentlemen's Magazine*, 1731-1765, volumes 1 to 35. See also John Duffy, *A History of Epidemics in the American Colonies*, doctoral dissertation, University of California at Los Angeles.

[7] The best study of this outbreak is Herbert U. Williams, " Epidemic among Indians, 1616-1620," *Johns Hopkins Hospital Bulletin*, XX, no. 224 (1909), pp. 340-49. Williams believes the infection was bubonic plague, but there is no agreement among the medical historians.

[8] Increase Mather, *A Relation of the Troubles*, etc., p. 23.

328   JOHN DUFFY

unburied, as appeared by the multitude of the bones up & down the countries where had been the greatest Numbers of them." [9]

By 1634 the infection had spread to the Narragansetts and the Con-
necticuts with similarly disastrous results. William Bradford asserts that
in this year the Indians near the Connecticut River " fell sick of the small
poxe, and dyed most miserably; for a sorer disease cannot befall them;
they fear it worse than the plague; for usually they that have this disease
have them in abundance . . . they dye like rotten sheep. . . . But by the
marvelous goodness and providens of God not one of the English was so
much as sicke, or in the least measure tainted with this disease." [10]   In
all likelihood previous exposure had made the English immune to the sickness, but to contemporary observers it seemed a miraculous preservation.

It is more than a coincidence that the Jesuits in Canada reported outbreaks of smallpox among the Indians in the same year that the infection
was plaguing the tribes in the Connecticut valley. The river provided
one of the easier routes to the St. Lawrence and the series of epidemics
which flared up in the Great Lakes and St. Lawrence region from 1634
to 1641 were undoubtedly a continuation of the New England epidemic.
The Montagnais around the St. Lawrence were infected in 1634, and the
disorder soon was passed on to the other tribes. [11]

The Hurons, who lived north of Lake Ontario, were particularly hard
hit in 1636 as indicated by the following graphic description:

Terror was universal. The contagion increased as autumn advanced; and when
winter came, far from ceasing as the priests had hoped, its ravages were appalling.
The season of the Huron festivity was turned to a season of mourning; and such
was the despondency and dismay, that suicides became frequent. The Jesuits
singly or in pairs, journeyed in the depth of winter from village to village, minister-
ing to the sick, and seeking to commend their religious teaching by their efforts
to relieve bodily distress. . . . No house was left unvisited. As the missionary,
physician at once to body and soul, entered one of these smoky dens, he saw the
inmates, their heads muffled in their robes of skins, seated around the fires in
silent dejection. Everywhere was heard the wail of the sick and dying children;
and on or under the platforms at the sides of the house crouched squalid men and
women, in all stages of the distemper. [12]

———————

[9] *Notebook*, Ebenezer Hazard MSS, Library of Congress.
[10] J. Franklin Jameson, ed., *Bradford's History of Plymouth Plantation, 1606-1646*,
Original Narratives of Early American History, American Historical Association (New
York, 1908), pp. 312-313.
[11] John J. Heagerty, *Four Centuries of Medical History in Canada* (Toronto, 1928),
I, 20.
[12] Francis Parkman, *The Jesuits in North America in the Seventeenth Century*
(Boston, 1888), p. 87.

Despite their ardent labors on behalf of the sick, the Jesuits found themselves objects of suspicion to the natives. Father Le Jeune reported: " They (the Indians) observed with some sort of reason that since our arrival in these lands those who had been the nearest to us had happened to be the most ruined by the disease, and that whole villages of those who had received us now appeared utterly exterminated." [18] Further along in his journal he noted sorrowfully that " it has happened very often, and has been remarked more than a hundred times, that where we were most welcome, where we baptized most people, there it was in fact where they died the most." [14] Le Jeune, like the other missionaries of his time, did not realize that although the Europeans had acquired some immunity to the infection, their ministrations to the sick and dying served to make them carriers of the disease.

Smallpox again returned to New England in 1638 and inflicted some casualties upon the English.[15] The following year a group of the Indians contracted the disease while trading with the Abenakis tribe of Maine who had probably acquired it from the New England settlers.[16] Subsequently a major outbreak developed which lasted well into 1640.

Little further is heard of the disease until the 1660's, when it exacted a heavy toll.[17] It struck the Iroquois in 1662-63 and evoked the following notation: " The small-pox, which is the American's pest, has wrought sad havoc in their villages and has carried off many men, besides great numbers of women and children; and as a result their villages are nearly deserted, and their fields are only half-tilled." [18] The disorder soon spread to the Indians in Canada, where it remained for several years.[19] A particularly virulent form of the contagion inflicted heavy casualties among the colonists in New England in 1666. According to one medical writer,

[18] Heagerty, *op. cit.*, I, 22.

[14] *Ibid.*, p. 23.

[15] Noah Webster, *A Brief History of Epidemic and Pestilential Diseases, etc.* (Hartford, Connecticut, 1799), I, 185.

[16] Reuben G. Thwaites, ed., *Jesuit Relations and Allied Documents* (Cleveland, 1896-1901), XVI, 101 (hereinafter cited as *Jesuit Relations*).

[17] The Stearns list an epidemic in Quebec in 1649 following an attack by an English expeditionary force. Their source is Chevalier de Callieres' report to M. de Seignelay, dated 1649, in E. B. O'Callaghan, ed., *Documents Relative to the Colonial History of the State of New York Procured in Holland, England, and France* (Albany, New York, 1856-1861), IX, 492 (hereinafter cited as *Doc. Rel. to Col. Hist. of N. Y.*). However, since the date 1689 appears in the content and reference is made to Count de Frontenac, this outbreak is undoubtedly the one which occurred in 1690. The date 1649 is probably a typographical transposition of 1694.

[18] Heagerty, *op. cit.*, I, 27.

[19] *Ibid.*

330   JOHN DUFFY

the infection was imported by sea,[20] but the prevalence of the sickness among the French and Indians during the preceding years makes the Indians a more likely source. As has been pointed out earlier, a mild type of the infection among the whites often gained in virulence when passed on to the Indians, and was then returned to the colonists in a more malignant form.

During the early years of the seventeenth century, nearly all evidence of smallpox among the Indian tribes relates to the northern regions. The first recorded epidemic in the southern colonies occurred in 1667, when a sailor, infected with the disease, landed in what is now Northampton County, Virginia, and conveyed the disease to some of the local Indians. The usual fatal results ensued, and it was reported that " they died by the hundred . . . in this way practically every tribe fell into the hands of the grim reaper and disappeared, the only exception being the Gengaskins." [21] Little more is heard of smallpox in the southern colonies until the end of the century when the disease once again made a destructive path through the various tribes.

In 1669-70, a severe outbreak affected the Indians in eastern Canada, New England, and upper New York. The Algonquins suffered most, but the Hurons, too, were affected.[22] Seven years later another major epidemic broke out on a wide front. William Hubbard in his narration of the Indian troubles states that " sundry diseases " weakened the Red Men in 1676 at a time when the whites were gradually gaining the upper hand in the bloody Indian struggle known as King Philip's War (1675-77).[23] Whether smallpox was one of these diseases is not known, but the infection did ravage all of New England, affecting both whites and Indians, in the following two years. Incidentally, this outbreak led to the publication of the first medical work in America, a broadside by Thomas Thacher entitled, *A Brief Rule to Guide the Common People of New England how to order themselves and theirs in the Small Pocks, or Measles.*

In addition to ravaging New England, smallpox caused a few deaths

[20] Francis R. Packard, *History of Medicine in the United States* (New York, 1931), I, 75.

[21] Thomas B. Robertson, " An Indian King's Will," *Virginia Magazine of History and Biography*, XXXVI (1928), 192-93.

[22] *Jesuit Relations*, LIII, 59 ff.

[23] William Hubbard, *A Narrative of the Troubles with the Indians in New-England, from the First Planting thereof in the Year 1607, to This Present Year 1677, etc.* (Boston, John Foster, 1677), p. 95.

among the Indians in the Great Lakes area,[24] and, according to the diary of Increase Mather, " destroyed a great part of the Indians of Delaware Bay." [25]

Next year, 1679, the Iroquois were decimated by the pestilence. Count de Frontenac declared of the Iroquois " that the Small Pox, which is the Indian Plague, desolates them to such a degree that they think no longer of Meeting nor of Wars, but only of bewailing the dead, of whom there is already an immense number." [26]   Three years later the disease struck the Indians at the Jesuit mission of Sillery near Quebec.[27]   However, the outbreak was localized, and the disease apparently subsided in North America for a brief period.

The years 1688 to 1691 saw smallpox prevailing extensively among both Indians and whites, French and British. Whether the disease origi- nated in the French or English settlements is not clear; possibly both regions may have been infected independently. In any case, the hostilities of King William's War broadcast the smallpox virus far and wide. Both sides suffered heavy casualties from the contagion since smallpox showed no partiality when Europeans fought each other. In fact, on more than one occasion well-planned military campaigns were thwarted by this unseen enemy. In 1690, the English, allied with the Mohegans and Iroquois, planned an assault on Quebec, but were foiled by an outbreak of smallpox. When British and Mohegan emissaries, still bearing the marks of the pestilence, were sent to the Iroquois, they were accused of bringing the plague. Subsequently the Iroquois became contaminated, about 300 died, and the rest refused to join the expedition.[28]   Father Michael DeCourvert reported to Count de Frontenac from Quebec in 1690, " A malady which was prevalent among the English having communicated itself to the Loups, and some of them having died, the Loups laid the blame upon the English." [29]   As a result the English abandoned the campaign. The next year, 1691, Father Millet, another Jesuit, stated specifically that the

[24] *Jesuit Relations*, LXIII, 205.
[25] Samuel A. Green, ed., *Diary by Increase Mather, March, 1675—December, 1676, Together with Extracts from Another Diary by Him, 1674-1687* (Cambridge, Massa- chusetts, 1900), pp. 20-21.
[26] Count de Frontenac to the King, Quebec, November 6, 1679, in *Doc. Rel. to Col. Hist. of N. Y.*, IX, 129.
[27] *Jesuit Relations*, LXII, 145.
[28] Count de Frontenac to Minister, December 12, 1690, in *Doc. Rel. to Col. Hist. of N. Y.*, IX, 460-61.
[29] Father Michael DeCourvert to Count de Frontenac, Quebec, 1690, in *Jesuit Relations*, LXIV, 47.

British had sent two armies against Quebec, adding that "smallpox stopped the first completely, and also scattered the second." [30]

Meanwhile the disease continued to rage among the Indians and whites in New York province. Major General Winthrop, in his journal of marches in the vicinity of Albany, New York, during these years often mentions the presence of smallpox among the troops and in the towns through which they passed.[31] As usual, the Indians were the chief sufferers. Robert Livingston reported the deaths of an entire group of Dovaganhae Indians who had come to Albany to trade in 1691.[32] In short, whether engaged in trade or in warfare, the Indian susceptibility to smallpox steadily reduced their numbers.

The southern provinces were the next to bear the brunt of smallpox attacks. An outbreak began in Jamestown, Virginia, in 1696 and gradually spread into the Carolinas, where it brought many fatalities to the whites, and even more to the Indians. One tribe, probably the Pemlico Indians, was almost completely destroyed. A correspondent from South Carolina reported in 1699 that smallpox was "said to have swept away a whole neighboring (Indian) nation, all to 5 or 6 which ran away and left their dead unburied, lying upon the ground for the vultures to devour." [33] The extermination of this tribe was described in 1707 by John Archdale, whose account subsequently was copied by John Oldmixon and many other eighteenth century writers.[34] The infection probably spread as far west as the Lower Mississippi valley for the tribes here were attacked at this time.[35]

The eighteenth century saw the decimation of the American Indian continue at an accelerated speed. Smallpox, which first became a serious problem in England and on the Continent around the time of the Stuart

---

[30] "Letter of Father Millet," 1691, in *Jesuit Relations*, LXIV, 97-99. Millet probably had in mind the two expeditions sent against Quebec in 1690: The New England and New York troops based at Albany attacked by land, and a naval force under the direction of Sir William Phips by sea.

[31] "Journal of Major General Winthrop's March from Albany to Wood Creek, July to September, 1690," *Doc. Rel. to Col. Hist. of N. Y.*, IV, 193-96.

[32] Letter from Robert Livingston, Albany, New York, June 4, 1691, in *ibid.*, III, 778.

[33] Mrs. Afra Coming to sister, March 6, 1699, quoted in Edward McCrady, *The History of South Carolina under the Proprietary Government*, 1670-1719 (New York, 1897), p. 308.

[34] John Archdale, *A New Description of that Fertile and Pleasant Province of Carolina* (London, 1707), in Bartholomew R. Carroll, *Historical Collections of South Carolina* (New York, 1836), II, 462-535. The account by John Oldmixon in his *British Empire in America* is identical with Archdale's.

[35] Stearn and Stearn, *op. cit.*, p. 33.

Restoration, grew steadily worse during the eighteenth century, tapering off only slightly during the last twenty years. The same held true in the American colonies although here the widespread use of variolation, or inoculation with smallpox, among the settlers greatly reduced the smallpox hazard by the 1760's.[36] For the Indians, however, there was no relief, and the higher incidence of the disease among the whites during the first half of the eighteenth century brought only further suffering and death to the Red Men.

In 1702 a mild form of smallpox was prevalent among the colonists in New York province. Governor Cornbury reported that the infection had been carried to the River Indians.[37] As so often happened, the disease spread north via the Indians and soon reached the town of Quebec which endured one of its most severe epidemics in the winter of 1702-1703. Heagerty estimates about 3,000 deaths from the contagion in Quebec alone.[38] Quite possibly the disease, which was relatively mild in New York, gained virulence as it progressed through the Indian tribes. Little evidence exists of its effect upon the Indians, but it doubtless took a heavy toll.

From 1703 to 1715 the English colonies gained relief from smallpox; but in the latter year it broke out anew and was to ravage all sections during the next seven years. The first reports of the sickness came from New Jersey in 1715.[39] By the following year, it was general throughout New York province. A missionary for the Society for the Propagation of the Gospel, a Church of England missionary society, wrote in October, 1716, " The Small Pox has been much among ye Indians here this last Summer & swept off a great many of ym & now it is got among ye other Nations beyond us, & Die as many there with it." [40] The disease continued to plague the Indians throughout 1716 and 1717, with few of the tribes in the Northwest escaping it.

In June, 1717, Governor Hunter of New York held a conference with the representatives of the Five Nations at Albany. In his opening address, he expressed sympathy " for the loss that has happened by the Small Pox

---

[36] Duffy, *op. cit.*; see chapter on variolation.

[37] Lord Cornbury to the Lords of Trade, New York, June 30, 1703, in *Doc. Rel. to Col. Hist. of N. Y.*, IV, 996-97.

[38] Heagerty, *op. cit.*, I, 67-68.

[39] Rowland Ellis to the Secretary, New Jersey, 1715, in S. P. G. MSS (L. C. Photo.), New York Letters, A 12, fp. 165.

[40] William Andrews to the Secretary, Fort by Mohawk Castle, October 11, 1716, in S. P. G. MSS (L. C. Photo.), London Letters, A 12, fp, 136.

JOHN DUFFY

to the bretheren, or any of your friends and allies." He pointed out, ". . . but we Christians look upon that disease and others of that kind as punishments for our misdeeds and sin, such as breaking of covenants & promises, murders, and robbery, and the like." [41] The Indians were not overly impressed and replied that they intended to dispatch someone to " Canistoge, Virginy, or Maryland " to find out who had been sending the contagion and to prevent them from so doing.[42] A French official who recorded the results of a meeting between the French and the Indians in October mentioned that the Iroquois were afflicted with the disease.[43]

The culmination of this widespread outbreak was an attack on Boston in 1721, which brought sickness to 60 per cent of the population and caused almost 900 deaths.[44] Following the Boston epidemic, the disease subsided for about nine years. In 1730, this city was again the scene of a major epidemic. On this occasion, some 4,000 cases developed and the death toll was approximately 500.[45] Neighboring towns such as Medfield and Cambridge reported additional cases, and a correspondent from Chatham noted that the disease was among the Indians, of whom, he said, " not so much as one has yet escaped." [46] The following spring the infection was reported among the Dutch around Albany and Schenectady, from whence it soon spread to the Indians in Eastern Canada.[47] By fall, the Senecas and other Iroquois tribes were victimized.[48] The infection continued to rage among the Indians in Canada throughout the winter, inflicting severe casualties. One tribe, the " Sounontonans," lost half their number.[49] Fear of the disorder in Canada drove many of the Indians into British territory, where they alarmed the frontier settlements.[50]

Meanwhile the tribes to the south of the Great Lakes-St. Lawrence

---

[41] Governor Hunter's Reply to the Five Nations at the Conference at Albany, New York, June 13, 1717, reported by Robert Livingston, Secretary of Indian Affairs, in *Doc. Rel. to Col. Hist. of N. Y.*, V, 485-86.

[42] Indian Reply to Governor Hunter, New York, June 13, 1717, in *ibid.*, p. 487.

[43] M. de Vaudreuil's Conference with Indians, October 24, 1717, in *Doc. Rel. to Col. Hist. of N. Y.*, IX, 877.

[44] See Duffy, *op. cit.*, p. 48 *passim*.

[45] William Douglass, *A Summary, Historical and Political, of the First Planting, Progressive Improvements, and Present State of the British Settlements in North America* (London, 1760), II, 396-397.

[46] Boston *Weekly Newsletter* (L. C. Photo), no. 1400, November 19-26, 1730.

[47] New York *Gazette* (L. C. Photo.), no. 248, March 26—April 5, 1731.

[48] M. de Beauharnois to Count de Maurepas, October 15, 1732, in *Doc. Rel. to Col. Hist. of N. Y.*, IX, 1035-1037.

[49] Heagerty, *op. cit.*, p. 35.

[50] *Belcher Papers*, Massachusetts Historical Society *Collections*, ser. 6, VI, 367.

region, too, paid toll to this grim pestilence. In September, Governor William Cosby of New York offered condolences to the Five Nations for the " great mortality among you by the small pox." [51] No statistics are available as to the number of cases or deaths in the various tribes, but the Indian susceptibility to the infection coupled with its widespread distribution must have produced some grim results.

The year, 1738, saw Charleston the victim of a major smallpox outbreak which sickened almost half the population. The neighboring Cherokee Indians, to whom the disease was carried, were devastated, losing fifty per cent of their members. Unable to explain this catastrophe, the Indians accused the English of poisoning them and threatened to trade with the French; this latter contingency was avoided only by careful diplomacy.[52] The Cherokees were estimated to have about 6,000 warriors prior to 1738 when the number was cut in half. Alexander Hewat, an eighteenth-century South Carolina historian, blamed smallpox for much of the decline in Indian population and asserted that by 1765 the Cherokees were reduced to less than 2,000 warriors.[53] In this same year, 1738, smallpox was transmitted to the Indians in the Hudson Bay region and spread widely in northern Canada.[54]

During the winter of 1746-47 the infection was again present in New York province and spread both north and south in the ensuing year. The governor of Canada was obliged to dispatch a message of condolence to the Onondagas for their sufferings from smallpox during the preceding winter.[55] In the American colonies, Maryland and Delaware were infected with the disease, but there is little evidence of it among the Indians. However, John Brainerd, a missionary in New Jersey, later spoke of a " Mortal Sickness," which may have been smallpox, carrying off many Indians in 1747.[56]

---

[51] *Doc. Rel. to Col. Hist. of N. Y.*, V, 963.

[52] " A Treaty Between Virginia and the Catawbas and Cherokees, 1756," *Virginia Magazine of History and Biography*, XIII (January, 1906), 227 fn.; see also Newton D. Mereness, *Travels in the American Colonies* (New York, 1916), p. 239. Captain James Oglethorpe met a delegation of Indians in September, 1739, and managed to allay their suspicions of the English.

[53] Alexander Hewat, *An Historical Account of the Rise and Progress of the Colonies of South Carolina and Georgia* (London, 1779), II, 279-80.

[54] Heagerty, *op. cit.*, I, 36-37.

[55] Colonel William Johnson to Governor Clinton, May 7, 1747, *Doc. Rel. to Col. Hist. of N. Y.*, VI, 362.

[56] John Brainerd to Mrs. Smith, Brotherton, New Jersey, August 24, 1761, in Simon Gratz Collection, Pennsylvania Historical Society MSS, American Clergymen.

The next smallpox epidemic among the Indians occurred in the Great Lakes region in 1752. The Miami tribe, to whom the French were looking for help, was completely routed by the infection. The French post at Detroit was attacked also, and one contemporary observer asserted that the sickness was " ravaging the whole of that Continent." [57] However, the Ohio valley and the areas to the East remained unaffected. Boston suffered a large scale outbreak in 1751, but the disease was sea-borne and does not seem to have spread beyond the city.

Three years later, 1755, the sickness reappeared. This time, contrary to its usual course, it began in Canada and then moved south into New York. Heagerty asserts that Canadians for years afterwards referred to 1755 as the year of the great smallpox epidemic, and that all activities, even the perennial warfare, ceased.[58] This disastrous plague in Canada did not wear itself out until late in 1757 after having swept through both French and Indian settlements. The epidemic first ravaged the French settlers and then spread to the Indian tribes. The Senecas were attacked in 1755 [59] and by the following spring nearly all of the Indians in Eastern Canada and the New England region were affected. In June, 1756, a French dispatch from Canada stated that the Indians on the borders of Acadia and New England were still hostile to the English, adding, however, ". . . unfortunately, they have not as yet been able to go on the war path, having been afflicted by the smallpox in all their villages." [60] Two months later a French official wrote of his difficulty in marshalling the Indians against the English because of their fears of the infection " at Niagara, Prequ'Isle and Fort Duquesne." [61]

The English settlements and the Indians to the south also were victimized in 1756. A report from Virginia stated that the contagion was raging among the Delawares who had caught the infection " in some Scalps they carried off from a place 20 miles above Bethlehem." [62] Meanwhile the infection manifested itself in the British armies, occasioning much alarm. The appearance of the disease in Albany, according to one writer, frightened the provincial troops more than the presence of Montcalm himself could have done, and made it necessary to garrison the town

[57] M. de Longueil to M. de Rouille, April 21, 1752, in *Doc. Rel. to Col. Hist. of N. Y.*, X, 246-50.

[58] Heagerty, *op. cit.*, I, 39-40.

[59] *Doc. Rel. to Col. Hist. of N. Y.*, X, 345.

[60] *Ibid.*, X, 408.

[61] *Ibid.*, X, 435-38; VII, 240.

[62] Boston *Weekly News-Letter* (L. C. Photo.), no. 2815, June 17, 1756.

entirely with British troops and to discharge all colonial soldiers there except one regiment raised in New York.[63]

Smallpox continued to flare up sporadically in most of the Middle colonies during 1757, and, as was usually the case, among the adjacent Indian tribes. A report to the French government in July asserted that the disorder was plaguing the English at Forts George and Lidius [Edward].[64] A month or two earlier a conference between the Indians and the English at Philadelphia had been disrupted when a number of the Indian representatives fell victim to smallpox. Soon the infection spread to the other Indians, who decided to return home immediately.[65] Subsequently the Governor's Council in Pennsylvania granted presents and extended condolences to the Indians for their heavy losses from the disease.[66]

In April, 1758, General Montcalm reported that a number of the Upper Country Indians were dying from smallpox " caught from the English on the expedition against Fort William Henry." [67] On this occasion, the garrison, hit hard by smallpox, surrendered to the French and their Indian allies. As was often the case, the Indians got out of control, murdered the sick, and in their quest for scalps, even dug up the bodies of those who had died.[68] Retribution was swift and severe for the Pandora's box, once opened, brought them far more death and suffering than they had inflicted upon the whites. In the long struggle between the Red Men and the colonists, the Indians, unfortunately, won far too many of these Pyrrhic victories.

The year 1758 again saw smallpox widespread in the provinces of New York and New Jersey. In December an S. P. G. minister wrote that the disease had " made dreadful havock . . . among thousands of white people and Indians when taken in the natural way." [69] His reference to " taken in the natural way " was to differentiate from smallpox inoculation which was then coming into general use. As a matter of fact, it was the indis-

[63] John Marshall, *A History of the Colonies Planted by the English on the Continent of North America* (Philadelphia, 1824), pp. 303-304.

[64] M. de Vaudreuil to M. de Moras, Montreal, July 12, 1757, in *Doc. Rel to Col. Hist. of N. Y.*, X, 579-580.

[65] Report of the Conferences with the Indians at Philadelphia, April 4, 1757, in *Minutes of the Provincial Council for Pennsylvania, Colonial Records*, VII, 517.

[66] " Minutes of the Council at Lancaster," May 21, 1757, in *ibid.*, p. 546.

[67] M. de Montcalm to M. de Paulmy, Montreal, April 18, 1758, in *Doc. Rel. to Col. Hist. of N. Y.*, X, 698-700.

[68] Francis Parkman, *Montcalm and Wolfe* (Boston, 1886), 11, 5.

[69] Colin Campbell to the Secretary, Burlington, New Jersey, December 20, 1759, in S. P. G. MSS (L. C. Photo.), London Letters, B 24, fpp. 151-153.

criminate use of variolation which not infrequently served to disseminate the infection among the settlers. The next section to feel the weight of smallpox was the southern colonies where the Indians in Georgia and South Carolina were devastated by the infection in 1759-60. The first notice of the outbreak occurred in a report from Georgia published in August, 1759, which stated that Savannah was exercising all precautions against the introduction of the disease; that Augusta was free of it; and that it had almost disappeared from among the Chickasaws [70] On December 15, the *South Carolina Gazette* commented editorially: " It is pretty certain that the Smallpox has lately raged with great Violence among the Catawba Indians, and that it has carried off near one-half of that nation, *by throwing themselves into the River*, as soon as they found themselves ill—This Distemper has since appeared amongst the Inhabitants of the *Charraws* and *Waterees*, where Many Families are down; so that unless special care is taken, it must soon [spread] thro' the whole country." [71]   Over a month later a correspondent in Augusta wrote: " The late Accounts from Keowee are, that the Small-Pox has destroyed a great many of the Indians there; that those who remained alive, and have not yet had that Distemper, were gone into the Woods, where many of them must perish as the Catawbas did." [72]   During the ensuing months smallpox continued its inexorable progress through the Indian tribes. On August 13, 1760, a *Pennsylvania Gazette's* correspondent reported from Augusta: " We learn from the Cherokee country, that the People of the Lower Towns have carried smallpox into the Middle Settlement and Valley, where that disease rages with great violence, and that the People of the Upper Towns are in such Dread of the Infection, that they will not allow a single Person from the above named Places to come amongst them." [73]   In October the Gazette noted that the " Cherokees had brought the Small-Pox into the Upper Creek Nation." [74]

To add to the Indian troubles, Governor Henry Lyttleton of South Carolina led an expedition against the Cherokees in 1759 which resulted in the Treaty of Fort St. George late in the fall. As the treaty was signed, smallpox, which had been raging in a nearby Indian village, broke out in the Governor's camp. The effect produced by the appearance of this dreaded plague among the colonial expeditionary force has been vividly

[70] Boston *News-Letter* (L. C. Photo.), no. 3021, August 2, 1759.
[71] *South Carolina Gazette*, no. 1321, December 15, 1759.
[72] *Pennsylvania Gazette*, no. 1625, February 14, 1760.
[73] *Ibid.*, no. 1654, September 4, 1760.
[74] *Ibid.*, no. 1662, October 30, 1760.

described by Dr. Alexander Hewat, a contemporary historian: " As few of his little army had ever gone through that distemper, and as the surgeons were totally unprovided for such an accident, his men were struck with terror, and in great haste returned to the settlements, cautiously avoiding all intercourse with one another, and suffering much from hunger and fatigue by the way." [75]   Despite all precautions, returning troops carried the infection into Charleston and the other towns.

Ordinarily the Indians were the chief victims of smallpox, but the South Carolina outbreak was an exception to the general rule.   The renewed virulence which often characterized smallpox after it had circulated among the Indian tribes held true of the virus which the Indians communicated to the troops in 1759.   During the winter that followed about 75 per cent of Charleston's inhabitants sickened with the infection and the ensuing deaths totaled well over 700.[76]   However, many of the smallpox cases resulted from the practice of inoculation, to which the people of Charleston resorted.   Augusta and Savannah, too, were infected, and like Charleston, bore heavy casualties.   The destruction among the whites was small consolation to the Indians whose already thin ranks were decimated, and who could ill afford such a depletion of manpower in the face of the steadily increasing European settlements.   The seriousness of the loss to the Indians is indicated in an article describing the Catawba Indians published in one of the colonial newspapers.   The account, written in 1760, declared that seventy years ago the Catawbas were a strong nation with four thousand members, but had been reduced since by " Rum, War and Small-Pox " to less than " 100 gunmen." [77]   Simultaneously with the major outbreak in South Carolina and Georgia, scattered epidemics occurred all the way to Canada.   Hostilities between the English and French widely disseminated the contagion, which seems to have been endemic among the troops.   The journals and diaries of soldiers in the field speak constantly of the omnipresent threat from smallpox.   And the Indians, either as allies or enemies, were even more susceptible to the disease than the colonial troops.   For example, a group of Dakotas, who journeyed to Quebec after its capture by the English, became infected, and the Menominee tribe in Wisconsin was greatly reduced by the ravages

[75] Bartholomew R. Carroll, *Historical Collections of South Carolina* (New York, 1836), I, 452.

[76] *Pennsylvania Gazette*, no. 1633, April 10, 1760; *South Carolina Gazette*, no. 1340, April 19, 1760.

[77] Boston *News-Letter* (L. C. Photo.), no. 2615, June 5, 1760.

of war and smallpox.[78] Sporadic outbreaks continued to develop through-out the war and few sections of British-controlled North America escaped.

The colonists were well aware of the potency of smallpox as a weapon against the Indians, and on several occasions deliberate efforts were made to infect the Red Men. One of these instances occurred during the Pontiac conspiracy in 1763. The British commander, Sir Jeffrey Amherst, added the following postscript to a letter to Colonel Henry Bouquet, " Could it not be contrived to send the small-pox among these disaffected tribes of Indians? We must on this occasion use every strategem in our power to reduce them." Bouquet replied on July 13, 1763, " I will try to inoculate the − − − − − with some blankets that may fall in their hands, and take care not to get the disease myself." [79] Just how successful Bouquet's experiment was is not known.

In the years 1764-65 smallpox flared up among the Indians in a number of widely separated regions. On July 30, 1764, the New York *Mercury* stated that " Smallpox has gone among the Creek Indians & carried off great Nos. of them." [80] The following spring the *Pennsylvania Gazette* reported that " 1,500 Choctaws and 300 Chicksaws had died from the infection." [81] Later in the summer, Cornelius Bennett, an S. P. G. mis-sionary among the Indians in the vicinity of Mohawk Castle, explained to the Society that the danger from smallpox had compelled him to return to Boston.[82] The notorious lack of enthusiasm among these missionaries for working with the Indians may have caused Bennett to overrate the danger; however, he did write the following year that he was ready to return to the mission field, which indicates that his concern over smallpox may have been justified.[83] Meanwhile the contagion was reported to be menacing the " Shawnese." [84] The settlers in Maryland were plagued with the infection in 1765, and Quebec suffered a major outbreak, but apparently these epidemics had little effect upon the Indians.

Smallpox subsided during the rest of the colonial period and did not constitute a serious threat to either the colonists or the Indians until the

[78] Francis Parkman, *History of the Conspiracy of Pontiac and the War of the North American Tribes against the English Colonies after the Conquest of Canada* (Boston, 1851), pp. 318 ff.

[79] Heagerty, *op. cit.*, I, 43.

[80] New York *Mercury* (L. C. Photo.), no. 666, July 30, 1764.

[81] *Pennsylvania Gazette*, no. 1901, May 30, 1765.

[82] Cornelius Bennett to Secretary, Boston, September 12, 1765, in S. P. G. MSS (L. C. Photo.), London Letters, B 22, fpp. 130-131.

[83] *Ibid.*

[84] Heagerty, *op. cit.*, I, 43.

opening hostilities of the Revolutionary War. As in previous wars, the troops carried the virus into all areas, infecting both civilians and Indians alike. By this time smallpox had already contributed much to the reduction of the Indian threat, but its task was still undone. Well into the nineteenth century smallpox continued its grim work of decimating the Indian tribes. In fact, it was not until the beginning of the present century that the infection was finally controlled.

The exact role played by smallpox in the settlement of North America is not easily determined. Certain tribes were literally wiped out, yet others survived many attacks, and were even, in the intervals between outbreaks, able to recoup their losses through a natural population increase. However, by eliminating a number of Indian tribes, smallpox cleared the way for white occupation in some areas with only a minimum of friction. Major epidemics among the surviving Red Men permitted easier advances into Indian territory, and often by the time the tribes had recovered enough to make an effective resistance, the whites were too well entrenched to be driven back. In times of war, smallpox, although a dangerous ally, was frequently a decisive factor in the victories of the Europeans over the Indians. The task of settling the New World was a difficult one at best. The enormous physical job of clearing forests and preparing land for cultivation combined with the constant menace of the Indians, always numerous, shrewd, and skillful adversaries, makes it apparent that the determination and courage of the early settlers has not been exaggerated.

11

The Significance of Disease in the Extinction of the New England Indians

Sherburne F. Cook

According to James Mooney (1928) there were originally about 36,500 natives living east of the Hudson River and within the present limits of the United States. In 1907, there were close to 2,400 left, many of them of mixed ethnic derivation. The loss in approximately 300 years, therefore, amounted to 93.5% of the initial value. Most of the loss occurred within the first century of European settlement.

Much has been written concerning the destruction of the red race, and much discussion has been devoted to the factors directly responsible for the catastrophic decline in numbers. One of these was admittedly the disease introduced by the white man. Among the many commentaries upon this subject are descriptions and accounts of epidemics written at the time the events took place, together with numerous recent essays which treat of the purely medical aspects of the more conspicuous maladies. There are few works, however, which attempt to assess quantitatively the severity of chronic and acute illness as a determinant in the demographic pattern.

Sherburne F. Cook

OPPORTUNITY FOR INFECTION

The first step in the evaluation of disease in the destruction of the red race must be to establish the opportunity for infection to occur. Subsequent to the foundation of permanent settlements at Plymouth and at New Amsterdam, at or near the year 1620, the white man was never absent, nor was there any cessation of the flow of commerce across the Atlantic Ocean. Any disease of a communicable nature consequently could very easily spill over into the new colonies. Prior to 1620 the intercourse was far more sporadic.

For practical purposes we may exclude the influence of the Vikings and place the beginning of European contact with North America at the time of Columbus, 1492. At the latitude of New England and eastern Canada the first discoveries date from the Cabots in 1497. Thereafter, contact became progressively closer. From the standpoint of the introduction of disease, two sources may be distinguished. The first is derived from the unknown ships and crews which pursued fishing off the coasts of Newfoundland and Nova Scotia during the entire sixteenth century. These men came predominantly from Spain, Portugal, France and England. Most of them never went ashore, but here and there must have occurred landings of which there is no record extant. The possibility can not be excluded that some types of pathogenic organisms may have been thereby communicated. However, there is no evidence from written record or oral tradition that serious harm to the natives resulted.

The second channel of transmission was provided by the numerous expeditions which moved along the coast or penetrated the interior between 1500 and 1620, most of them subsequent to 1600. For the details of their wanderings and the shores they visited, the reader may turn to the many histories of New World Exploration. It is sufficient to point out here that not merely from 1620 but from the beginning of the seventeenth century, no impediment existed to the introduction of any European disease to the colonies of New England or Canada.

RECORDED EPIDEMICS

With the exception of minor and local outbreaks of already established contagions, two pestilences of wide, severe, epidemic proportions struck the New England natives in the early years of settlement by the English. They stand out as of particular importance as agents destructive to the Indian population. Indeed, there never was complete, or even substantial recovery from their lethal effect. The first was the so-called plague of 1616-1619.

The exact date at which this epidemic began its ravages is not certain. There is no doubt, however, that it was at full intensity in 1617 and persisted in its initial fulmination until 1619. The introduction is ascribed, at least by implication, to a group of French sailors who were shipwrecked in Massachusetts Bay. They were captured by the local Indians who boasted that their number was too great ever to be conquered. Then, according to Thomas Morton (1632), "in a short time thereafter, the hand of God fell heavily upon them, with such a mortall stroake, that they died on heaps. . . ." Whether or not these Frenchmen were the agents, it is probable that the first onset was in Massachusetts Bay. This area remained the focus from which the disease spread southward to Cape Cod and northward to Maine.

Concerning the nature of the infection we are obliged to rely upon a few rather cursory statements made by contemporaries. All comment since the middle of the seventeenth century, and there has been a great deal, reflects only interpretation based upon modern advances in medical knowledge. Starting from unanimous agreement that the epidemic was enormously destructive in many areas, two principal theories have been developed, that the malady was bubonic or pneumonic plague (H. U. Williams, 1909), or small pox (Shrewsbury, 1949). A third possibility suggested by Hoyt (1824), and by others in the early nineteenth century, is that it was yellow fever. C. F. Adams (1903) excluded yellow fever and small pox, but otherwise remained non-committal. Recently, Duffy (1951, 1953) excluded yellow fever but made no further attempt to identify the epidemic.

The yellow fever theory was derived from a statement of Daniel Gookin, who wrote in 1692, seventy five years after the epidemic. As quoted by H. U. Williams (1909), he said: "I have discoursed with old Indians who were then youths, who say that the bodies all over were exceeding yellow, describing it by a yellow garment they showed me, both before they died and afterwards." Williams (1909, page 348, footnote 41) also cites J. H. Trumbull who pointed out that the Indian name of the plague—quite different from that of the small pox—meant literally "a bad yellowing." There is no reason to deny the veracity of these witnesses, or to doubt that, at least in some cases, there was a marked degree of jaundice. However, yellow fever can not be held responsible because the epidemic persisted throughout the year, and no mosquito-borne infection can survive the New England winter. The possibilities, therefore, narrow down to plague and small pox.

Two arguments have been advanced against the small pox theory. The first is that the English colonists were thoroughly familiar with the symptoms and appearance of small pox, and could diagnose the disease without hesitation. The contention of Shrewsbury (1949) that the settlers would not recognize small pox in a non-immune population is nonsense. Europeans had seen small pox spread among Indians since 1519, the year Cortez invaded Mexico. It was described by many chroniclers of the early explorations, and indeed is the one disease among the natives which was universally recognized as a pathological entity.

A convincing bit of evidence is the statement of Bradford in 1634 (edition of 1901, page 387). Regarding the Indians in the Connecticut Valley he wrote: ". . . for it pleased God to visite these Indians with a great sickness. . . . This Springe, also, those Indians that lived about their trading house there fell sick of ye small poxe, and dyed most misearably: for a sorer disease can not befall them; they fear it more than ye plague. . . ." A similar piece of evidence that the Indians knew both small pox and plague and distinguished between them is presented by Roger Williams in his *Key into the Language of America* (1643, page 157). Under the heading of sickness he gives nine words or phrases in the language of the Narragansetts. In a parallel column he translates these as follows:

> "I have a swelling
> He is swelled
> All his body is swelled
> He hath the Pox
> The Pox
> The last Pox
> He hath the plague
> The plague
> The great plague"

Finally, we may quote a modern writer, Charles Fancis Adams (1903), who sums up the case of Deacon Samuel Fuller: "Dr. Fuller could hardly have seen the Indians dying of 'an infectious fever,' and then have died of it himself among his dying neighbors, and never have identified the malady as small-pox, if it had been small-pox."

The second argument relates to symptoms. We have mentioned jaundice, which certainly seems to have been present, although perhaps not universal in occurrence. Sir Ferdinando Gorges (1658) describes the experience of Vines at Sagadahoc, who with his men inhabited cabins where Indians had died, and says that "not one of them ever felt their heads to ache while they stayed there." Johnson (1654) refers to "Their disease being a sore Consumption, sweeping away whole families . . ." Bradford describes the death of the Indian Squanto, who "fell sick of an Indian feavor, bleeding much at ye nose (which ye Indians take for a simptome of death). . . ." This disease, however, may or may not have been identical with the plague of 1617. Dermer, in a letter of 1619 to Purchas (quoted by Williams, 1909, page 344) describes the Maine coast: ". . . in other places a remnant remaines, but not free from sicknesse. Their disease the plague, for we might perceive the sores of some that had escaped, who described the spots of such as usually die." We have then jaundice, nose bleed, head ache, lung congestion, and superficial spots or sores. None of these are clear symptoms of small pox.

The argument in favor of plague is less clear. It is true that the colonists were familiar with plague in both bubonic and pneumonic forms. It is also true that the word plague was used to designate almost any highly contagious febrile infection which resulted in quick demise. Yet reference is constantly made to *the* plague as if it were a well recognized entity. The few symptoms which we have described could pertain to plague. The headache in the early phases, the bleeding from the nose, the "sores" or "spots" which were probably sub-epidermal hemorrhages, could indicate, but do not necessarily impose acceptance of plague. Winter infection is possible with the pneumonic form by direct person-to-person contact. The transmission by rats and fleas is likewise possible. That the Indians were overrun by fleas is attested by all contemporary observers. The invasion of the mainland by rats from ships is described by Lescarbot (1612) as being noted in the time of Champlain, 1603-1606. In sum, although there is little solid evidence in favor of the theory, there are no facts that clearly negate the possibility that the epidemic of 1616-1619 was some type of bubonic or pneumonic plague.

The center of the epidemic was along the shore of Massachusetts Bay, in the territory of the tribe of that name. It was particularly violent in the region of Boston Harbor and southward through Plymouth where the native inhabitants were virtually exterminated. The details, as recounted by Smith (1622, 1631), Bradford (edition of 1901), Morton (1632), and many others, need not be repeated here. To the southward

490 *Sherburne F. Cook*

it attacked the Wampanoags. Edward Johnson (1654) refers to the epidemic as ". . . chiefly desolating those places where the English afterward planted the countrey of Pockanocky (Wampanoag), Agissawamg (Agawam). . . ." Mourt (1622) in his *Relation* tells of a trip down the Taunton River, in Plymouth and Bristol counties. He says: "Thousands of men have lived there, which died in a great plague not long since . . . ", and "As we passed along we observed that there were few places by the river but had been inhabited; by reason whereof much ground was clear. . . ." The infection, however, did not cross Narragansett Bay and affect the inhabitants on the west side, in the present State of Rhode Island, a point concerning which all writers are in agreement.

To the northward the plague reached southern Maine. Gorges (1658) is explicit in his statement that Vines found plague at Sagadahoc. He also says (1658, page 57): ". . . for that war had consumed the Bashaba and most of the great Sagamores . . . and those that remained were sore afflicted by the plague so that the country was in a manner left void of inhabitants." The reference is to the region between the Kennebec and the Penobscot Rivers. Capt. John Smith (1631) refers to "three plagues in three years successively neere two hundred miles along the sea coast. . . ." Among more modern writers, Samuel Drake (1851, page 80) says of the plague: "The extent of its ravages, as near as we can judge, was from Narragansett Bay to Kennebeck or perhaps Penobscot. . . ."

Intermediate points along the coast are frequently mentioned. Johnson (see above) specifies Agawam, or Cape Ann as being attacked. According to Drake (1867, page 53) the Pawtucket, a tribe near Lowell, Massachusetts, had a considerable population, but the pestilence "almost totally destroyed them" (quoting Gookin). Morse (1822) refers to the Pemaquid tribe, who had been probably the chief group among the Tarrantines ". . . till the great and mortal sickness among the natives along the whole coast, from the Penobscot to Narragansett, A.D. 1617". The modern ethnographer Willoughby (1935) says that the pestilence reduced the numbers of the Pennacook as well as of the Massachusetts and Wampanoag.

There can be little doubt, therefore, that the plague of 1616-1619, although sharply circumscribed in the south by Narragansett Bay, spread continuously north as far as the Kennebec Rivers and perhaps to Penobscot Bay and decimated all native tribes in its path. It is a significant fact that, as was pointed out by White (1630), this plague "nor then raged above twenty or thirty miles up into the land. . . ." It is true that the heaviest native population lived along the coast, but the interior was by no means uninhabited. There is no immediate explanation why the infection did not move up the rivers, or why it failed to cross the head of Narragansett Bay near Providence and spread among the Indians of the western shore.

Subsequent to 1620, with a few exceptions, the plague assumed a minor role in the disease pattern of both the native and the European races in the northeastern United States. The outstanding exception is the outbreak of what was called the plague in the Connecticut Valley in 1633-1634, and which was discussed under this name by Bradford. Locally it was highly lethal, but unless it moved into unknown areas up the river, it did not affect more than the population of the valley between Hartford and Springfield. Other instances of "putrid" or "malignant" fevers were recorded but there is no clear evidence which equates them with the plague of 1616-1619. If the great epidemic of these years was indeed the only significant appearance of the disease, and if it was really the bubonic or pneumonic plague, then its failure to break out again is an indication that the causative organism could not establish itself in the New England environment among the rodent population as it has on the Pacific Coast. Its introduction in 1616 must be regarded as a one-time event, which, fortunately, was not repeated.

In view of the universal occurrence of small pox, in both the Old and the New World, it is surprising that the disease did not appear in New England prior to 1633.[2] The Spanish colonies in Mexico and the Caribbean had been the scene of disastrous epidemics for a century, and there had been some movement of shipping between them and the northern coasts for decades. Even the ships from England were loaded with infection. Thus Hubbard (1680) relates that in 1630 the ship *Talbot* arrived from England in Boston. She "had been sore visited with smallpox in her passage, and whereof fourteen died in the way." Josselyn (1673) states that on his voyage to Boston in 1638 many passengers were ill with the disease and several died. Nevertheless, among the Indians the first great outbreak took place in 1633.

This epidemic and its offshoots was so wide spread as to become almost universal. It is first reported from the Boston area where it was described in detail by John Winthrop in his *Journal* (edition of 1908).

[2] The extent and distribution of small pox in the English and French colonies is discussed extensively in the book by Stearn and Stearn (1945). Reference may also be made to the study by Duffy (1951).

In November, 1633, he records: "A great mortality among the Indians. Chikatabot, the Sagamore of Neponset, died and many of his people. The disease was the smallpox." On December 5 he wrote: "John Sagamore died of the smallpox and almost all of his people; (above thirty buried by Mr. Maverick of Winesemett in one day). The towns in the bay took away many of the children; but most of them died soon after.

"James Sagamore of Sagus died also, and most of his folks. . . . The English ministered to them, yet only two families were infected." Later he says: "This infectious disease spread to Pascataquack, where all the Indians (except one or two) died." Pascataquack undoubtedly is a spelling variant of Piscataqua (see Hodge, 1907, Vol. II, page 262). The name is repeated in the entry for January 20, 1634 in which Winthrop states regarding deaths from small pox: ". . . but beyond Pascataquack none to the eastward." Since the village of Piscataqua was on the river of that name, near the coast, the eastern limit of the epidemic at that time is established.

Meanwhile it had reached the Narragansetts, who suffered heavily, and crossed over into the region beyond. Winthrop entered in his journal on January 20, 1634 that a certain Hall and two others who had returned from Connecticut ". . . informed us that the small pox was gone as far as any Indian plantation was known to the west, and much people died of it. . . ." At that time "Indian plantations" were known to the English as far as western Connecticut and Massachusetts. Bradford (edition of 1901) has left us the most circumstantial and authoritative account of the progress of the disease in that area up to the late winter of 1633-1634. He first described the effect of an epidemic which appears to have been very similar to, if not identical with the plague of 1616-1619, and which was lethal in its intensity. Then he went on to outline the effect of small pox as it raged among the Indians. (The distinction which he drew between the two epidemics has already been mentioned.)

Before the end of the same year small pox was present among the Indians to the west of the Hudson River. An anonymous author (1634) mentions in a journal of a visit to the Mohawks, under the date of December 13, 1634, that ". . . a good many of the savages here in the castle died of small pox." Within three or four years not only the Iroquois but the Hurons, Ottawa and other tribes were involved. Stearn and Stearn comment (1945, page 24): "During the period between the years 1633 and 1641 there seems to have been an almost unbroken series of smallpox epidemics through the Great Lakes-St. Lawrence River region. It seems quite probable that the different reported outbreaks in the different years and in different parts of the general region affected are aspects of the same general epidemic." Whether these outbreaks extending a thousand miles to the interior were actually touched off by the New England epidemic is a debateable question. Intercommunication between New England and both the Hudson and the St. Lawrence valleys was sufficiently free and copious to account for the rapid extension of the disease. On the other hand it is very difficult to find the necessary documentation for a point-to-point dating of the spread of the epidemic.

After the decade 1630-1640, small pox was never absent among the populations of eastern North America. At intervals it flared into epidemic proportions as it reached new Indian tribes, or attacked the non-immune younger generations in older territory. In New England it became almost endemic among the residue of the native race, and occasionally achieved the magnitude of an epidemic. For instance Eliot (1651) commented that in the winter of 1649-1650 "it please God to work wonderfully for the [Christian] Indians who call upon God in preserving them from the small pox, when their prophane neighbors were cut off by it." Potter (1835) states that in October, 1664, small pox swept away many Massachusetts Indians. Ruttenber (1872) recounts an epidemic among the Montauks of Long Island in 1658, when "the small pox destroyed more than half the clan." A very adequate summary of outbreaks of small pox in New England, New York, and lower Canada has been given in the study by Duffy (1951). For the present purpose it is sufficient to emphasize the fluctuating but continuous drain upon the vitality of the native population caused by small pox throughout the seventeenth century.

ENDEMIC AND CHRONIC DISEASE

Apart from the ravages of the conspicuous, destructive plague and small pox, the natives of New England were subjected to uninterrupted attrition from infections of many other types. Some of these may have reached the level of true epidemics, but have gone unrecorded; others exacted their toll almost without notice as individual pathological entities. Their effect can be estimated only in the aggregate, although some specific diseases were sufficiently widespread and damaging to warrant special mention by contemporary writers.

Of these perhaps the outstanding example is tuberculosis. Its importance was early recognized by Gookin (1692) who wrote: "Of this dis-

494   *Sherburne F. Cook*

ease of consumption sundry of these Indian youths died, that were brought up to school among the English. The truth is that this disease is frequent among the Indians; and sundry die of it, that have not been with the English. A hectick fever, issuing in a consumption, is a common and mortal disease among them." A century later Bennet (1794) described the surviving Indians in the town of Middleborough, Massachusetts. "They are subject to hectical complaints, for more than half that are born are carried off young with consumptions." General Lincoln (1795), in a letter published by the Massachusetts Historical Society, remarks: "Their tender lungs are greatly affected by colds, which bring on consumptive habits; from which disorder, if my information is right, a large proportion of them die."

Together with tuberculosis other respiratory complaints, such as pneumonia and influenza, must have been common. Hubbard (1680) relates that: "In the year 1647, an epidemical sickness passed through the whole country of New England, both among Indians, English, French and Dutch. It began with a cold, and in many was accompanied by a light fever." It spread through the whole coast, all the English plantations in America, even to the West Indies. "Whether it might be called a plague or pestilential fever, physicians must determine." It may very well have been influenza. More recently Ellis and Morris (1906) wrote concerning the condition of the Indians during King Philip's War: "Disease . . . had been rife during the winter and the Indians, weakened by privations, had fallen easy victims to colds and malignant fevers, to whose ravages among the settlers Mather bears mournful testimony."

Specific non-respiratory diseases are occasionally mentioned. M. de Denonville wrote in 1687 (Docs. Rel. Hist. New York, vol. IX, page 354) that a ship which recently arrived in Canada brought the measles and the spotted fever. As a result there had been several hundred cases in the Christian Indian villages. Thus the possibility exists that an epidemic of typhus occurred, although the writer does not specify whether the deaths resulted from measles or from the fever.

Dysenteries were frequent, not only among the natives but also among the colonists. In a document entitled "Confession of Ephraim", found in the Collections of the Massachusetts Historical Society, Series III, vol. 4, page 259, we find that "This Spring, in the beginning of the year 1652, the Lord was pleased to afflict sundry of our praying Indians with that grievous disease of the Bloody-Flux, whereof some with great torments in their bowels died. . . ." He then describes the death of a mother and two children which was highly edifying in the religious sense. That dysentery was not confined to Christian Indians is attested by the fact that the Narragansetts had a word for the malady in their language, given by Roger Williams in the *Key* (1643) together with its English equivalent "I have the bloody Flixe".

In view of the controversy concerning its ultimate origin, syphilis among the Indians in the Colonies is of considerable interest. It was present in North America early. Charlevoix states (1743) that at the time of Cartier's voyages in 1534 and 1535, the French crews had had venereal disease. This was only 40-odd years after Columbus, but by that time Europe had become thoroughly infected. Whether or not it had existed in the New World previously, upon its introduction, or reintroduction, from European sources, it attacked the natives with augmented severity. Lescarbot (1612) described in detail Cartier's difficulty with scurvy and discussed a cure for the ailment. Apropos of the cure Lescarbot wrote: ". . . insomuch that some of the crew who had had the French pox for five or six years were clean cured by this medicine."

Since relations between all European crews and native women were notorious, there can be no doubt that infection was introduced wherever the ships landed on the American coast. The presence of syphilis is confirmed by Josselyn (1673) who says: "There are not so many diseases raigning amongst them as our Europeans. The great pox is proper to them. . . ." Roger Williams (1643) adds a word when he describes the sweating technique. The treatment is ". . . doubtlesse a great meanes of preserving them, and recovering them from diseases, especially from the French disease, which by sweating and some potions, they perfectly and speedily cure. . . ."

One significant implication of these citations is that syphilis was not particularly virulent among the natives of northeastern America. If so, the contrast is striking with the Indians of Mexico and California, who suffered severely from the disease. Nevertheless considerable damage must have been unavoidable, particularly in the form of congenital defects and even reduction in procreative capacity. We have no direct evidence concerning these conditions and can merely speculate from general knowledge of venereal disease.

EPIDEMIC DISEASE AND POPULATION LEVEL

The introduction of new, lethal diseases could affect the native population by reducing the birth rate or increasing the death rate, or both. Concerning the former we have very little information. From New

496

Sherburne F. Cook

England, New York, or even the St. Lawrence Valley, I have encountered no serious attempt on the part of contemporary observers to evaluate the reproductive potential of the native peoples. It is of course permissible to adopt the working hypothesis that within the pre-contact environment the birth rate exceeded the death rate, and, that, in the absence of external restraint such as intertribal warfare, the population would increase up to the subsistence limit of the area. The rarity of indigenous epidemics and the general high level of health among the Indians drew the comment of many Europeans. Hence, even with constant attrition due to warfare and its attendant disturbance, the mean number of children produced per reproductive female should have reached at least three.

As to whether this goal was attained there is conflicting opinion. It may have been if Roger Williams (1643) was correct in his statement: "They commonly abound with children, and increase mightily; except the plague fall amongst them, or other lesser sicknesses, and then having no means of recovery, they perish wonderfully." On the other hand Isaac de Rosières (1628) wrote with reference to the region of New Amsterdam, before any destructive epidemic had reached the natives: "It would seem that they are very libidinous . . . whence it results that they breed but few children, so that it is a wonder when a woman has three or four children, particularly by any man whose name can be certainly known." Probably neither Williams nor de Rosières had more than a subjective impression upon which to base his statements. Williamson (1839) in his History of Maine felt that there was a significant upward population pressure. He said regarding the matter: "War is always a heavy tax upon the population of the Indians. Fights, fatigue, famine and sickness, occasion wastes which the *natural increase among them in seasons of tranquility never repair.*" (Italics mine).

If we asume that the replacement rate was adequate to maintain, or even augment the population under aboriginal conditions, we still face the question how far introduced diseases reduced that rate below the pre-contact level. Here we are without any concrete data whatever. Furthermore we have to interpret any suggestions of reduced number of children in the light of undoubted increased rates of infant mortality. Moreover, if we established child-woman ratios, as might in some cases be possible, they would have no value as indices to actual reproduction. We can therefore only postulate that the birth rate did not rise, but either remained constant or diminished in the face of the white man's epidemics.

This assumption is consistent with general experience among the native races of America. Not only disease but physical dislocation and unrest, coupled with an extremely adverse reaction to foreign invasion, caused the Indian women throughout the hemisphere to resent the giving birth to more children. This reaction expressed itself frequently in abortion and infanticide, although I have seen no mention of these acts in the accounts by European settlers of New England. Nevertheless they may have occurred without exciting comment. With the exception of a few earnest workers such as John Eliot, the English and Dutch were notoriously indifferent to the social status of the indigenes.

The effect of disease upon the death rate was clear and unequivocal. It was exerted through rapid destruction of large numbers by deadly epidemics, and through relatively slow attack by less violent maladies over a considerable period of time. The epidemic crises were sufficiently severe to attract the attention of the colonists.

Proportionate mortality is stated for several cases. The most widely quoted is that of the Massachusetts during the plague of 1616-1619. Capt. John Smith (*New England's Trials*, 1622, page 12) says ". . . for where I had seene 100 or 200 people there is scarce ten to be found." If the initial number was 150 and 140 of them died the factor of reduction would have been 93.5%. In the *Advertisements* (1631) he makes two more estimates. In the first he says: ". . . of five or six hundred about the Massachusetts, there remained but thirty, on whom their neighbors fell and slew twenty-eight. . . ." The factor of reduction here is from an average of 550 to 30, or 94.5%. The second estimate is: "for where I have seene two or three hundred, within three years after remained scarce thirty." The factor of reduction is 88%.

White (*The Planter's Plea*, 1630) refers to the plague: ". . . which swept away most of the inhabitants all along the sea coast, and in some places utterly consumed man, woman and childe, so that there is no person left to lay claim to the soyle which they possessed; in most of the rest, the contagion hath scarce left alive one person of an hundred." Here the factors are 100 and 99%. Morton (*New English Canaan*, 1632) says: "For in a place where many inhabited, there hath not been but one left alive, to tell what became of the rest. . . ." The factor of reduction is again 99%. With regard to Patuxet (Plymouth), according to Mourt's Relation (1622), the Indian Samoset said: "all the inhabitants died of an extraordinary plague". The factor is 100%.

Here are seven estimates of mortality, ranging from 88 to 100% of the affected population. They were to be sure approximations, but they were offered by reasonably responsible men who were present at the scene or shortly thereafter. There may have been error, but not deliberate falsification. To claim this would be to demand an incomprehensible motivation and a grand conspiracy on the part of individuals who never came in contact with one another.

The error, if present, would have resulted from the fact that the writers cited saw, or were told about only the most extreme cases. Back from the coast, and in scattered spots along the coast, the mortality may have been less. Certainly the plague did die out in the interior. Furthermore, the natives, in their ignorance and terror, very probably fled to points of greater security and thus escaped infection. Some of the areas later found completely vacant may have simply been abandoned by survivors who took refuge with friendly neighbors. If these suggestions are valid then the reduction in population was not quite as great as has been in good faith reported.

The Wampanoags were also attacked by the plague. Mourt's description of the valley of the Taunton River indicates almost total depopulation. However, the chief, Massasoit, appeared at Plymouth with 60 men, undoubtedly his entire group of adult males. The unknown in the equation is pre-plague population. That it was large is demonstrated by the figures of the conservative Mooney (1928) who allows the tribe 2,400 persons. Nevertheless, Bradford (1901 edition) described Massasoit's village thus: ". . . ye people not many, being dead and abundantly wasted in ye late great mortalitie . . . wherein thousands of them dyed." Perhaps thousands of them did die. Sixty men implies a total population of about 240. This is one tenth of Mooney's estimate of 2,400 and would yield a reduction factor of 90%.

Beyond the Massachusetts to the northeast many tribes were invaded by the epidemic. Most of the statements concerning them are general in nature, rather than specifically numerical. However, the Pawtucket along the Merrimac River, with several subtribes, were "almost totally destroyed" by the pestilence of 1617, according to Drake (1867) who quotes Gookin. Gorges (1658) describes the situation on the lower Maine coast in 1616-1617: ". . . for that war had consumed the Bashaba and the most of the great Sagamores . . . and these that remained were sore afflicted with the plague so that the country was in a manner left void of inhabitants."

Mooney's (1928) figures for the population of the New England tribes are probably too low. However, there are no others available. We may therefore accept them provisionally and subject to future revision.

He gives for the Wampanoag, Massachusetts, Pennacook, and Abnaki in Maine a total of 10,400 souls. Of these the interior Pennacook and all but the lower coastal Abnaki must be deducted, say 3,000. The remainder is 7,400. If the Massachusetts and Wampanoag values are taken as typical, then a minimum of 90%, or 6,650 died in the epidemic. If we concede a certain degree of exaggeration, and likewise remember that the extreme virulence may have been somewhat erratic in occurrence, we may reduce the factor to 75%, with a mortality of 5,550. To lose even this number struck a mortal blow to the Indians of the central New England coast from which they never were allowed to recover.

For estimates of fatality in the small pox epidemic of 1633-1634 we depend entirely upon the accounts of Bradford and of Winthrop. The latter, in his journal for December 5, 1633 wrote that the disease spread to Pasacataquack (Piscatagua) River "where all the Indians (except one or two) died." On the same day he tells how the mortality was extremely heavy around Boston Bay. Here lived the remnants who had survived the plague of 1616-1617. The Narragansetts were spared this plague but were attacked by the small pox seventeen years later. Winthrop notes on January 20, 1634 that "at Narraganset, by the Indians report, there died seven hundred." Mooney's figure for the aboriginal tribe is 4,000. Hence, if 700 died the factor of reduction was 17.5%, a very low value for the initial onset of small pox. Nevertheless there is no evidence, direct or indirect, that the mortality was greater. Evidently the Narragansetts escaped the worst of the infection.

On the contrary the natives of the Connecticut Valley were badly hit, according to Bradford (1901 edition), by both plague and small pox. In the first epidemic, probably the plague, they lost 950 people out of 1,000, and the dead could not be buried. In the subsequent small pox, the chief and "almost all his friends and kinred" died. Bradford's statement can be understood to mean literally that there were 1,000 Indians of whom 950 died. It may also be interpreted as indicating that the proportion of deaths was 950 out of 1,000. Either alternative yields a factor of reduction of 95%. As to the absolute number, Bradford (1901 edition, pages 387-388) tells of a company of English who had established a trading house on the river (not far from Windsor, Connecticut). They were afraid of the Indians for "About a thousand of them had inclosed them selves in a forte, which they had strongly palissadoed about." This is presumably the thousand of whom 950 died in the plague epidemic, which in turn was followed by the small pox. The total number is probably exaggerated, although the proportion of deaths may be nearly cor-

Sherburne F. Cook

rect. However, if we allow for both types of disease, and for their spread beyond the point occupied by the English at their trading house, an aggregate of 950 may be accepted.

The experience of the French a few years later on the St. Lawrence is worth noting, particularly since the French were far more accurate in the records of Indian affairs than were the English. Charlevoix (edition of 1743, Vol. III, page 153) describes the Jesuit mission at Sillery, near Quebec. In 1670 it contained about 1,500 converted Indians, mostly local Algonquins. At or near 1670 small pox utterly destroyed the town. "Fifteen hundred Indians were attacked and not one recovered." Thereafter (see Charlevoix, 1743, Vol. IV, page 44, footnote) "Abenaquis were received in such numbers as to make it an Abenaquis mission". In 1684 (or 1687) there was another epidemic, recounted by Maurault (1866, page 233) which was brought by the Abenaquis from the Iroquois, this time of "fievres" in which "presque tous" were affected. M. de Denonville, in a letter to M. de Seigneley (Docs. Rel. Hist. New York, Vol. IX, page 354) said there were 130 deaths at Sillery out of a population of 500 to 600. The factor of reduction for the earlier epidemic is 100% and for the later one about 25%.

The best analysis of mortality among the Indians caused by an epidemic in colonial New England is that by Zaccheus Macy (1810) concerning a disease among the surviving Indians on the Island of Nantucket in 1763. The island had originally contained about 3,000 natives, but they had been seriously depleted. ". . . in the year 1763 there were but three hundred and forty eight left on the island. In that year an uncommon mortal distemper attacked them. It began the 16th of the eighth month 1763 and lasted till the 16th of the second month 1764. During that period two hundred and twenty two died. Thirty four were sick and recovered. Thirty six who lived among them escaped the disorder. Eight lived at the west end of the island, and did not go among them; none of them caught the disease. Eighteen were at sea. With the English lived forty of whom none died." We deduct 66 who were not exposed, leaving 282. Of these 256 had the disease, 91%. Those who died, 222, were 87% of those who were sick, 79% of those exposed, and 64% of the total Indian population of the island.

In spite of the statements by seventeenth century colonists which imply mortalities of 90 to 100% of the total Indian population, it is likely that the Nantucket experience is more or less typical. As we have suggested previously, the exceptions would be aggregations in restricted areas, such as the village of Patuxet or the congregation at Sillery, when a completely unfamiliar disease arrived. These calamities, in turn, would impress the Europeans and would be noted in the writing of the time. It will not be unreasonable to consider 75 percent as the mortality, or the factor of reduction, associated with the epidemics of the early seventeenth century which affected the total population over a substantial expanse of territory.

CHRONIC DISEASE AND LONG TERM EFFECTS

In addition to the devastation wrought by sudden, catastrophic epidemics, the natives suffered even more severely from endemic disease such as tuberculosis or dysentery, together with sporadic, local flare-ups of small pox. It is difficult to assess what might be called the basal level of attrition due to long-term illness because of frequent physical disturbance and civil disorder during the first century of white occupation. We are fortunate, therefore, in finding two areas which were quite free from both intertribal raiding and warfare with the settlers. These are the two large islands off the southern New England coast, Martha's Vineyard and Nantucket. Here we may observe in a relatively pure form the effect of chronic disease and its antecedent causes upon the level of population.

An anonymous document, entitled *A Description of Duke's County*, in the Massachusetts Historical Society Collections, Series 2, Vol. III, pages 38-94, 1815, states that in 1642 the Indian population of Martha's Vineyard was 3,000 souls. The people had not suffered from the plague in 1616 nor the small pox in 1633, although the document says that "In 1643 and at several other times they were visited by a general disease." However, "In 1674 they were reduced to five hundred families, or about fifteen hundred souls." A letter by Thomas Mayhew, quoted by Gookin (1693, page 205) says there were 300 families in 1674, but if we allow 5 persons per family, the total is still somewhere near 1,500.

In 1698 the document in the Historical Society Collections says there were 1,000 and that in 1720 there were 800. The first of these figures is substantiated by Rev. Mr. Hawley (1698), a missionary at Marshpee. He says that there were 956 Indians on the island. The second figure is confirmed by a footnote in Gookin (page 205) to the effect that in 1720 there were 145 families. At the ratio of five to one, this means 725 people. In 1764 there were 313 persons by actual count. These, however, were racially mixed with both blacks and whites.

We may calculate roughly and by stages the reduction per year from 1642 to 1764. To do so we take the population loss between each two dates and divide by the number of years represented. Then we divide the result by the average of the population at the two dates, so as to get an expression in units of percentage. The essential data are in Table 1.

The average of the four percentages is 1.69. If we use the entire interval, 122 years, and the average population, $(3,000 + 313)/2$, or 1,656, we get an annual loss of 1.33%. However, it is highly probable that the loss was an exponential function of the population, and that to get the true value of the annual loss we should calculate the value of k in the equation:

$$p_t = p_o - kt,$$

where p_o is the beginning population, p_t is the population after time t in years, and k is the average annual loss in decimals, not in units of percentage. When we solve for the data from Martha's Vineyard, we get 0.0185 for k, that is 1.85%. The percentages obtained with the three methods by no means coincide precisely, yet the range, 1.33 to 1.85%, with the midpoint at 1.59%, can not be far from the actuality.

Table 1

Mean Annual Loss of Population on the Island of Martha's Vineyard between 1642 and 1764. See Text for Sources

Period	Reduction From	To	Number Persons Lost per Year	Persons Lost per Year as Percent of Average Population
1642-1674	3,000	1,500	47	2.09
1674-1698	1,500	1,000	21	1.68
1698-1720	1,000	800	9.1	1.01
1720-1764	800	313	11.1	1.98

The island of Nantucket contained two Indian groups, or tribes, which were not always friendly, but between whom there is no record of outright warfare. Macy (1792) says that in 1659 there were "near three thousand Indians on Nantucket." There certainly must have been 3,000 in 1620. In 1674, Rev. Thomas Mayhew made a count and found 300 families, or close to 1,500 souls. In 1698 Rev. Mr. Hawley reported a visitation to Nantucket by two other missionaries. They found five congregations with 500 adults. An adult was a person ten to twelve years or older. Perhaps half the total population was included. If so, the aggregate would have been approximately 1,000. Macy is very explicit that before the epidemic of 1763 there were 348 souls of Indian origin on Nantucket, and also that at the time of writing, 1792, there were just twenty. We can therefore estimate the percentage reduction per year for four periods, as was done with Martha's Vineyard. The results are in Table 2.

Table 2

Mean Annual Loss of Population on the Island of Nantucket 1659-1792. See Text for Sources

Period	Reduction From	To	Number Persons Lost per Year	Persons Lost per Year as Percent of Average Population
1659-1674	3,000	1,500	100.1	4.45
1674-1698	1,500	1,000	21	1.68
1698-1763	1,000	348	10.1	1.50
1763-1792	348	20	11.1	6.35

The average of the four periods is 3.50% of the population lost per year. However, this value is far too high and certain adjustments are required. In the first place, if 3,000 was close to the aboriginal population, and it could scarcely have been less, the date 1659 is too late. We would be quite justified in moving it back 30 years, to 1629. Then the first period is not 15, but 45 years in duration, and the mean annual reduction becomes 1.48%. In the second place, the fourth period includes the deadly epidemic of 1763, which reduced the number from 348 to 126 within six months. During the following 28 years the population fell from 126 to virtual extinction by 1792. These abnormalities created a very uncharacteristic decline, one which is probably best deleted completely from the record. If this period is omitted the three remaining percentages are 1.48, 1.68 and 1.50. The average is 1.55. If we use the entire interval, from 1629 to 1763, 134 years, the mean annual loss is 1.18. If we consider that the loss was exponential over the 134 years and apply the equation previously stated, the value is 1.61% of the existing population. The three methods yield a range of from 1.18 to 1.55%, with the midpoint near 1.45%.

If the mean annual loss was 1.59% of the population on Martha's Vineyard and 1.45% on Nantucket an overall value of 1.5% is acceptable. It must be remembered, however, that the error inherent in the data and in the modes of calculation is very considerable, at least plus or minus 20%. This means that the annual average loss of population under the conditions in existence was somewhere between 1.2 and 1.8%.

If a reduction of approximately 1.5% of the population per year is allowed for the two islands, the question arises concerning the transfer of this factor to the mainland. Such a transfer is probably possible because we have excluded from the island figures warfare and physical violence. These were at the vanishing point, together with the sudden effects of known serious epidemics. If, on the mainland, from the Hudson to the St. Croix, we likewise eliminate the effect of warfare and physical destruction, and leave out of consideration the epidemics of plague, small pox and "malignant fevers", the residue of attrition caused by chronic illnesses and their sequelae must be substantially the same throughout the entire region. There is certainly no evidence that health conditions among the Indians were materially different in Connecticut, on Cape Cod, or along the coast of Maine than they were on Martha's Vineyard or Nantucket.

It is possible now to formulate some sort of estimate of the degree to which the Indian population of New England and eastern New York was reduced by disease. We exclude as far as we can the casualties due to warfare both in battle and from exposure and famine resulting from military operations. The base figure is the aboriginal population, which, for want of a better value, we take from Mooney (1928) as 36,500. Since, with the exception of small settlements at Plymouth, Manhattan, and elsewhere, the contact with the whites was light prior to 1630, we take that year as the starting point for all diseases except the plague.

The only epidemics of great magnitude appear to have been the plague in 1616-1619 and small pox in 1633-1634. The effect of these was immediate and definitive. We have estimated 5,550 deaths from the first. For the second we add 700 in Rhode Island and 950 in Connecticut. The Massachusetts fatalities can not be evaluated. The total is, then, 7,200 which must be subtracted from the initial number. The remainder is 29,300, who were subjected to the attrition of chronic maladies and minor epidemics. The period of exposure is a matter of arbitrary selection. Purely as an example, let us take the year 1730. If we apply the exponential formula discussed previously, and set $-k$ equal to 1.5% loss per year, we have t equal to 100. The residual population in 1730 is 6,540 souls. This is no precise figure. It indicates merely that after the first century of European occupation, the introduced diseases would have shrunk the aboriginal population to somewhere near one fifth of its original strength.

ASSOCIATED FACTORS

The mortality which we attribute to endemic disease was in fact associated also with other factors. It is relatively easy to state the proximate cause of death: tuberculosis, dysentery, pneumonia, an occasional eruption of small pox. It is much more difficult to assess the ultimate causes, such as exposure to weather, malnutrition or outright starvation, bad sanitation, and an all-pervasive feeling of despair. Nevertheless, these forces operate powerfully to predispose a population to the onset of infection.

It should be emphasized that the aboriginal Indian was physically and culturally adjusted to his environment and that intertribal warfare was the only real obstacle to population increase, or at least maintenance. Under these circumstances even introduced epidemics would probably not have brought about more than temporary setbacks, had they not been accompanied by the invasion of European colonists. The white incursion produced bitter warfare which seriously depleted the native population, but this warfare itself was generated by a conflict of cultures which the Indian could not withstand.

In terms of subsistence economy alone, the struggle was mortal. The northeastern Indians utilized a great range of territory, including arable land for corn agriculture, forests for hunting, coasts for fishing and shellfish gathering. It was a type of variable land use which required complete freedom of movement over a large region. The Englishman and the Dutchman were sedentary. They required a small, permanent area for planting crops, pasturing live stock, and building towns. The two systems could not exist together. War provided the decision, in favor of the settlers. The Indian was forced to conform to the European pattern. This he could not do, physically or psychologically. Therefore, once the supremacy of the white was established by war, the red man was relegated to a position at the foot of the social scale, where he could not provide himself with adequate food, shelter and clothing. As a result he succumbed to every infection that came his way.

It is not necessary to describe in detail the social and moral plight of the New England Indian during the colonial period. But it is necessary to realize that the fraction of the population decline which was not

506 *Sherburne F. Cook*

caused by actual warfare, or by sudden epidemic catastrophes, was referable only in part to the pathogenic organisms so widely disseminated through the entire environment. Disease, therefore, which accounts for much more than half the gross reduction in numbers, acted essentially as the outlet through which many other factors found expression.

Received: 30 January, 1973.

Literature Cited

ADAMS, CHARLES FRANCIS 1903 Three Episodes of Massachusetts History. Reprint, 1965, Russell and Russell, New York.

ANONYMOUS 1634 Narrative of a Journey into the Mohawk and Oneida Country, 1634-1635. *In:* Narratives of New Netherland, 1609-1664. J. Franklin Jameson, (ed.), Scribner's Sons, New York, 1909, pages 135-162.

ANONYMOUS 1807 A Description of Duke's County. *In:* Massachusetts Historical Society, Collections, series 2, vol. 3, pages 38-94, 1815.

BENNET, NEHEMIAH 1794 Description of the Town of Middleborough, in the County of Plymouth. *In:* Massachusetts Historical Society, Collections, Series 1, vol. 3, pages 1-3.

BRADFORD, WILLIAM 1620-1647 History of Plymouth Plantation. Edition authorized by the Massachusetts Legislature, 1897. Wright and Potter Printing Co., Boston, 1901.

CHARLEVOIX, REV. P. F. X. DE 1743 History and General Description of New France. Translated by John Gilmary Shea. Francis A. Harper, New York, 1900. This published translation is in six volumes. The original work consisted of twenty books.

DENONVILLE, M. DE 1687 Letter to M. de Seigneley. *In:* Documents Relative to the Colonial History of the State of New York, Albany, 1855, Volume 9, page 354.

DRAKE, SAMUEL G. 1851 Biography and History of the Indians of North America, from its First Discovery. Eleventh edition, B. B. Mussey and Co., Boston, 720 pages.

—— 1867 The Old Indian Chronical. Samuel A. Drake, Boston. We use the introduction, entitled Origin of Indian Wars, pages 1-118 of the volume.

DUFFY, JOHN 1951 Smallpox and the Indians in the American Colonies. Bulletin of the History of Medicine, **25:** 324-341.

—— 1953 Epidemics in Colonial America. Louisiana State University Press, 274 pages.

ELIOT, JOHN 1651 Letter, Feb. 28, 1651. *In:* Massachusetts Historical Society, Collections, series 3, vol. 4, pages 165-168, 1834.

ELLIS, GEORGE W. and JOHN E. MORRIS 1906 King Philip's War. Grafton Press, New York.

FORCE, PETER 1838 Tracts and Other Papers, Relating Principally to the Origin, Settlement, and Progress of the Colonies of North America. Volume II. Washington, 1838. This volume contains several papers. Some of them are cited here under the individual names of the authors.

GOOKIN, DANIEL   1693   Historical Collections of the Indians of New England. *In:* Massachusetts Historical Society, Collections, series 1, vol. 1, pages 141-232, 1792.

GORGES, SIR FERDINANDO   1658   A Briefe Narration of the Original Undertakings . . . etc. *In:* Massachusetts Historical Society, Collections, Series 3, vol. 6, pages 45-94, 1837.

HAWLEY, REV. MR.   1698   Account of an Indian Visitation A.D. 1698, copied for Dr. Stiles, by Rev. Mr. Hawley, Missionary at Marshpee, from the Printed Account Published in 1698. *In:* Massachusetts Historical Society, Collections, series 1, vol. 10, pages 129-134, 1809.

HODGE, FREDERICK W., editor   1907-1910   Handbook of America Indians North of Mexico. Bureau of American Ethnology, Bulletin No. 30, 2 volumes, Washington, D.C.

HOYT, EPAPHRAS   1824   Antiquarian Researches: A History of the Indian Wars in the Country Bordering the Connecticut River. Greenfield, Mass.

HUBBARD, WILLIAM   1680   A General History of New England. Published by the Massachusetts Historical Society in its Collections, series 2, volumes 5 and 6, pages 1-676, 1815.

JOHNSON, EDWARD   1654   Wonder-Working Providence of Sions Saviour in New England. *In:* Massachusetts Historical Society, Collections, series 2, vol. 2, pages 49-96, 1819.

JOSSELYN, JOHN   1673   An Account of Two Voyages to New England. *In:* Massachusetts Historical Society, Collections, series 3, vol. 3, pages 211-354, 1883.

LESCARBOT, MARC   1612   L'Histoire de la Nouvelle France. Translated by W. L. Grant and H. P. Biggar under the title The History of New France. Published by the Champlain Society in its series, volume VII, Toronto, 1907-1914.

LINCOLN, GENERAL   1795   Observations on the Indians of North America . . . etc. *In:* Massachusetts Historical Society, Collections, series 1, vol. 5, pages 6-12.

MACY, ZACCHEUS   1792   A Short Journal of the First Settlement of the Island of Nantucket . . . etc. *In:* Massachusetts Historical Society, Collections, series 1, vol. 3, pages 155-160, 1810.

MAURAULT, JOSEPH A.   1866   Histoire des Abenakis, depuis 1606 jusqu'a nos jours. Printed by "Gazette de Sorel", Quebec.

MOONEY, JAMES   1928   The Aboriginal Population of America North of Mexico. Smithsonian Institution, Miscellaneous Publications, vol. 80, No. 7, pages 1-40.

MORSE, JEDEDIAH   1822   A Report to the Secretary of War of the United States, on Indian Affairs. . . . etc. S. Converse, New Haven.

MORTON, THOMAS   1632   New English Canaan. *In:* Peter Force, Tracts and Other Papers, Vol. II, No. 5.

MOURT   1622   Relation or Journal of a Plantation Settled at Plymouth in New England, and Proceedings Thereof. *In:* Massachusetts Historical Society, Collections, series 1, vol. 8, pages 203-239, 1802.

POTTER, ELISHA R. JR.   1835   The Early History of the Narragansett Country. *In:* Rhode Island Historical Society, Collections, vol. 3, pages 1-315.

RASIERES, ISAACK DE   1628   Letter to Samuel Blommaert. *In:* Narratives of New Netherland, 1609-1664. J. Franklin Jameson, editor. Scribner's Sons, New York, 1909, pages 97-115.

508   *Sherburne F. Cook*

RUTTENBER, EDWARD M.   1872   History of the Indian Tribes of Hudson's River. J. Munsell, Albany, 415 pages.

SHREWSBURY, J. F. D.   1949   The Yellow Plague. Journal of the History of Medicine, 4: 5-47.

SMITH, CAPT. JOHN   1622   New England's Trials. *In:* Peter Force, Tracts and Other Papers, vol. II, No. 2.

———   1631   Advertisements for the Inexperienced Planters of New England, or any where . . . etc. *In:* Massachusetts Historical Society, Collections, series 3, vol. 3, pages 1-53, 1833.

STEARN, E. WAGNER AND ALLEN E. STEARN   1945   The Effect of Smallpox on the Destiny of the Amerindian. Bruce Humphries, Inc., Boston, 153 pages.

WHITE, JOHN   1630   The Planters Plea. *In:* Peter Force, Tracts and Other Papers, vol. II, No. 3.

WILLIAMS, HERBERT U.   1909   The Epidemic of the Indians of New England, 1616-1620, with Remarks on Native American Infections. Johns Hopkins Hospital Bulletin, 20: 340-349.

WILLIAMS, ROGER   1643   A Key into the Language of America; or an Help to the Language of the Natives in that Part of America, called New England. *In:* Rhode Island Historical Society, Collections, vol. 1, 1827.

WILLIAMSON, WILLIAM D.   1839   The History of the State of Maine. 2 volumes. Hallowell, Maine.

WILLOUGHBY, CHARLES C.   1935   Antiquities of the New England Indians. Publication of the Peabody Museum of American Archaeology and Ethnology, Cambridge, Mass.

WINTHROP, JOHN   1630-1649   Winthrop's Journal, "History of New England". *In:* Original Narratives of Early American History, J. Franklin Jameson, editor, Barnes and Noble, New York, 1908.

12
Smallpox in Aboriginal Australia, 1829–1831

Judy Campbell

The epidemic of smallpox among Aborigines in eastern Australia between 1829 and 1831 was the second of three smallpox epidemics seen in Aboriginal Australia between 1788 and 1870.[1] The first was seen on the east coast at Port Jackson, Botany Bay, Broken Bay and on the Hawkesbury in 1789; the third occurred in the 1860s on the northwest coast, inland and in South Australia. There are inevitable gaps in the history of the epidemics which has received little attention since the pioneering studies of an earlier generation of eminent medical scholars, but surprisingly little ambiguity in the evidence: the epidemics were of smallpox and their effects were profound.[2]

Because the second epidemic in Aboriginal Australia occurred when colonial settlement was expanding in eastern Australia, there is more evidence of the presence of smallpox then than there is of its presence in 1789. It is possible to investigate the introduction of smallpox to Aboriginal populations at that time, its geographical incidence, and its spread among them. The mortality caused by smallpox during the second epidemic, its possible effects on the size of affected groups and their capacity to sustain their accustomed traditional life can be examined. The morale of survivors and their subsequent relations with colonists can also be explored.

Various diseases contributed to Aboriginal depopulation after 1788. Scholars refer to the inroads of acute infections such as measles, whooping cough and influenza among Aborigines as one result of European occupation,[3] but they do so without reference to their incidence, to their unexpected absence in the British population of the new colonies or to their transmission to Aborigines.[4] Among

[1] This article is part of an extended study of the second epidemic, and deals with smallpox north of the settled districts of NSW 1829-31. A subsequent article will deal wtih smallpox in the settled districts and to the south and southwest in 1831 and later. I am indebted to Professor F. Fenner, John Curtin School of Medical Resarch, ANU, for his generous assistance on medical questions.

[2] E.C. Stirling, 'Preliminary Report on the Discovery of Native Remains at Swanport, River Murray; With an Inquiry into the Alleged Occurrence of a Pandemic Among the Australian Aborigines', *Transactions and Proceedings of the Royal Society of South Australia*, vol. xxxv, 1911, esp. pp. 15-45; J.H.L. Cumpston, *The History of Smallpox in Australia, 1788-1908*, Commonwealth of Australia, Quarantine Service Publication No. 3, Melbourne 1914, esp. pp. 1-8, 147-182; Cumpston's reprinted historical sources remain useful, but he used edited versions of some documents now available; J.B. Cleland, 'Diseases Among the Australian Aborigines', *Journal of Tropical Medicine and Hygiene*, vol. xxxi, 1928, esp. pp. 54-55, 67-70. For a modern bibliography see P.M. Moodie and E.B. Pedersen, *The Health of Australian Aborigines: An Annotated Bibliography*, Commonwealth Department of Health, School of Public Health and Tropical Medicine Service Publication No. 8, Canberra 1971.

[3] E.g., D.E. Barwick, 'Changes in the Aboriginal Population of Victoria, 1863-1966', in D.J. Mulvaney and J. Golson (eds), *Aboriginal Man and Environment in Australia*, Canberra 1971, pp. 303-309; H. Reynolds, *The Other Side of the Frontier*, North Queensland 1981, p. 102.

[4] W.C. Wentworth, *A Statistical Historical and Political Description of the Colony*, London 1819, p. 44; P. Cunningham, *Two Years in New South Wales*, 2 vols, London 1827, vol. I, pp. 183-185; R. Dawson, *The Present State of Australia* (second ed.), London 1831, pp. 322-324. Buckley saw no European contagious disease between 1803 and 1835 on the Barwon in Victoria (J. Morgan, *Life and Adventure of William Buckley*, London 1967, p. 68.) See also J.H.L. Cumpston, *The History of Diptheria, Scarlet Fever, Measles and Whooping Cough in Australia 1788-1925*, Commonwealth of Australia, Dept. of Health Service Publication No. 37, Canberra 1927.

chronic infections seen among Aborigines and attributed to contact with Europeans, tuberculosis has been recognised as a significant lethal disease. Its history in Europe between the eighteenth and twentieth centuries suggests that emigrants to Australia normally included apparently healthy but infectious sufferers. It is probable that tuberculosis, which was not obvious among Aborigines when colonists first saw them, was transmitted during contact with Europeans. But, except in the records of Aboriginal settlements, the previous incidence of the disease is uncertain.[5] Syphilis was also ascribed to European contact by colonists who were unaware of the existence of two related Australian treponemal infections. These were common diseases in traditional Aboriginal society, were not usually lethal, and childhood infection protected against the sexually transmitted syphilis of European adults. Some scholars have accepted nineteenth-century misinterpretations of the relevant evidence and still assume that colonists were accurate in their descriptions of syphilis introduced by Europeans. The further confusion in historical records caused by the presence of other venereal diseases, old and new, has also been largely unnoticed.[6] One scholar has recently described syphilis and tuberculosis as the two major causes of death among Aborigines in New South Wales.[7] But smallpox was in fact the most lethal of acute infections and perhaps the most widespread of either acute or chronic new diseases during the century after 1788. It was also the most lethal of several new diseases that were not necessarily introduced by colonists, though it coincided with their presence and was well-known by them.[8]

The history of smallpox among Aborigines has been relatively neglected for 50 years for various reasons. There were and are statistical problems, as illustrated by the estimates by the anthropologist Radcliffe-Brown of the size of the original Aboriginal population. He suggested an estimate of between 250,000 and 300,000, still in use today as a safe though questionable minimum figure.[9] A contemporary of Cleland, Stirling and Cumpston, Radcliffe-Brown acknowledged only some of the available evidence of smallpox in his population estimates for Western Australia, South Australia, Victoria and Queensland. Nor did he refer to its presence in New South Wales, where the epidemics of 1789 and 1829-31 were widespread, well-known and much written about, or the Northern Territory where the evidence of several past epidemics was apparent until this century. Radcliffe-Brown did not even explain how he estimated mortality. The historical evidence suggests that it varied considerably. There were few survivors in some affected

---

[5] Barwick, *op.cit.*, esp. pp. 305, 308, 309; Reynolds, *op.cit.*; R. & J. Dubos, *The White Plague*, London 1953; P.M. Moodie, *Aboriginal Health*, Canberra 1973, pp. 142-151, esp. 1864-99 at Point McLeay and 1880-99 at Point Pearce, SA, p. 148.

[6] C.J. Hackett, 'A Critical Survey of Some References to Syphilis and Yaws among Australian Aborigines', *The Medical Journal of Australia*, vol. I, 1936, pp. 733-745; C.J. Hackett, 'Treponematoses (Yaws and Treponarid) in Exhumed Australian Aboriginal Bones', vol. 17, no. 27, 25 July 1978, pp. 387-405, Records, SA Museum; Moodie, *op.cit.*, pp. 165-168.

[7] L.R. Smith, *The Aboriginal Population of Australia*, Canberra 1980, pp. 93-94.

[8] Cf. leprosy, Moodie, *op.cit.*, pp. 151-154.

[9] A.R. Radcliffe-Brown, 'Former Numbers and Distribution of the Australian Aborigines', Official Yearbook of the Commonwealth, No. 3, 1930, pp. 687-696; cf. D.J. Mulvaney, *The Prehistory of Australia*, London 1969, p. 40, and Smith, *op.cit.*, pp. 68-77.

Judy Campbell

groups at Port Jackson in 1789, but sometimes in later epidemics the fatal impact of the accompanying economic and social crisis was mitigated by the prior exposure and experience of older people, and occasionally by the provision of food and shelter by settlers. It seems that Radcliffe-Brown was unable to determine the statistical effects of smallpox in his estimate. Birdsell, who referred in 1953 to one epidemic of smallpox and its possible importance for population studies, considered that 'the magnitude of its impact cannot now be estimated', a judgement which Radcliffe-Brown's arbitrary references to the disease anticipated.[10]

Changing attitudes towards Aborigines in this century have helped to limit modern interest in the smallpox epidemics. In the 1830s, after the second epidemic, references to smallpox among Aborigines coincided with the belief that their extinction was inevitable.[11] In the nineteenth century the smallpox experience seemed to be another example of 'a law of nature' which made it easy for coloured races to contract diseases from whites, but difficult for whites to contract diseases from coloured races.[12] At the end of the century a scientific paper suggested that the 'race tolerance' of whites, as well as vaccination, had protected them from smallpox in Australia.[13] But more recently the persistent image of Aborigines as 'a dying race' has been attributed to the need of some nineteenth-century colonists to mask the inhumanity of their relations with Aborigines.[14] Historical evidence of smallpox, which lent some substance to nineteenth-century opinion, was easily ignored by scholars who were both unfamiliar with the disease and sceptical of the motives of those who wrote the records. The freedom of most twentieth-century Australians from smallpox, its deaths and its scars, may be one reason for their ignorance of its history.

During the past 20 years Australian scholars have evinced a renewed interest in the role of diseases such as smallpox in the destruction of Aboriginal society. The resulting discussion has been in some instances accurate but brief and has referred only to evidence of limited or local significance. In other instances writers do not cite historical sources and the accounts of several are misleading.[15] In addition, the

[10] J.B. Birdsell, 'Some Environmental and Cultural Factors Influencing the Structure of Australian Aboriginal Populations', *American Naturalist*, vol. 87, 1953, p. 197.
[11] E.g., in the Aborigines' Protection Society pamphlet 'England and Her Colonies Considered in Relation to the Aborigines with a Proposal for Affording Them Medical Relief', London 1834(?).
[12] E.M. Curr, *The Australian Race*, 4 vols, Melbourne 1886, vol. I, pp. 221-224.
[13] F. Tidswell, 'A Brief Sketch of the History of Smallpox and Vaccination in New South Wales', *Australasian Association for the Advancement of Science*, vol. VII, Sydney 1898, p. 1060.
[14] See discussion by Reynolds, who considers that nineteenth-century argument about the importance of disease in the decline of the Aboriginal population contained 'an element of truth' (Reynolds, *op.cit.*, p. 103).
[15] E.C. Black, 'Population and Tribal Distribution', in B.C. Cotton (ed.), *Aboriginal Man in South and Central Australia*, part I, Adelaide 1966, pp. 101-102; Barwick, *op.cit.*, p. 307; Moodie, *op.cit.*, pp. 156-157; M. Kamien, 'The Aboriginal Australian Experience', in N.F. Stanley & R.A. Joske (eds), *Changing Disease Patterns and Human Behaviour*, London 1980, pp. 256-257; Reynolds, *op.cit.*, pp. 47, 72-73 and notes; C.D. Rowley, *A Matter of Justice*, Canberra 1978, p. 38; J. Wright, *The Cry for the Dead*, Melbourne 1981, pp. 23, 30, 38, 39, 171; E.G. Docker, *Simply Human Beings*, Brisbane 1964, pp. 51-52; A. Moorehead, *The Fatal Impact*, London 1966, pp. 145, 171; A.T.A. & A.M. Learmonth (eds), 'Smallpox', *Encyclopaedia of Australia*, London 1968; A.A. Abbie, *The Original Australians*, Sydney 1969, p. 92.

need for a reappraisal of the history of smallpox among Aborigines is obvious in the context of New World history. The usual neglect of epidemiology by historians has been remedied in recent years except in the case of Australia.[16] The impact of smallpox in the Americas is well-established.[17] McNeill considers that epidemics of lethal infections in general reduced populations in North America to as little as one twentieth of the pre-Columbian totals within 130 years of Cortes' arrival in Mexico. In Brazil, where smallpox in particular along with other diseases and causes reduced the Indian population catastrophically, estimates of the pre-conquest population of 1500 A.D. vary from well under 1,000,000 to almost 5,000,000, and the relative significance of various causes of depopulation is a matter of opinion only.[18] By comparison, the colonial evidence of smallpox among Aborigines is more amenable: it is as much as three centuries more recent than some American evidence, it covers a shorter period of time, fewer introductions of the disease, smaller populations and one smaller continent.

The historical evidence of smallpox can now be interpreted alongside the definitive findings of the Global Commission for the Certification of Smallpox Eradication, which resulted from the successful global eradication programme carried out between 1967 and 1979. Smallpox was caused by a virus known as smallpox or variola virus.[19] The effective transmission of the virus to a new susceptible host was followed by an incubation period which was usually 10 to 12 days long, but very rarely was as short as a week or as long as 17 days. During that time the victim was not infectious and was apparently well. At the end of the incubation period the pre-eruptive stage of the illness started abruptly, with fever, headache, muscular aching, prostration, and often nausea and vomiting. After 2 to 3 days the rash began to appear and the sufferer became infectious. The rash developed over about a week, changing from macules to vesicles to pustules. About a week later scabs formed and fell off within another week or 10 days everywhere except from the soles of the feet and the palms of the hands, where hardened skin prolonged the scabbing process. A case fatality rate between 25 per cent and 30 per cent was usual in unvaccinated persons where smallpox was endemic.[21] Pregnant women were severely affected and very often died.[22] In each Australian epidemic,

---

[16] W.H. McNeill, *Plagues and Peoples*, Oxford 1977; 'Migration Patterns and Infection in Traditional Societies', in Stanley and Joske, op.cit., pp. 27-36.

[17] E.W. Stearn & A.E. Stearn, *The Effect of Smallpox on the Destiny of the Amerindian*, Boston 1945; W.H. Oswalt, *This Land Was Theirs: A Study of the North American Indian* (second ed.), New York 1973; J. Duffy, 'Smallpox and the Indians in the American Colonies', *Bulletin of the History of Meidcine*, vol. 25, 1951, pp. 324-341; S.F. Cook, 'The Significance of Disease in the Extinction of the New England Indians', *Human Biology*, vol. 45, 1973, pp. 485-508.

[18] McNeill, 'Migration Patterns and Infection', p. 32; J. Hemming, *Red Gold*, London 1978, pp. 487-501, *passim*; cf. Smith, *op.cit.*, pp. 226-229 and N. Butlin, 'Close Encounters of the Worst Kind: Modelling Aboriginal Depopulation and Resource Competition 1788-1850', *Working Papers in Economic History*, Department of Economic History, ANU, no. 8, 1982.

[19] Variola and smallpox are synonyms. During the twentieth century, two varieties of smallpox were recognised, variola major, with case fatality rates in unvaccinated patients of 25-30 per cent, and variola minor, with case fatality rates of less than 2 per cent. Only variola major was konwn before 1890. (Personal communication, Frank Fenner, 5 July 1983).

[20] World Health Organisation, *The Global Eradication of Smallpox*, Geneva 1980, p. 19.

[21] *Ibid.*, pp. 68-69.

[22] A.R. Rao, *Smallpox*, Bombay, 1972, pp. 120-129.

Judy Campbell

accounts by eyewitnesses who saw sick Aborigines are consistent with the Commission's findings about sickness and mortality.

The retrospective diagnosis of smallpox during the eradication campaign was used by the Commission as one method of determining when smallpox last occurred in places where it had been endemic. The presence of five or more depressed facial scars greater than one millimetre in diameter was accepted by the Commission as being virtually diagnostic of a previous attack of smallpox. Experienced observers, including older people in formerly endemic areas, recognised smallpox easily and distinguished between the facial pockmarks of smallpox and other facial scarring. The faces of many victims showed heavy diffuse scarring that could be observed at a distance of five metres; lesser degrees of scarring could only be detected by close inspection. Among victims of severe smallpox, 85 per cent of unvaccinated survivors had 5 or more facial pockmarks; the pockmarks were permanent in about 70 per cent of those cases.[23] The past presence of smallpox was associated with blindness in some victims.[24]

After the second epidemic, colonists described pockmarks and blindness among Aboriginal survivors and referred to their accounts of past disaster. The only source of confusion in the records is the opinion of several contemporary medical men who did not see sick Aborigines and the hearsay of laymen that the disease seen in 1831 was chickenpox, or in colloquial terms 'native pock'.[25] Similar opinions, revived in 1962 by Dixon and in 1979 by Urry, are inconsistent with the reported presence of chickenpox as a mild disease among both white and black populations in the colony earlier in the nineteenth century;[26] more importantly, modern knowledge of smallpox establishes that descriptions of the same disease and its scars by other contemporary medical and lay observers were, as they said, descriptions of smallpox.[27] The Global Commission's successful use of facial

[23] World Health Organisation, *op.cit.*, pp. 19-20; F. Fenner, 'Smallpox and Its Eradication,' in Stanley and Joske, *op.cit.*, pp. 225-229.
[24] World Health Organisation, *op.cit.*, p. 16; Fenner, *op.cit.*, p. 229.
[25] E.g., J. Bowman, Medical Department, Sydney, to Colonial Secretary, 10 Oct. 1831; G. Busby, Bathurst, to the Inspector of Colonial Hospitals, Sydney, 19 Oct. 1831; Bowman to Col. Sec., 14 Nov. 1831, in A.O. ref. 4/2130, A.O. ref. 31/10001 with 32/34, Archives Office of NSW (hereafter referred to as A.O. 4/2130). See also D.J. Thomas, *Australian Medical Journal*, vol. x, 1865, pp. 78-80; *Australian Medical Journal*, 1846, p. 53, cited in Cumpston, *op.cit.*, p. 6; Aaron in 'Local Items', *NSW Medical Gazette*, vol. II, 1871-72, p. 352; T. Strode, *Argus*, 8 Feb. 1877; G.W. Rusden, *Argus*, 22, 24, 25 and 29 Jan. 1877.
[26] C.W. Dixon, *Smallpox*, London 1962, pp. 205-206; J. Urry, 'Beyond the Frontier', *Journal of Australian Studies*, no. 5, 1979, p. 7; cf. Mair to Col. Sec., 14 Feb. 1831, Bowman to Col. Sec., 10 Oct. 1831, A.O. 4/2130.
[27] J. Mair, Assist. Surgeon, 39th Regiment, to Col. Sec., 26 Sept. 1831; A.C. Imlay, Staff Assistant Surgeon, 39th Regiment, to Bowman, 5 Oct. 1831; Mair to Col. Sec., 10 Dec. 1831, with enclosure 'Observations on the Eruptive Febrile Disease which Prevailed among Several Tribes of the Aborigines in New South Wales During the Year 1830 and 31', pp. 1-26; Mair and Imlay to Col. Sec., 24 Dec. 1831, with enclosure; Capt. Smyth, Port Macquarie, to A. Hamilton, 20 Dec. 1831 (abstract), A.O. 4/2130; recent comment: 'I have not the slightest doubt that the disease described by Mair was smallpox ... there are so many features that are characteristic of smallpox and of no other disease' (F. Fenner, 21 April 1983). Sections of Mair's report, *op.cit.*, were edited and used by G. Bennett in his journal, *Wanderings in New South Wales ... During 1832, 1833 and 1834*, 2 vols, London 1834, and Facsimile, Adelaide 1967, vol. I, Chap. VIII; Extracts from Bennett, with additional note, in *NSW Medical Gazette*, vol. I, 1870-71, pp. 215-219, and in Cumpston, *op.cit.*, pp. 150-154.

pockmarks to diagnose smallpox retrospectively has implications for historical evidence about smallpox.[28] Not only do the Commission's conclusions clarify the interpretation of historical evidence, but it is now possible to trace the past incidence of smallpox through descriptions of pockmarks in historical sources. By comparison, the past presence of other introduced diseases such as measles and whooping-cough which left no traces on survivors cannot be identified beyond the settled districts or with any certainty there.

Knowledge of the infectivity of smallpox and how it was transmitted from person to person was similarly central to the work of the Commission during the eradication programme. The sufferer remained infectious during the illness, especially in the first week. Secretions from his oropharynx contaminated his face and body. Droplet infection during face to face contact, physical contact with the sick and with contaminated articles were frequent sources of infection. People who had close personal contact with the sick and their immediate surroundings were at great risk; so were people who handled corpses or cleansed them for burial. But without close physical contact, susceptible people usually escaped infection. Matter from ruptured pustules and from scabs contained virus, but was not a common source of infection.[29] The survival of the virus depended on person to person transmission among human hosts: there were no animal hosts, there were no long-term carriers and one attack usually conferred life-long immunity. Chains of person to person infection required a continuing supply of people who had not previously been exposed to smallpox. It has been estimated that the measles virus can persist indefinitely in populations of over 200,000; a similar situation existed with smallpox.[30]

Historically the infectivity of smallpox and its means of transmission had significance for the origin of the disease, its introduction to susceptible populations and its world-wide spread. Smallpox probably evolved in the ecology of the relatively dense agricultural populations of the last 10,000 years: it was first known among the inhabitants of Eurasia, in northeast Africa or India, where it became endemic.[31] In large populations exposure to infection usually occurred during childhood, and immunity was common among older people. Continuing chains of infection became normal in the large and relatively mobile populations of Eurasia and parts of Africa. Smallpox spread to islands and other continents only when infectious travellers from Europe, Africa or Asia arrived and had sufficiently close contact with local inhabitants to transmit infection. In populations of low immunity lacking prior experience of smallpox, its relatively low communicability and long incubation period, followed by a similarly long period when it was possible for infection to be transmitted in various ways, resulted in protracted epidemics.[32] In small populations, such as the populations of some

[28] 'Smallpox was unique in the ease of making retrospective diagnoses of its presence many years after an epidemic, because of facial pockmarks' (F. Fenner, 21 Jan. 1983).
[29] World Health Organisation, *op.cit.*, p. 22.
[30] F.L. Black, 'Modern Isolated Pre-Agricultural Populations', in Stanley and Joske, *op.cit.*, pp. 43-44; F. Fenner, 'Sociocultural Change and Environmental Disease', in Stanley and Joske, *op.cit.*, p. 15.
[31] Fenner, 'Smallpox and its Eradication', in Stanley & Joske, *op.cit.*, pp. 216-217; World Health Organisation, *op.cit.*, p. 16.
[32] *Ibid.*, p. 22.

542   *Judy Campbell*

islands or geographically remote areas, epidemics occurred rarely or often, depending on the frequency of close contact with infectious people from outside. After smallpox had run its course through the susceptible population, it died out and remained unknown until the next introduction gave rise to new chains of infection among a new generation of susceptible people.[33] When introductions were infrequent, perhaps only once or twice in the lifetimes of most people, the ages of pockmarked survivors and of those with no pockmarks were a guide to the date of the last epidemic.[34]

Smallpox had not evolved as a human infection before the human settlement of Australia, and Aborigines, like Amerindians, were free of smallpox until it was introduced by travellers from Africa and Eurasia in the sixteenth century in the Americas and probably later in Australia. The possibility that smallpox was introduced to Australia through outside contact before the eighteenth century cannot be dismissed, but it is improbable that the coincidences necessary for its transmission happened when small numbers of casual or accidental visitors from the north happened to arrive.[35] On the east coast there was no sign of smallpox, past or present, at Endeavour River in 1770 or at Port Jackson in 1788.[36] Its absence suggests that there had been no introductions of smallpox there or elsewhere during the lifetimes of Aborigines then living: subsequent history showed that the size and distribution of Aboriginal populations didn't prevent the spread of smallpox among them when it arrived. Observers' descriptions of 1789 show that local populations lacked immunity and that smallpox was new to them. In later epidemics it was still unknown to most, though by 1870 Aboriginal populations had been exposed, but patchily, to infection 3 times in 80 years during Asian or European contacts.

The introduction of smallpox to Aborigines in the late 1820s and the subsequent epidemic among Aboriginal populations was not caused by the European presence on the east coast. Although many ships reached Australia after infection with smallpox during voyages from Europe and Asia, both colonists and Aborigines were protected from introductions of smallpox by people on those ships after 1788. Sometimes infection that started in Europe died out during the long voyage before passengers disembarked; more importantly, as many vessels arrived more quickly from Asia or Africa, those arriving in colonial ports were quarantined if smallpox had occurred or was suspected on board.[37] And after Jenner's discovery in 1796, vaccination was used where possible to prevent and contain smallpox in the colonies. The earliest cases of smallpox among colonists were the few resulting from contact with infectious Aborigines in 1831. No other cases occurred among

---

[33] Cf. measles epidemics in small remote or island populations. D. Morley, 'Severe Measles', in Stanley and Joske, *op.cit.*, pp. 116-117.
[34] World Health Organisation, *op.cit.*, p. 54.
[35] Mulvaney, *op.cit.*, chap. 1.
[36] J. Hawkesworth, *An Account of the Voyages*, 3 vols, London 1773, vol. III, p. 230; J.C. Beaglehole (ed.) *The Endeavour Journal of Joseph Banks*, 2 vols, Sydney 1962, vol. II, p. 126; Letter and Journal of G.B. Worgan, 1788, typescript, p. 14, Mitchell Library; J. Hunter, *An Historical Journal of the Transactions at Port Jackson and Norfolk Island*, London 1793, p. 134.
[37] Cumpston, *op.cit.*, chaps X and XII.

colonists until 1857 when a small epidemic at Gisborne, Victoria followed the arrival of an infectious ship's passenger. One Aborigine contracted the disease. It was unusual for Aborigines to be infected in later outbreaks caused by infectious shipboard arrivals because their contact with new arrivals and infected colonists was so limited.[38]

But as Blainey suggested recently, a virus that entered Australia in the Gulf of Carpentaria might eventually have reached the Great Australian Bight through a network of Aboriginal connections. In 1911 Stirling speculated that smallpox seen among Aborigines at three different periods was Asian in origin and was introduced by 'Malay trepang fishers' who paid annual visits to the north coast. In 1967 Cleland similarly attributed the first and second epidemics of smallpox to 'Malays' in the north.[39] What is known of the circumstances of the introduction of the second epidemic and its spread supports these hypotheses.

Later in the century after Europeans had arrived in the Northern Territory and New Guinea, they realised that smallpox was sometimes introduced from Asia by infectious travellers on colonial, Asian and indigenous shipping. Colonial authorities in the Territory checked introductions from Chinese sources at Darwin: P.M. Wood, Colonial Surgeon and Protector 1885-89, undertook the mass vaccination of Aborigines there and infectious arrivals were quarantined. Quarantine was again used among pearlers at Broome in 1904.[40] Epidemics of smallpox in German New Guinea and New Britain in the 1890s illustrated the vulnerability of inexperienced populations of low immunity; local inhabitants were severely affected and the disease spread easily except where hostility between coastal and highland people, or vaccination by Wesleyan missionaries, broke the chains of infection.[41]

Before Europeans arrived in the Territory and in New Guinea there had been recent outbreaks of smallpox in both places that could only have resulted from the arrival of infectious people among indigenous traders from the archipelago when the disease was prevalent there. In the Territory, Foelsche saw pockmarked and blind survivors when he was sent to Darwin as sub-inspector of police in 1870; in New Guinea in 1871 the Russian scientist Mikloucho-Maclay saw survivors at Astrolabe Bay who said the disease had come from the northwest of the island.[42] The collection of items for trade linked Australia and New Guinea with Island

[38] *Ibid.*, chaps III-VI, esp. p. 27; 2 Aboriginal cases in the variola minor epidemic in NSW 1913-18; J.H.L. Cumpston and F. McCallum, *The History of Smallpox in Australia 1909-23*, Commonwealth of Australia Department of Health, Service Publication No. 29, Melbourne 1925, p. 49.
[39] G. Blainey, *Triumph of the Nomads*,Melbourne 1975, p. 103; Stirling, *op.cit.*, pp. 30-33; J.B. Cleland, 'Ecology Environment and Disease' in Cotton, *op.cit.*, pp. 155-156.
[40] C.E. Cook, 'Medicine and the Australian Aboriginal: A Century of Contact in the Northern Territory', *Medical Journal of Australia*, vol. I, 1966, pp. 561-562; Cumpston, *op.cit.*, pp. 70, 76, 79, 85, 86-87.
[41] P. Sack and D. Clark (eds), *German New Guinea, The Annual Reports*, Canberra 1979, pp. 81, 101; P. Sack and D. Clark (eds and trs), Albert Hahl, *Governor in New Guinea*, Canberra 1980, pp. 13-14.
[42] P. Foelsche, Inspector of Police, 'Notes on the Aborigines of North Australia', *Transactions and Proceedings of the Royal Society of South Australia*, vol. V, 1881-82, pp. 7-9; C.L. Sentinella (tr.), M.N. Mikloucho-Maclay, *New Guinea Diaries, 1871-1883*, Madang 1975, pp. 91, 179.

Judy Campbell

Southeast Asia, and indirectly with the endemic centres of smallpox in Asia. After living at Darwin for ten years, Foelsche associated smallpox among Aborigines in northern Australia with the visits of the trepang collectors from Macassar, whom he described as 'Malays' a term used loosely by his contemporaries and later by Stirling and Cleland. According to Foelsche, about 30 'Malay prahus' from Macassar visited the coast from Port Essington to Blue Mud Bay in the Gulf of Carpentaria every year from early January until late May. During that time,

they employ all the coast tribes trepanging for them, and they all live together; and I think there can be no doubt as to smallpox having been brought to these shores by them,

at earlier times 'and on the last occasion' in the 1860s.[43] For obvious reasons there is no contemporary evidence of the introduction of smallpox on the north coast in the 1780s, and except for Foelsche's account, little evidence about the origins of smallpox in northern and northwestern Australia in the 1860s. But for various reasons it is likely that Macassans transmitted smallpox to Aborigines in the 1820s.

Macassans came to collect trepang and other items. In the eighteenth century and perhaps slightly earlier trepang, or sea slugs, became a valuable commodity and its collectors frequent visitors to Australia.[44] The Chinese appetite for trepang stimulated its collection. Indigenous traders gathered sea slugs from remote parts of the archipelago and sold them to China. The Australian voyage was possible and profitable. By the second half of the nineteenth century, about a quarter of all trepang sold in China came from northern Australia. The port of Macassar in South Celebes was the centre for Australian trepang and its export: Macassar traded with Canton and Amoy.[45] Crewmen and praus from other islands were sometimes seen on the northern Australian coast, but those from Macassar were pre-eminent. They dominated the industry between the Cobourg Peninsula and the Wellesley Islands in the Gulf of Carpentaria during the nineteenth century when colonial observers were present.[46]

The sheer scale of the Macassan enterprise and the susceptibility of some crewmen to smallpox meant that the necessary coincidences of infectivity, monsoon and contact would probably happen in the course of their Australian visits. By the nineteenth century between 30 and 60 praus with about 30 men on each sailed to the Cobourg Peninsula and beyond each year: between 1,000 and 2,000 men collected trepang between the Peninsula and the Gulf.[47] And though most fishermen from densely populated islands such as modern Java where smallpox was endemic were immune, the immunity of Macassans was less predictable.[48] Some were immune through prior exposure: in 1803, on Flinders' voyage, Robert Brown described traces of smallpox on the faces of Pobassoo's

[43] Foelsche, *loc.cit.*; C.C. MacKnight, *The Voyage to Marege*, Melbourne 1976, pp. 1-2.
[44] *Ibid.*, pp. 42-47, 96-97.
[45] *Ibid.*, chap. I, esp. pp. 12-16.
[46] *Ibid.*, pp. 17, 18, 36.
[47] *Ibid.*, pp. 27-29.
[48] P. McDonald, 'An Historical Perpsective to Population Growth in Indonesia', in J.J. Fox (ed.), *Indonesia: Australian Perspectives*, vol. 1, Canberra 1980, p. 86.

crew.[49] Others were probably susceptible. Most were Macassarese or Bugis, but a few came from more remote islands such as Ceram or New Guinea. Aborigines too, who sometimes visited Macassar, travelled in the praus.[50] Some crewmen from Celebes itself might have been susceptible. In South Celebes the total poulation of the peninsula in the nineteenth century was 1,000,000 or less, and was mostly a static agricultural population that probably included pockets of both immunity and susceptibility. The towns were small; in 1838 the largest town was the port of Macassar, with a population of 23,575.[51] In such a small community smallpox was not endemic, but was introduced occasionally through outside contacts. In that setting some adults perhaps remained susceptible. But the most important fact is that many of the crews were young: boys as young as ten years old sailed and childhood susceptibility to infections made them unpredictable workers.[52]

The fleet left Macassar with the monsoon between late November and mid-January. If smallpox was prevalent in the archipelago when the wind blew to the southeast, susceptible crewmen apparently well but already incubating the virus if they had been exposed to it before departure would sicken, and become infectious on the voyage. On the praus, crowded quarters and close contact encouraged the spread of infection to other susceptible crewmen. The praus arrived on the Cobourg Peninsula during December and January, after voyages via Timor that took as little as 10 to 15 days, roughly the same time as the incubation period for smallpox. The protracted period of incubation and infectivity of smallpox meant that a succession of sick and infectious crewmen might be present for weeks or even months after the fleet's arrival in Australia. The praus did not leave for home until the wind changed in April and May.[53] And so, from December to May, some Aborigines had close personal contact with Macassans who set up camps on shore to process trepang. Sometimes local Aborigines met Macassans when they arrived on the Peninsula; they visited praus and camps; they helped to collect and process trepang; they talked and traded, ate and sometimes slept with Macassans. The cultural influence of Macassans, especially on Aboriginal language, was profound. Relations between Aborigines and Macassans, though unpredictable, were more often familiar than uneasy or distant. Day-to-day contact was intimate enough for the transmission of smallpox.[54]

The recollections of a Port Essington Aborigine, Jack Davis, suggest that smallpox was prevalent on the Cobourg Peninsula on one occasion well before the second epidemic. In about 1880 Davis, who was well known and respected by European visitors to the Peninsula, recalled that very old people had told him that when they were children, smallpox, which they called *meeha-meeha*, 'killed plenty blackfellows'. Davis was born around 1830. The childhood memories of his very

[49] C.C. Macknight, 'Macassans and Aborigines', *Oceania*, vol. XLII, 1972, p. 292.
[50] Macknight, *The Voyage*, pp. 17-18, 85-87.
[51] C.W.M. van der Velde, *Gezigten uit Neêrlands Indie*, Amsterdam 1844-45, republished Buijten & Schipperheyn 1979, p. 56. I am indebted to Dr Macknight, the Faculties, ANU for this information.
[52] Macknight, *The Voyage*, p. 29.
[53] *Ibid.*, pp. 24-25, 32-37; cf. incubation and infectivity of smallpox, above, pp. 9, 14.
[54] *Ibid.*, chaps 4, 6 and plates, *passim*; cf. above, pp. 14-16.

Judy Campbell

old people could well refer to the period when the inroads of smallpox among Aborigines were witnessed on the east coast by many of the First Fleet.[55] Observers who were occasionally present on the north coast after that time did not refer to smallpox among Aborigines. The shipwrecked lascar De Sois remarked on the absence of diseases among Aborigines on the east coast of Cape York Peninsula, where he lived with them for some years until 1827.[56] The British themselves were troubled by scurvy but suffered no epidemic or contagious disease at Raffles Bay.[57]

But while the British were at Raffles Bay in the trepang seasons of 1827-28 and 1828-29, their records showed unexplained deaths among Macassans. The evidence suggests a severe infection among susceptible crewmen. Of acute infections, smallpox was the most likely to be associated with severe mortality. On 21 February 1828, Captain Smyth of Fort Wellington, Raffles Bay, interviewed Daeng Riolo, the captain of a Macassan prau, through an interpreter. Daeng Riolo had left Macassar, with 41 other praus, on 22 December 1827: the complement of his prau was 14, 3 of whom died after leaving Macassar.[58] There is no record of other crews that season, nor of causes of death on Daeng Riolo's prau. A fuller record of praus at Raffles Bay the following season, the single surviving document of its kind, suggests that the deaths among Daeng Riolo's crew were not unusual.[59] In 1828-29, 1046 men left Macassar on 34 praus. By June, 1005 men had returned to Macassar. During voyages lasting between 3 and 6 months, 41 men died, nearly 4 per cent of those who sailed. In 36 cases, causes of death were unspecified: the record states only that the men 'died on the passage'. The distribution of these deaths between praus was uneven: there were no unspecified deaths on the passage on 16 of the 34 praus, 18 recorded deaths, and on 13 of these praus between 5 and 10 per cent of the crews 'died on the passage'. There were twice as many deaths among Macassans that year than was usual on convict ships sailing from Britain to Australia at that time.[60]

In 1829, two medical officers at Raffles Bay saw unmistakable evidence of recent smallpox among Aborigines. Davis of the 39th Regiment described deep circular impressions in particular on the faces of several people, 'as if caused by the small-

---

[55] Foelsche, *op.cit.*, p. 8; Macknight, *op.cit.*, p. 101. That smallpox introduced on the north coast in the late eighteenth century had spread to the east coast by 1789 is a more feasible explanatin of the origins of the first epidemic than that 'variolous matter in bottles' brought out by the First Fleet surgeons was responsible; for W. Tench's description, see L.F. Fitzhardinge (ed.), *Sydney's First Four Years*, Sydney 1961, p. 146. Before Jenner's discovery of vaccination, variolous matter, or virus taken from the pustules of sufferers, was used for the deliberate inoculation, or variolation, of susceptibles to induce immunity by a less severe infection. The practice was widespread in England by the 1780s and was most frequently used when smallpox threatened (World Health Organisation *op.cit.*, p. 17); P. Razzell, *The Conquest of Smallpox*, Sussex 1977, chaps 4 and 5. It was to be expected that First Fleet surgeons were equipped with variolous matter; its hypothetical theft and misuse early in 1789 by whites or blacks, without the knowledge of Governor Phillip, John White or his colleagues is possible, but unlikely.

[56] E.g., P.P. King, *Narrative of a Survey of the Intertropical and Western Coasts of Australia*, 2 vols, London 1827; T.B. Wilson, *Narrative of a Voyage Round the World*, London 1855, pp. 143-145.

[57] *Ibid.*, pp. 149, 151, 157.

[58] Capt. Smyth to Col. Sec. Macleay, 20 March 1828, Historical Records of Australia, series III, vol. VI. p. 790.

[59] Macknight, *The Voyage*, pp. 129-132.

[60] Wilson, *op.cit.*, p. 334.

pox'. Braidwood Wilson also recorded his own observations:

The natives described, in language, or rather, by signs sufficiently significant, the history of the malady, which they called *oie-boie*, and which appears to be very prevalent among them. It evidently bears a resemblance, both in its symptoms and consequences, to smallpox, being an eruptive disease, attended with fever, and leaving depressions. It frequently destroys the eyes, and I observed more than one native who had thus suffered. Mimaloo's left eye was destroyed by this disease.[61]

The colonists had not seen active cases of smallpox; the 60 or so Raffles Bay Aborigines had kept away from the settlement during 1828.[62] The British heard that their relations with 'the Malays' were particularly hostile during the year.[63] By contrast and despite the spearing and shooting in 1827, from the end of 1828 British and Aborigines enjoyed cordial, frequent and familiar contact until the settlement was abandoned in August 1829. Local people came into the settlement and slept in a tent pitched for them by Captain Barker; the rapprochement was reminiscent of the changed relations that followed smallpox at Port Jackson in 1789.[64] Later, at Port Essington in 1838, when soldiers gave the young Jack Davis his English name, Captain Bremer confirmed that smallpox was known to Aborigines there.[65]

The Raffles Bay people were one group of Aborigines who had contracted smallpox by the late 1820s. When smallpox was active in the archipelago, opportunities for its transmission probably extended over several years and to various parts of the long northern coastline. There were perhaps enough contacts between infectious visitors and susceptible Aborigines to start more than one chain of infection. Within Australia in the late 1820s and the early 1830s, various chains of infection reached the east coast, the Murray-Darling Basin and the south coast. Fragmentary evidence of smallpox has survived from south and east of the Gulf of Carpentaria, through the hot and often dry country beyond districts that were explored or settled at the time of the sickness. The past presence of smallpox was observed where watercourses and rainfall allowed human settlement; where Aboriginal populations were relatively dense and survivors were seen for up to 50 years, and where colonists eventually attempted to use the land and wrote about its pockmarked people.

Near the Gulf of Carpentaria, pockmarked Aborigines were seen in the 1860s when colonists settled the Cloncurry River about 100 miles south of the Gulf in

[61] *Ibid.*, p. 170; cf. pockmarks and blindness, above, p. 11.
[62] Smyth to Col. Sec., 17 July 1827, HRA, series III, vol. VI, p. 772; *ibid.*, Smyth to Col. Sec., 30 Oct. 1827, pp. 776-777; *ibid.*, Smyth to Col. Sec., 12 Feb. 1828, pp. 781-789; *ibid.*, Lieut. Sleeman to Col. Sec., 4 June 1828, pp. 798-799; *ibid.*, Sleeman to Col. Sec., 4 Sept. 1828, pp. 816-817; *ibid.*, Capt. Barker to Col. Sec., 21 Sept. 1828, p. 819; *ibid.*, Smyth to Col. Sec., 20 March, 1828, p. 790.
[63] Wilson, *op.cit.*, pp. 149, 155.
[64] Barker to Col. Sec., 26 Feb. 1829, *HRA* series III, vol. VI, pp. 826-828; *ibid.*, Barker to Col. Sec., 22 Aug. 1829, p. 837. Cf. events at Port Jackson, described by W.E.H. Stanner, *After the Dreaming*, ABC, Sydney 1969, p. 9.
[65] Bremer to Beaufort, 7 Dec. 1838, cited in F.J. Allen, *Archaeology, and the History of Port Essington*, Ph.D. Thesis, ANU 1969, vol. I, p. 399.

Queensland. Edward Palmer, an early settler, informed Curr that when he first knew the Miappe tribe, some were lightly pitted with smallpox and a few survivors were still alive in the 1880s. Other causes resulted in further catastrophic depopulation.[66] In the eastern coastal ranges smallpox was described among the Breeaba tribe at the headwaters of the Burdekin River some 300 miles east of the Cloncurry and about 100 miles inland from Townsville. An Aboriginal woman, Wonduri, told a local Warden of Goldfields that smallpox, *chin-chin*, proved fatal to many at some recent period. According to Wonduri, the tribe decided at the time of the scourge that anyone it attacked should be killed without delay whilst asleep, and this plan was carried out.[67] North of the Burdekin, Curr found no evidence of the past presence of smallpox on the east coast; similar negative evidence suggested that there was no trace of smallpox for 300 miles south of the Burdekin on the east coast.[68]

About 300 miles southeast of the Cloncurry, colonists moved into the Torraburri tribe's territory on the upper Barcoo River and its tributary the Ravensbourne Creek by 1862. In the 1880s, a local trooper of the Native Mounted Police knew 4 or 5 pock-marked Aborigines about 50 years old who had suffered from smallpox, *weeteen*, before he was born.[69] By the 1860s, colonists occupied country further east over the coastal range towards Rockhampton. Some 200 miles east of the Barcoo, and 100 miles west of Rockhampton, at the head of the Comet River, was a cave full of bones, the remains of people who died 40 years earlier according to Curr's Aboriginal informant. Pockmarks were still to be seen on local people.[70] Another account of deaths and pockmarks came from the upper Dawson River 100 miles southwest of Rockhampton.[71]

Near Rockhampton among the Byellee tribe on the Calliope River, at Keppel Bay and on Curtis Island, an early settler recalled seeing pockmarks when colonists arrived in 1855: he said many had died of smallpox, called *wanboy*. There were about 300 people in the tribe then; 32 remained in 1882. South of Rockhampton, smallpox was present before colonial settlement in the 1850s on the rivers of the coastal range, the Burnett and the Boyne. In the 1870s, the Brisbane Commissioner of Police informed Curr that many of the Boyne River Toolooa tribe over 40 years old were pockmarked as a result of smallpox, *deeum*, said to have reached them

[66] Curr, *op.cit.*, vol. II, pp. 330-334. In the course of his enquiries, Curr collected extensive evidence of the past presence, or absence, of smallpox among Aborigines from his informants. They appear to have based their observations on the presence or absence of pockmarks among local people; most Europeans were familiar with the disease in the nineteenth century. For an example of Curr's questions about Aborigines and the answers of one informant, see his correspondence with G.N. Teulon, vol. II, p. 186 ff. Cf. above, p. 11, and note 28 above. Curr's informants' evidence about the past presence of smallpox is acceptable (see *p. 13* above). But his interpretation of the introduction and spread of smallpox before 1845 (vol. I, p. 226), is not easily reconciled with epidemiological data (see pp. *14-17* above), or with the history of 1789 (c.f. note 55 above).
[67] Curr, *op.cit.*, vol. II, p. 432.
[68] *Ibid.*, pp. 389, 394, 400, 402-403, 424-425, 465, 474, 486; *ibid.*, vol. III, p. 91.
[69] *Ibid.*, pp. 78-79.
[70] *Ibid.*, p. 97.
[71] 'W.', *Argus*, 25 Jan. 1877.

about 1835 when the Burnett tribes visited them. Survivors were unable to bury the many dead. East of those rivers the disease reached Many Peaks Range and the coast; over 60 miles north of Bundaberg at Bustard Bay and Rodd's Bay it was known as *tingal*. South of Bundaberg the evidence was similar. Perhaps from the coast, or from the ranges to the west, smallpox spread to the headwaters of the Mary River and the Bunya Bunya country. Offshore near the mouth of the Mary, on Fraser Island which was occupied in 1849, there were 2,000 Aborigines in the 1870s; smallpox was known by a number of distinct names among them.[72]

The information Curr received from far west Queensland was negative: no signs of smallpox were observed on the Georgina or the lower Diamentina Rivers, or at the junction of the Thomson and the Barcoo.[73] Nor were pockmarks seen in the northwest corner of New South Wales.[74] But the Barcoo and the Ravensbourne, where pockmarks were seen, rise in the Warrego Range in Central Queensland; and on other rivers that rise there and flow south to the Darling and Barwon, some pockmarked survivors were seen and memories of smallpox persisted throughout the century. To the west, on the lower reaches of the Paroo, the colonists moved in about 1860. According to Curr's informant, G. Scrivener, 'there are undoubted signs of smallpox having visited this tribe about 30 years ago, and ... is said to have half exterminated it'.[75] That had happened before the tribe dwindled for other reasons. Further east on the Maranoa, in the country near Roma, several Aborigines pitted with smallpox were seen late in the century.[76] South of the Maranoa, on the Narran as it flowed towards the Barwon, the Euahlayi people still spoke of smallpox at the end of the nineteenth century. According to their white historian, there were ghastly traditions of the time when *dunnerh-dunnerh*, the smallpox, decimated their ancestors. Terror-stricken tribesmen did not stay to bury their dead, and 'flying even from the dying, a curse was laid on them, that some day the plague would return, brought back by the Wundah or white devils'.[77]

North of the settled districts in 1829, colonists saw active cases of smallpox among Aborigines for the first time since 1789. In February 1829 Sturt and his party, including Hamilton Hume, travelled west from the Macquarie River to the Darling. Here they met diseased and distressed Aborigines. A melancholy old man tried to explain the afflication: 'a violent cutaneous disease raged through the tribe, that was sweeping them off in great numbers'. He showed the explorers several young men who had been ill:

Nothing could exceed the anxiety of his explanations, or the mild and soothing tone in which he addressed his people, and it really pained me that I could not assist him in his distress.[78]

---

[72] Curr, *op.cit.*, vol. III, pp. 114, 121-122, 126, 152, 144-145.
[73] *Ibid.*, vol. II, pp. 366, 371, 374.
[74] *Ibid.*, p. 159.
[75] *Ibid.*, p. 182.
[76] *Ibid.*, vol. III, p. 252.
[77] K. L. Parker, *The Euahlayi Tribe*, London 1905, p. 39.
[78] C. Sturt, *Two Expeditions into the Interior of Southern Australia During the Years 1828, 1829, 1830 and 1831*, 2 vols., London 1833, and Facsimile, Adelaide 1965, vol. I, p. 93.

Further upstream, about 70 Aborigines visited the explorers' camp; Sturt wrote that:

Several of them carried firesticks under the influence of the disease I have already noticed, while others were remarked to have violent cutaneous eruptions all over the body. ... They appeared to be strangers who had come from a distance.

He also thought that the Darling population had been thinned.[79] Hamilton Hume agreed that when they arrived at the Darling, Aborigines were suffering severely from 'this eruptive malady': numbers had died, and many more were still dying.[80] Returning soon after, past the Castlereagh, Sturt remarked that 'the natives were dying fast, not from any disease, but from the scarcity of food'; he blamed the drought. On the Macquarie, approaching the Wellington Valley in April, Sturt saw people who were 'actually starving, and brought their children to us to implore something to eat'.[81]

Sturt's observations were substantiated when six years later Mitchell saw pockmarked people on the Darling. They remembered Sturt. Near Fort Bourke in May 1835, Mitchell met 12 men, women and children, most of whom were pockmarked. Mitchell thought these people were the remains of a tribe, and that smallpox had almost depopulated the Darling. Further downstream the explorers met a group of 17 men: almost all were pockmarked. Lower on the river people deeply marked by smallpox were seen. A party of children and adults was encountered, and these people:

as well as most others seen by us on the river, bore strong marks of the smallpox, or some such disease, which appeared to have been very destructive among them.

Mitchell described deep scars and grooves prominent on the noses of these people. Dr Souter, a convict member of the expedition, called this confluent smallpox. On the same stretch of the river, Mitchell described deserted huts, and what he beleived to be three large tombs which covered 'the remains of that portion of the tribe, swept off, by the fell disease, which had left such marks on all who survived'.[82] Nearly 50 years later it was said that the pockmarked survivors of *mungga* were still to be seen in the Bourke district, and that many Aborigines believed that the white man introduced it.[83]

The year after Sturt's expedition to the Darling, Andrew Brown, a Wallerowang settler, travelled through some of the same country. On the Castlereagh in August 1930, he saw five Aborigines sick with smallpox. He later saw one of these men, pitted with smallpox, and ascertained that the other four had died. Six months earlier, Brown had heard that the disease was prevalent to the north. He also visited

---

[79] *Ibid.*, p. 105.

[80] Later consultations between Hume, the visitor Dr George Bennett and Dr Mair, Assistant Surgeon 39th Regiment, established that the disease on the Darling, like the disease seen among Aborigines in the Bathurst district and officially investigated by Mair in 1831, was indeed smallpox (Bennett, *op.cit.*, vol. I, p. 153, and note 27 above).

[81] Sturt, *op.cit.*, vol. I, pp. 137, 149-150.

[82] T.L. Mitchell, 'Second Expedition to the River Darling in 1835'. *Three Expeditions into the Interior of Eastern Australia* (second edition), 2 vols, London 1839, vol. I, pp. 218, 240-241, 257, 261-263, 307.

[83] Curr, *op.cit.*, vol. II, p. 194.

the Wellington Valley where the disease broke out between October and December 1830. Mair, who interviewed Brown, wrote that 'The poor creatures blamed Captain Sturt for its introduction, were much alarmed about it, and ... anticipated some grievous calamity ... which would ... destroy them', as one of their sages predicted.[84]

During that time of exploration north of the settled districts, an escaped convict was living among the Kamilaroi on the Namoi, about 100 miles southeast of the Darling. George Clark alias the Barber was recaptured in October 1831 and interviewed at Bathurst Jail by Mair. In 1825 after 6 months in Australia the 19 year old convict escaped from assigned service and joined Aborigines north of the Liverpool Range. By 1831 he looked Aboriginal, stained his skin, used ochre and clay markings, had cicatrices and a possum skin cloak. He spoke Aboriginal dialect and was accompanied by Aboriginal women. He saw smallpox, called *boulol*, among the Kamilaroi in October 1830, not long after Brown saw the sickness. Clarke spoke of a traditional healer, a *kradjee*, who was present.[85]

After interviewing Clarke and others, Mair described the sickness in terms characteristic of smallpox, referring to pre-eruptive symptoms and to eruptions that commenced on the face and particularly affected the head, breast and extremities, including the soles of the feet which were numerously studded with lesions; the tongue and lips were also involved. The illness lasted two or three weeks. The eyesight of some was affected, some had ulcers and abscesses and were debilitated and emaciated. Survivors could not walk for a long time owing to the tenderness of their feet from which the cuticle had entirely separated. Death came early in severe cases, at the onset of sickness before any eruptions occurred. The disease was chiefly fatal to adults and old people, seldom to children. Except for those with old pockmarks, few were exempt. Mair reported the case fatality rate seen by Clarke as one in six, a more conservative estimate than estimates by other colonists, and not easily reconciled with Clarke's other information. The Namoi *kradjee* had 'treated' five victims by immersion in cold water: four of them died. He then tried other remedies:

scorching the hair from the head and pricking the pustules with a sharp pointed fish bone, then squeezing out the fluid contained in them with the flat part of the instrument:

only one of six of these victims died. According to Clarke the infectivity of the disease was recognised: they 'sometimes bury alive those whom he [the *kradjee*] has abandoned — they believe the disease to be infectious but do not shun one another on that account'. Clarke described particularly severe illness among tribes to the northwest of the Liverpool Plains: symptoms were extreme, and fluid discharged with difficulty from the mouth appeared bloody. Mair recognised confluent smallpox in Clarke's account.[86]

Sick Aborigines were seen by Mitchell when, in search of the Kindur, he explored the upper Hunter River in December 1831. Just over the summit of the Liverpool

[84] Mair, *op.cit.*, pp. 2-4.
[85] D. Boyce, *Clarke of the Kindur*, Melbourne 1970, esp. chaps 4 and 5; Mair, *op.cit.*, pp. 4-7.
[86] Mair, *op.cit.*, pp. 5-11; footnote p. 24; cf. above pp. 9-11 and note 27.

Range, the source of the Namoi and the Hunter, which then divided the colony from the unexplored country, Mitchell's party camped

beside the natives from Dart Brook, who had crossed the range before us, apparently to join some of their tribe, who lay at this place extremely ill, being affected with a virulent kind of smallpox. We found the helpless creatures, stretched on their backs, beside the water, under the shade of the wattle or mimosa trees, to avoid the intense heat of the sun. We gave them from our stock some medicine; and the wretched sufferers seemed to place the utmost confidence in its efficacy ... I found that this distressed tribe were also "strangers in the land", to which they had resorted. Their meekness, as aliens, and their utter ignorance of the country they were in, were very unusual in natives, and excited our sympathy.[87]

Exploring the country between the Liverpool Plains and the Hunter in about 1832, Breton heard of 'Corborn Comleroy' and 'frequently observed the skin [of Aborigines] much scarred and also raised in blisters or vesicles.'[88]

Reece has suggested that attacks on surveying parties on the Gwydir described by Mitchell in 1832 were motivated by the desire for rations. That situation was not unlike what Sturt saw in the wake of smallpox. On the Liverpool Plains, it was followed by the prolonged and bitter conflict of the 1830s, when rapid pastoral expansion caused the loss of traditional Aboriginal lands.[89] Estimates of the affected Kamilaroi population are obscure, firstly because early observations such as Mitchell's of the size of local groups before confrontation were made when the second smallpox epidemic was prevalent.[90] It is not clear whether the groups described had avoided smallpox, or whether they were depleted groups which had amalgamated to maintain traditional life. The anomalies of population estimates of the 1840s reflect the inroads of smallpox as well as the movements of seasonal migrations and the impact of colonists.[91] The history of the area was complex. But traces of smallpox were still to be seen 20 years or more after the second epidemic. When Frank Bucknell first met some Kamilaroi in 1853, he saw several pockmarked people who called the disease *booert*. It was said to have cut off many about 1830.[92]

An explanation of the presence of smallpox beyond colonial settlement was given by George Clarke who stated that 'The disease proceeded from the North West coast, and spared none of the tribes as far as Liverpool plains, attacking 20 and 30 at a time — none escaping its fury'. Clarke told his captors that at different times he had lived with eight or nine 'tribes', had travelled some hundreds of miles through the northern parts of the colony towards the coast, and had met coastal Aborigines who told him of strangers who came across the sea from the north in praus to collect scented wood and sea slugs. He told Mair that the Namoi *kradjee* 'had previously been with a tribe situated near the Sea, and it is probable may have seen the disease before, although he disclaimed any but *supernatural* knowledge of

[87] Mitchell, *op.cit.*, vol. I, pp. 25-26.
[88] Lieut. Breton, *Excursions in New South Wales, Western Australia and Van Dieman's Land During the Years 1830, 1831, 1832 and 1833* (second ed.), London 1834, cited in P.A. Conlon, *The Other Side of the Mountains*, M.A. Honors Thesis, Sydney University 1973, pp. 91, 187.
[89] R.H.W. Reece, *Aborigines and Colonists*, Sydney 1974, pp. 25, 28-52.
[90] Boyce, *op.cit.*, p. 45.
[91] I. McBryde, *Aboriginal Prehistory in New England*, Sydney 1974, pp. 6-10.
[92] Curr, *op.cit.*, vol. III, p. 305.

it'.[93] Clarke's descriptions of the interior were received in the colony with scepticism: he spoke of a great river, the Kindur, which Mitchell was never able to find.[94] But Mair saw no reason to disbelieve Clarke's account of smallpox, and his own enquiries in the settled districts complemented Clarke's description of a spread from the northwest. Mair concluded that the disease had been 'communicated by contagion from the inhabitants of some other country ... or ... if the disease originated in this continent it most probably arose in a very distant part of it'.[95] Those who disbelieved Clarke's claims were probably equally sceptical of other curious reports by colonial visitors. Peron, at Sydney in 1802, wrote that Aborigines there asserted that on the other side of the Blue Mountains 'there is an immense lake, on the banks of which live white people, like the English, who dress in the same manner, and have large towns, with houses built of stones'. Peron himself doubted the existence of 'this sort of Caspian Sea'.[96] Inland 30 years later, Breton was told by Aborigines west and northwest of Wellington Valley about an inland sea with salty water and whales; the inland Aborigines imitated whales spouting water, which Breton thought they could only have done from observation.[97]

Later reports of the past presence of smallpox in Queensland, its recognisable recent presence at Raffles Bay in 1829, and its appearance on the upper Darling early that year are consistent with Clarke's account of its spread from the northwest coast. But as smallpox travelled towards the settled districts of New South Wales, the spread of infection was mostly unobserved by colonists until 1831, when chains of infection extended east and south down the coast as well as west and south into the Murray-Darling Basin. The reasons why the disease spread within traditional society, beyond the observation of colonists, are necessarily speculative. That it spread at all is contrary to an older interpretation of disease in Aboriginal society.[98] It was thought that the small and scattered population was protected from the introduction of infectious diseases by 'Malay traders' or early British settlers by both their 'lonely wandering existence' and a quarantine barrier imposed by respect for tribal boundaries.[99] As Blainey suggested recently, acute infections, for instance arboviruses transmitted by mosquitoes from other animals, were not unknown: Australian encephalitis (Murray Valley encephalitis) might have occasionally given rise to sudden unexpected deaths in particular localities.[1] But the slower pace of transmission and spread of chronic infections which did not kill their victims was probably typical of diseases experienced among nomads. Local groups have been described as the really effective social units, and usually the

---

[93] Mair. *op.cit.*, pp. 4-5; Boyce. *op.cit.*, pp. 36-37.
[94] Boyce, *op.cit.*, chaps 1, 6, 7; D.W.A. Baker, 'Mitchell, Sir Thomas Livingstone'. *ADB*, vol. 2. pp. 238-242.
[95] Mair. *op.cit.*, p. 14.
[96] M.F. Peron, *A Voyage of Discovery to the Southern Hemisphere ... During the Years 1801, 1802, 1803 and 1804* (translated from the French). London 1809. pp. 290-291.
[97] Breton. *op.cit.*, p. 139.
[98] Blainey, *op.cit.*, pp. 102-104; notes pp. 264-265 for older anthropological view.
[99] Cook. *op.cit.*, p. 560.
[1] Blainey, *op.cit.*, pp. 104-105, N.F. Stanley, 'Man's Role in Changing Patterns of Arbovirus Infections', in Stanley and Joske, *op.cit.*, esp. pp. 164-171.

effective political and economic units as well.[2] Such groups sometimes had reasons for close contact with other local groups. Through those groups and so through the wider organisation of traditional society, goods and rituals were exchanged to an extent not recognised until recently.[3] Those occasions of economic and spiritual life were sufficient to maintain yaws and treponarid, the two chronic treponemal infections which have a long history in Australia.[4]

Aboriginal encounters with smallpox, which evolved as a human infection elsewhere in the world, differed from previous Aboriginal encounters with any known Australian infections. Experiences of smallpox among Aborigines also differed from modern experience of the disease in that the relatively low communicability of the virus apparent during the eradication campaign was offset in Aboriginal Australia by conditions that did not apply in most modern countries. The uniformly low immunity of Aborigines and their lack of experience of smallpox meant that it spread within and between groups more easily in parts of Aboriginal Australia than in most modern communities; and it spread in more spectacular fashion than accustomed chronic infections had done. In some groups the lack of immunity and experience, still significant in the second epidemic, was slightly modified by prior exposure to infection. Pockmarked people over 40 were immune, and the spread of the disease might have been limited by some recognition of its infectivity; there was some such knowledge on the Namoi, and the radical action described by Wonduri implied similar knowldge. Nevertheless, when smallpox was introduced to a local group, its high incidence among them during the second epidemic was obvious. Among nomads, the usual daily activities of food-getting, eating, sleeping, sheltering and caring for children, which all entailed physical contact, made opportunities for infection. Those opportunities were possibly even greater among nomads than in the nucleated villages of early agrarian society or in pastoral hamlets. The high incidence of disease within local groups and the easy transmission of infection among susceptible nomads made it likely that any contact between affected groups and others would spread infection.

Death and its associated rituals were normally occasions of contact between groups. Within the deceased's group, the bereaved embraced the dying person and attended to his corpse. They then left the camp where the death had occurred. The movement of people associated with the death was not confined to the immediate family of the deceased; messengers were sent with news of imminent death to summon kinsmen, and later took the deceased's possessions to distant kinsfolk. The bereaved delegated the necessary tasks to appropriate kinsfolk: the corpse was prepared for disposal according to local rites. Inquests into the cause of death, perhaps sorcery, which might involve examination of the corpse, were held and retribution for the death was occasionally pursued.[5] The smallpox epidemics would have set in motion the traditional network of connections between groups.

[2] R.M. Berndt and C.M. Berndt, *The World of the First Australians*, Sydney 1964, pp. 39-41.
[3] *Ibid.*, p. 19, (map-diagram); D.J. Mulvaney, '"The Chain of Connection": The Material Evidence', in N. Peterson (ed.), *Tribes and Boundaries in Australia*, Canberra 1976, pp. 72-94.
[4] Hackett, 'Treponematoses (yaws and treponarid)'.
[5] Berndt and Berndt, *op.cit.*, Chap. XIII, esp. pp. 386-412; Chap. IV, esp. p. 108; Chap. IX.

But the effects of smallpox were exceptionally alarming. As well as the high incidence of sickness within affected groups, there was the gradual awareness of infectivity. Most alarming were the many deaths, the blindness of some survivors and the scarring of most. Nor did the traditional beliefs in sorcery necessarily offer satisfactory explanations of what had happened. In such circumstances the patterns of contact were possibly not simply the usual ones. Historical precedents from the Old World suggest that one common human reaction to the disasters of unfamiliar, acute, lethal epidemics was to move out from affected neighbourhoods. This was evident during the fourteenth century plague in Europe. In that situaiton, as Boccaccio explained, 'there was no medicine for the disease superior or equal in efficacy to flight'.[6] In that way the lives of the healthy might be saved. However Aborigines already infected with smallpox who moved away from the source of infection could spread it further. The incubation period allowed the still-healthy to travel; whole families might move, and men, for instance messengers without families, could walk several hundred miles before sickness made them stop. In those circumstances, smallpox spread in Australia.

From Watkin Tench to James Urry, doubts have been raised about whether the disease seen among Aborigines was *really* smallpox, and questions have persisted about its origins. The disease was unquestionably smallpox; in the late 1820s it was transmitted to Aborigines not by European colonists but by Asian visitors, probably Macassans, on the north coast. Smallpox, said to have been recently active at Raffles Bay in 1829, spread through Queensland, east to parts of the coast, and southeast into the Murray-Darling Basin where it was seen first on the northern fringes of the settled districts between 1829 and 1831, and by settlers in 1831; evidence of its past presence was subsequently common knowledge among southeast Australian colonists. Except for the experiences of the first epidemic in parts of eastern Australia 40 years before, the impact of smallpox in traditional communities during the late 1820s and early 1830s was unprecedented. The alarm it caused and the movement of people it provoked expedited the spread of infection; in the more densely populated regions, the accustomed chains of connection became the chains of infection as the disease spread away from affected areas to susceptible groups further south and east.

The first observers of the epidemic beyond the settled districts referred to the high incidence of disease within affected groups. The case fatality rate of smallpox of 25-30 per cent in unvaccinated populations might have been exceeded in some Aboriginal groups in the second epidemic. Except among survivors of the first epidemic, immunity and experience were lacking. Death inevitably followed the abandonment of the sick and their unsuccessful treatment. Hunter-gatherers could not get food during acute illness, and the lack of food continued into convalescence because of painful feet and the deaths of pregnant women food-gatherers;

---

[6] G. Boccaccio, *The Decameron*, 2 vols, London 1930, vol. I, p. 7; J. Nohl, *The Black Death* (abridged ed.), London 1961, p. 58.

Judy Campbell

starvation was possible. The failure of traditional medicine, bereavement and melancholy, the fear of impending disasters and fears about unfulfilled obligations to the dead all suggest a devastating loss of morale in affected groups.

In more densely populated regions, where natural resources attracted pastoralists, the demise and demoralisation of many Aborigines beyond the settled districts before colonists arrived made the occupation of Aboriginal lands easier when settlers came. In less densely populated regions, as Sir Keith Hancock found in Monaro, pastoralists could simply ignore surviving hunter-gatherers. When whites like Sturt appeared during the smallpox epidemic, Aboriginal beliefs in sorcery predisposed them to blame the whites for the sickness and deaths as well as for taking land. Elsewhere, Aboriginal experiences of smallpox and their beliefs about it were not necessarily connected with the presence of whites, and their subsequent relations with colonists did not directly reflect the smallpox experience. But notwithstanding such local variations in beliefs about smallpox, its effects on Aboriginal numbers and morale as colonists moved into their country were profound.

13

Disease and Infertility:
A New Look at the Demographic
Collapse of Native Populations in
the Wake of Western Contact
David E. Stannard

During the past fifty years few subjects of historical consequence have been more controversial than that of the population history of the American Indian. At one extreme, in 1939 Alfred L. Kroeber estimated the population of pre-Columbian North America at about 900,000. At the other extreme, in 1983 Henry F. Dobyns estimated it at about 18,000,000. Since the total North American Indian population by the early twentieth century was no more than 350,000 to 450,000, the human question concealed in the statistical controversy is staggering: did the North American Indian population decline by a ratio of about 2 to 1 between the end of the fifteenth century and the end of the nineteenth century – or did it decline by 50 to 1? Or more?[1]

Today, no scholars any longer accept Kroeber's low estimate. But Dobyns's high estimate, along with his more commonly cited 1966 estimate of roughly 10,000,000 to 12,000,000, also continues to meet

[1] Alfred L. Kroeber, *Cultural and Natural Areas of Native North America*, University of California Publications in American Archaeology and Ethnology, Volume 38 (Berkeley: University of California Press, 1939), Section 11; Henry F. Dobyns, *Their Number Became Thinned: Native American Population Dynamics in Eastern North America* (Knoxville: University of Tennessee Press, 1983), 42.

resistance among many scholars working in the field. The estimates of most writers now range from slightly more than 2,000,000 to just over 7,000,000.[2]

The reasons for the controversy range from the narrowly technical to the broadly political, and usually contain a combination of both. But also at the core of the skepticism regarding Dobyns's high estimates is, as one of his critics has bluntly put it, "the problem of explaining how so many people could seemingly disappear so fast."[3]

Dobyns's response, in part, has been to argue that the disease epidemics that followed in the wake of European contact with American Indians – including smallpox, influenza, measles, bubonic plague, diphtheria, typhus, and (later) cholera – were so devastating that "the aborigines collectively could not have survived" unless the population at contact were as large as he suggests. His calculations show that "a serious contagious disease causing significant mortality invaded North American peoples at intervals of four years and two and a half months, on the average, from 1520 to 1900." Some of these epidemics, which Dobyns calls "the true shock troops with which the Old World battered the New," spread across the entire continent. "Yet," he adds, "the relatively long intervals between invasions by the same disease prevented Native Americans from acquiring much immunity for well over three centuries." Thus, the same disease returned again and again, driving the native population down at a nearly extermination-level rate: "To employ a very simple numerical device to emphasize the amount of depopulation that appears to have occurred," Dobyns writes, "one Native American lived early in the twentieth century where about seventy-two had existed four centuries earlier."[4]

It is precisely, however, that matter of "relatively long intervals between [disease] invasions" that has caused at least one critic, sociologist Russell Thornton, to contend that Dobyns's population decline trajectory

---

[2] For the lower range of current estimates, see Douglas H. Ubelaker, "Prehistoric New World Population Size: Historical Review and Current Appraisal of North American Estimates," *American Journal of Physical Anthropology*, 45 (1976), 661–66. For the higher range, though still well short of Dobyns, see Russell Thornton, *American Indian Holocaust and Survival: A Population History Since 1492* (Norman: University of Oklahoma Press, 1987), 32.

[3] S. Ryan Johansson, "The Demographic History of the Native Peoples of North America: A Selective Bibliography," *Yearbook of Physical Anthropology*, 25 (1982), 137.

[4] Dobyns, *Their Number Become Thinned*, 43, 24, 343. The discrepancy in Dobyns's 72:1 ratio and the 50:1 ratio noted earlier derives from Dobyns's acceptance in his more recent work of a lower population nadir ("about one quarter to one third million") in the late nineteenth century than in his earlier work.

is too extreme. As Thornton has pointed out, populations tend to rebound upward once an epidemic has passed. Thus, while not denying that the post-Columbian population history of American Indians was nothing short of a holocaust, Thornton argues that it was less disastrous demographically than Dobyns suggests.

Whereas Dobyns's graph of the Indian population decline resembles a staircase, with population *stability* characterizing the periods between epidemics, Thornton claims that the more correct graph should resemble a downward-pointing lightning bolt, with short upward strokes of population *growth* characterizing the intervals between plagues.[5] Dobyns's large pre-Columbian population estimate is, in this reasoning, not supported by his argument from necessity – that is, that a population on the order of magnitude that Dobyns suggests was essential for the Indians to have survived the European epidemiological assault. On the contrary, says Thornton, the tendency of populations to rebound upward once an epidemic has dissipated argues for a lower pre-Columbian population estimate than Dobyns has advanced.

Thornton, of course, has no direct evidence of Indian population growth during non-epidemic years. The data simply are not available. But there is a good deal of evidence from other populations that the rebound pattern Thornton describes is common in the wake, not only of epidemics, but of other demographic assaults such as warfare and natural disaster. However, a contrary pattern also exists – that of continuing *de*population following epidemics because of disease – induced infertility and sub-fecundity.[6] Again, as Thornton elsewhere notes, there is no direct evidence of increased infertility or subfecundity among American Indians following the waves of European-introduced epidemics, because the first reliable tabulations of native death- and birth-rates were made only centuries after initial European contact. In response to this lack of evidence for either population growth *or* decline between epidemics, Thornton opts for the growth intervals scenario and assumes that while, overall, "the American Indian decline was due to both increases in death rates [primarily from disease] and decreases in birth rates ... it is clear that the increased death rates were of primary importance."[7]

---

[5] Russell Thornton, unpublished commentary at annual conference of the American Society for Ethnohistory, Williamsburg, Virginia, 1988.

[6] Note: The term *infertility* refers to a diminished ability to bring about conception or to conceive; the term *subfecundity* refers to a diminished capacity to reproduce because of coital inability, pregnancy loss, conceptive failure, and other factors.

[7] Thornton, *American Indian Holocaust*, 53, 43.

In fact, it is not so clear at all. One of the best comparative situations for which data are presently available – the post-European population history of native Hawaiians – suggests that the cataclysmic population decline of American Indian populations may well have been the result *primarily* of infertility and subfecundity arising from the disease, stress, and malnutrition that followed in the trail of the European invasion. To the extent that there is some comparability between the native Hawaiian and native American disease histories, these data suggest that American Indian populations may well have been in a downward free-fall – not a "staircase" or "lightning bolt" patterned decline – even during the interstices between epidemics. If so, Dobyns's posited pre-Columbian population level for North America that is considered by many to be too high may one day be considered, as Wilbur R. Jacobs once observed, "the tip of an iceberg of tremendous proportions."[8]

II

The islands of Hawai'i constitute the most isolated archipelago on earth. First discovered by humans no later than the first century A.D., the islands remained virtually free of other outside human contact until 1778 when they were encountered by Captain James Cook as he sailed north from Tahiti in search of a western terminus for the long-sought northwest passage.[9]

For nearly two thousand years, then, Hawai'i's native people had lived in separation from the rest of the world. Moreover, it had been at least several thousand additional years since their ancestors' last contact with a mainland population. That great time and vast distance had an epidemiological effect on the Hawaiians not unlike the even greater time and distance that separated fifteenth and sixteenth century American Indians from their Asian ancestors: the diseases that were found among them were relatively mild or had their main impact late in life and none of them were epidemic "crowd-type" ecopathogenic diseases such as

---

[8] Wilbur R. Jacobs, "The Tip of an Iceberg: Pre-Columbian Indian Demography and Some Implications for Revisionism," *William and Mary Quarterly*, 3rd Series, 31 (1974), 132.

[9] For the best concise discussion of the evolution of Hawaiian society prior to Western contact – including the matter of earliest settlement dates – see Matthew Spriggs, "The Hawaiian Transformation of Ancestral Polynesian Society: Conceptualizing Chiefly States," in John Gladhill, Barbara Bender, and Mogens Trolle Larsen (eds.), *State and Society: The Emergence and Development of Social Hierarchy and Political Centralization* (London: Unwin Hyman, 1988), 57–73.

smallpox, typhoid, yellow fever, measles, or malaria. While debate continues over the existence of treponemic infections (such as syphilis) and tuberculosis among pre-Columbian American Indians – and among them, among *which* American Indians on the enormous North American continent – all the historical and paleopathological evidence indicates the absence of these afflictions from pre-1778 Hawai'i.[10] As a consequence, again like most such contagions among the American Indians, the Hawaiians had no immunity to these and other epidemic infectious diseases when they were introduced. Thus, as with other so-called "virgin soil" populations, the new diseases wreaked havoc almost immediately upon first contact.

Syphilis, gonorrhea, tuberculosis, and more – including, perhaps, influenza – tore through the Hawaiian population as soon as their barrier of isolated was penetrated.[11] Even before Cook's ships departed from Hawai'i after their brief sojourn, the surgeons and others aboard recorded the presence among the natives of the diseases the ships had brought. The Hawaiians became infected "in a violent degree," wrote the *Discovery's* surgeon's second mate William Ellis, as he acknowledged that it was the Europeans who "had been the cause of this irreparable injury."[12] Indeed, less than a decade after that first contact with the West the natives of a remote and isolated part of Maui, an island not even visited by the first Europeans, were found to be horribly affected by the diseases Cook and his crews had left behind. Writing in 1786, the surgeon on board the French ship *Boussole*, commanded by Captain J. F. G. de la Pérouse, observed of this area:

The beauty of the climate, and fertility of the soil, might render the inhabitants extremely happy, if the leprosy and venereal disease prevailed among them less generally, and with less virulence. These scourges, the most humiliating and most destructive with which the human race are afflicted, display themselves among these islanders by the following symptoms: buboes, and scars which result from their suppurating, warts, spreading ulcers with caries of the bones, nodes,

---

[10] See summary treatments in Marshall T. Newman, "Aboriginal New World Epidemiology and Medical Care, and the Impact of Old World Disease Imports," *American Journal of Physical Anthropology*, 45 (1976), 667–72, and David E. Stannard, *Before the Horror: The Population of Hawai'i on the Eve of Western Contact* (Honolulu: University of Hawai'i Press, 1989), 69–78.

[11] For an exchange on the possibility that influenza was among the early diseases introduced to Hawai'i by Europeans, see Francis L. Black's review of Stannard's *Before the Horror* and Stannard's reply in *Pacific Studies*, 13 (1990), 274, 292–94.

[12] William Ellis, *An Authentic Narrative of a Voyage* (London: G. Robinson, 1782), 73–74.

exostoses, fistula, tumors of the lachrymal and salival ducts, scrofulous swellings, inveterate ophthalmiae, ichorous ulcerations of the tunica conjunctiva, atrophy of the eyes, blindness, inflamed prurient herpetic eruptions, indolent swellings of the extremities, and among children, scald head, or a malignant tinea, from which exudes a fetid and acrid matter. I remarked, that *the greater part* of these unhappy victims of sensuality, when arrived at the age of nine or ten, were feeble and languid, exhausted by marasmus, and affected with the rickets.[13]

The journals of subsequent explorers to Hawai'i echoed these observations. Thus, the English Captain George Vancouver (who had been with Cook in 1778–79) noted upon his return in the 1790s that he now found previously well-populated areas "entirely abandoned" and other places "reduced at least two-thirds" their earlier size. Added the Russian Captain I. F. Kruzenshtern in 1804, "there was hardly a single [Hawaiian]" whose body did not show traces of the "disease of lasciviousness." Others routinely commented that "the depopulation is evident...[diseases] brought to these islands a few years ago...make dreadful havoc among the natives."[14]

By the dawn of the nineteenth century – less than twenty-five years after Cook's initial visit – the Hawaiians reported and modern evidence seems to confirm that "the majority of the people from Hawai'i to Ni'ihau [that is, at least 400,000 people on all the inhabited islands] had died."[15] *Then*, in 1804, the islands were hit with a disastrous epidemic of typhoid fever. In 1848–49 epidemics of measles, influenza, whooping cough, and dysentery descended on the islands, and finally, in 1853, smallpox appeared, while the ever-present syphilis, gonorrhea, and tuberculosis continued to bore away at those who remained alive.

Ghastly as this scenario is, it is far from unique. On the contrary, it is typical of what happened to many communities of American Indians in the immediate wake of Western contact. In Hawai'i, however, there was one small but significant difference: because of its relatively late discovery

---

[13] M. Rollin, M.D., "Dissertation on the Inhabitants of Easter Island and the Island of Mowee," in J. F. G. de la Pérouse, *A Voyage Round the World Performed in the Years 1785, 1786, 1787, and 1788* (London: A. Hamilton, 1799), Vol. II, 337. The reference to leprosy, which also appears in other eighteenth and early nineteenth century commentaries, is an error. The symptoms observed were probably attributable to syphilis.

[14] George Vancouver, *A Voyage of Discovery...Round the World* (London, 1789), Volume I, 158–60, 187–88; I. F. Kruzenshtern, "Journal," in Glynn Barratt (ed.), *The Russian Discovery of Hawai'i* (Honolulu: Editions Limited, 1987), 88; Isaac Iselin, *Journal of a Trading Voyage Around the World, 1805–1808* (New York: McIlroy and Emmet, n.d.), 68, 73–4.

[15] David Malo, "On the Decrease of Population in the Hawaiian Islands," *Hawaiian Spectator*, April, 1839, 125; see also Stannard, *Before the Horror*, 45–58.

by Western explorers, within half a century of initial contact with Europeans Hawai'i was filled with Protestant missionaries determined to record – and to count – everything that they encountered. By the early 1830s the missionaries had fanned out and established mission stations on all the major inhabited islands, mission stations that were required to file annual reports – often including enumerations of births and deaths in the individual districts – to the central office in Honolulu. Nothing even resembling such a relatively sophisticated system of data collection and storage existed in North America until long centuries after Western contact – long centuries of hidden devastation.

By coincidence, the mission stations in Hawai'i were established, and for their first decade and a half existed, during a time when major epidemics were absent from the islands. As the Hawaiian chronicler David Malo wrote in 1839: "There have been no seasons of universal sickness since [the typhoid epidemic of 1804]; men have died, but not in an uncommon degree, but from that time to this it is clear that there has been a steady decrease of the people."[16] Thus, it is particularly striking to encounter the first annual (1835) census report from the Reverend W. P. Alexander in the district of Wai'oli on the island of Kaua'i:

What we do for the people must be done quickly, for they are rapidly melting away. – During the 8 months from September to May [1834–35] the proportions of deaths to births within my bounds was, as 2 to 1 – the number of deaths 122; & of births 61. The whole population of the district according to a census taken last April is 3603.[17]

Projected out for the year, this was a crude death rate of about 50 per thousand and a birth rate of about 25 per thousand. A year later, in 1836, the Reverend Alexander reported: "During the past year, affliction has often reminded those of us who live on Kaua'i, that our breath is in our nostrils & our days like a shadow." The numerical reports showed the following:

From May 1835 to September 1835 – 40 deaths, 26 births
From September 1835 to January 1836 – 51 deaths, 22 births
From January 1836 to May 1836 – 43 deaths, 25 births
Total for 1 year ———— 134 deaths, 73 births

---

[16] Malo, "On the Decrease of Population," 125.

[17] Wai'oli, Kaua'i Mission Station Report, 1835 – on file at the Hawaiian Mission Children's Society Library (HMCS) in Honolulu. Subsequent references to and quotations from mission station reports refer to the same archival source.

In the years that followed, whenever a census was mentioned the pattern was the same:

1837 – Deaths 84, Births 60
1840 – "Death is still making ravages among the people.... Since the first of January last, five deaths to one birth! If this or any thing like it be the ratio of decrease, it is evident that what we do for the nation we must do quickly."
It was the same in other districts.

Island of Kaua'i, district of Waimea:

1835 – Ratio of ten deaths for every birth "for a few months past." Population, by census count, has fallen from 4,297 in 1831 to 2,222 in 1835.
1836 – Deaths 160, Births 75
1840 – Population of district has decreased by 453 in past two years.
1841 – Deaths 78, Births 39

Island of Maui, district of Lahaina:

1835 – "The station at Lahaina has been in deep affliction the past year."
1836 – Population of Maui is now 24,248 "instead of 35,000 as published in the Geography." On Lana'i the death rate is reported to be double the birth rate.

Island of O'ahu, districts of Waialua and Wai'anae:

1835 – "Births in Waialua alone during the past 10 months 37, deaths 115. Deaths of children 45, of adults 69."
1836 – Deaths (Waialua only) 67, Births 24
1837 – Deaths 119, Births 42 – "And yet Waialua for ought I know is about as healthy as any station on the islands."
1839 – Deaths in 1838 – 143, Births 64
1840 – Deaths 185, Births 56

Island of O'ahu, district of 'Ewa:

1835 – "The people of 'Ewa are a dying people.... There have been as many as 8 or 10 deaths to one birth. I have heard of but 4 births in Waiawa during the year, & all of these children are dead."
1836 – Deaths 130, Births 41
'Ewa population has declined by 592 in 4 years. Wai'anae population has declined to 214 in 4 years. "The facts are alarming & cause the missionaries at 'Ewa to feel that what they do must be done quickly."

Island of O'ahu, district of Kane'ohe:

1836 – Deaths past 5 months–38, Births 14
1841 – Population down to "about 4,000" from 4,636 in 1836
1846 – Deaths per 1,000 population last six years 314, Births 126

Island of Hawai'i, district of Waimea:

1835 – "I have been called to attend many funerals–The number I cannot recollect–Nor am I acquainted with the number of births–But I infer from what little knowledge I have that the number of deaths is by far the greatest.... The total population is declining."

1841 – Deaths–more than 300, Births about 90
Population of the district has fallen by almost 5% in one year.

1842 – Deaths 207, Births 121

1843 – Deaths 434, Births 98

1844 – Deaths 277, Births 106

In district after district, on island after island, the pattern was the same: the population was collapsing despite the absence of major epidemics during the 1830s and early 1840s. A retrospective survey of the overall population characteristics of the islands during the non-epidemic years of 1834 to 1841 has produced a median crude death rate of 47·3 per 1,000 inhabitants and a median birth rate of only 19·3.[18] In sum, despite the absence of major epidemics (there were occasional local outbreaks of "fever," "catarrh," and "croup"), the population of Hawai'i was decreasing during this time at a median annual rate of 2·6 percent – a rate sufficient to cut the population in half in less than twenty years and fully to exterminate it well within the lifetime of a single individual.

What was happening? The first clue comes from the extraordinarily low birth rate and the consequently low proportion of children in the general population – in Honolulu a ratio of 5·28 adults for every child – a fact that the missionaries termed "astonishing," "alarming," and without parallel "in any other nation."[19] Whether without parallel in any other nation, the relative absence of children was indeed without parallel in Hawaiian history prior to Western contact. Indeed, the most assiduous note-takers among Captain Cook's crews in 1778–79 never failed to observe, among the extraordinarily strong and healthy natives, the "abundant stock of Children" encountered everywhere in the islands, a greater number of such "fine lively" creatures than they had encountered "at any other place during this voyage."[20]

[18] Robert C. Schmitt, *The Missionary Censuses of Hawai'i* (Honolulu: Bishop Museum Pacific Anthropological Records, Number 20, 1973), 13.

[19] Samuel Whitney, Waimea, Kaua'i, Mission Station Report, 1840 (HMCS); Robert C. Wyllie, "Notes," *The Friend*, 2 (2 December, 1844), 115; Asa Thurston, *Missionary Herald*, 1836, 385, cited in Schmitt, *Missionary Censuses of Hawai'i*, 12.

[20] Captain Charles Clerke, "Journal," in J. C. Beaglehole (ed.), *The Journal of Captain James Cook* (Cambridge: Hakluyt Society and the University Press, 1967), Volume III, Part One, 593; Lieutenant David Samwell, "Some Account of a Voyage to the South Seas," in ibid., Volume III, Part Two, 1182.

Yet, by the time the missionaries were in place in Hawai'i, reaping their harvests of souls, Hawaiian women were desperate to have children – and more desperate still to keep what few children they did have from dying. In 1851, for example, the Reverend Dwight Baldwin reported from Lahaina on Maui that during the last six months of 1849 there had been 132 deaths and only 24 births in the district. And of those few live infants, many were dying before reaching their first or second birthdays, in part Baldwin wrote, because – paradoxically – of "the *eagerness* of parents, that their children should live": "As many are living childless, there seems to be an increasing desire in those who have children to save them. They are more ready, therefore, to stuff them with food and medicine." Too often, said Baldwin, the result of this was the death of the child from excessive solicitude. "There are many signs among us," he lamented, "that seem to show that the native race is going out of existence."[21]

Three years earlier a succession of epidemics had literally decimated the native population: about 10,000 people, out of the then-surviving population of well under 100,000, died during 1848 and early 1849 from waves of measles, whooping cough, influenza, and an unspecified intestinal disease described simply as "diarrhea." During that time, according to the official census, the death rate was 98 per 1,000 inhabitants and the birth rate only 16 per 1,000. After the worst of the epidemics had passed, the death rate dropped to about 70 per 1,000 and then back down to about 35 per 1,000 – somewhat lower than the rate during the epidemic-free decade and a half preceding the 1848 epidemics.[22] (For the sake of comparison, this "normal" death rate, during non-epidemic years – a rate that the Hawaiian writer Malo, who was born in 1793, had in 1839 described as "not...an uncommon degree" of death in the context of his experience – was two to three times the death rate of military-age American males during the concluding year of World War I and the devastating world-wide influenza pandemic.) But the birth rate hardly budged: between 1848 and 1852 it averaged barely 21 per 1,000.

Then in 1853 the death rate soared to over 105 per 1,000 – smallpox had hit – and the birth rate remained at about 19 per 1,000. By 1860 the native Hawaiian population had fallen to around 66,000, almost exactly half of what it had been just thirty years earlier. By 1870 it was down to about 52,000. But barely one-third of that drop was attributable to the epidemics

---

[21] Dwight Baldwin, Lahaina, Maui, Mission Station Report, 1851 (HMCS).

[22] Robert C. Schmitt, *Historical Statistics of Hawai'i* (Honolulu: University of Hawai'i Press, 1977), 43; Eleanor C. Nordyke, *The Peopling of Hawai'i*, Second Edition (Honolulu: University of Hawai'i Press, 1989), 23.

of 1848 and 1853. The other two-thirds was caused by a birth rate that, in the best of years, barely crept above 22 per 1,000.[23]

By the middle of the 1850s Hawai'i's mission outposts were beginning to close. The statistics coming from them were more irregular than in the past and the overall official Hawai'i birth and death rate statistics during this time did not make racial distinctions. Hawaiians still constituted about 95 percent of the population, however, and in only one year between 1852 and 1865 did the overall Hawai'i birth rate exceed 24 per 1,000; moreover, the overall birth rate in the islands *never* exceeded the death rate until 1889 – more than a century after initial contact with the West – by which time the Hawaiians represented only a dwindling 45 percent of the population and both the birth and death rates combined for all races hovered at about 22 per 1,000. For Hawaiians the death rate exceeded the birth rate into the twentieth century.[24]

In the latter 1850s the missionaries reporting from the field mentioned few epidemics, but continued to comment, as Reverend Baldwin did in 1860, on the "unusual number" of deaths among the natives "mainly because there have been an unusual number in the church who were enfeebled by age." In that year there were 139 deaths and 78 births in Baldwin's district of Lahaina. Two years later he reported 139 deaths again, but only 58 births. "One half" the people in his district, he reported, "are getting to be old men and women."

The same reports were coming out of other districts. The population in O'ahu's Waialua district had fallen by half in 24 years, wrote Reverend John Emerson in 1857, but the number of *students* was down to between one-sixth and one-eighth of what it had been in the early 1830s. The population decline was primarily caused by so few births and a high child mortality rate in the district. "We now have in the church quite a number of aged and infirm people," Emerson noted, "and a few drones." But very few children.

The same year found Reverend Bishop reporting from the 'Ewa district on O'ahu that "there are but few births...and of those born, the greater part die early." Ten years earlier, he noted, there were eighteen schools in his district; now he had only eight, so few were the children to fill them.

In part the small number of children reported by all the missionaries who filed reports was due to the extraordinarily low birth rate. In part it was also due to a very high infant and child mortality rate. Unlike the crude birth and death rates, on infant and child mortality there exists only

---

[23] Schmitt, *Historical Statistics*, 43.   [24] Ibid.

anecdotal information from the missionaries. But all of it points to alarmingly high rates. "We have mothers among us who have had 10, 12, 16 and 18 children each, who are now almost as desolate as those who have had none," wrote Baldwin in 1860, adding: "we have one who has borne 36 children, and has now but one left."

Improbable as this last example may seem, there is some striking statistical confirmation of a high infant and child mortality rate from a very different source. In the same year that Baldwin's report was filed, 1860, the Hawai'i Legislature had ordered that physical examinations be made of all the prostitutes in Honolulu. The required report found 257 women, all Hawaiian, identified as prostitutes. Together they had given birth to a reported 170 living children (less than seven children for every ten adult women) of whom 115 of the offspring – two out of every three – had died. Overall, it took about five of those sexually very active women to produce a single living child.[25]

By 1885 the native population of Hawai'i was down to about 44,000 – compared with 130,000 just fifty-five years earlier and probably at least 800,000 in 1778. It continued to decline. By 1893, when American Marines and local white sugar planters toppled the government, it was less than 40,000. By the 1890s, however, a distinction between Hawaiian and "part-Hawaiian" was becoming statistically significant. For thirty years – from 1890 to 1920 – the Hawaiian (including part-Hawaiian) population held at about 40,000, although in that mix the part-Hawaiian component was increasing at an average rate of slightly more than 3 percent per year, while the so-called "pure" Hawaiian numbers continued to decline. Today, the part-Hawaiian population exceeds 200,000; the pure Hawaiian population is less than 8,000 and still declining.

III

Clearly, in Hawai'i, the great population collapse of the eighteenth and nineteenth centuries was caused by a combination of high death rates from epidemics and from other diseases – such as syphilis and tuberculosis – that became endemic, *and* by a birth rate that remained extremely low during all the years for which we have reasonably reliable data. Census reports from 1831 to 1890 show a steady decline in the native population during that time from about 130,000 to less than 40,000 – a decline of 70 percent in sixty years. *Never* during those sixty years did the native population of Hawai'i increase or even hold steady; it was in a perpetual

[25] *The Polynesian*, Volume 17, Number 36 (5 January, 1861), 2.

state of diminishment, varying in intensity from year to year, but never failing, in any given year, to be lower than in the years preceding. It probably had taken the Hawaiian population about seven centuries to grow from 40,000 to 800,000 in 1778; it took only a little more than one century to bring it back down to 40,000.

While epidemic and endemic diseases certainly caused high levels of death during the era of the great population collapse, the unwavering downward trajectory of the population was in fact principally a secondary consequence of the newly-introduced diseases: low birth rates and high infant mortality rates were the primary causes. This becomes evident from an examination of the complications that commonly result from the diseases known to have been transmitted by Europeans and Americans to the non-immune Hawaiian population in the eighteenth and nineteenth centuries.

Gonorrhea: Gonorrhea and syphilis traveled together throughout the Pacific in the eighteenth century – and the Hawaiians had no history of, and therefore no resistance to, either one. While not itself a killer, gonorrhea can have an extremely depressing effect on the reproductive rates of untreated peoples. The principal problem occurs when the disease in female hosts spreads upward from the urethra and cervix to invade the uterus and the fallopian tubes. The result is pelvic inflammatory disease (PID). A single episode of PID may result in tubal occlusion and sterility in almost 12 percent of cases; two episodes triple the risk; and three or more episodes cause tubal occlusion and sterility in up to 75 percent of cases. The likelihood of infertility also increases with the severity of the disease. And the studies leading to these conclusions were, of course, conducted in the post-antibiotic era. It is now believed that 60 to 70 percent of women who have any episode of PID and go untreated (as all the thousands of eighteenth and nineteenth century Hawaiian women with gonococcal PID did) will become sterile.[26]

In those women for whom sterility does not result directly from PID, there remains the danger of ectopic pregnancy or spontaneous abortion. Even in the post-antibiotic era ectopic pregnancies have been shown to occur in more than 4 percent of women with PID who become pregnant;

[26] L. Westrom, "Effect of Acute Pelvic Inflammatory Disease on Fertility," *American Journal of Obstetrics and Gynecology*, 127 (1975), 707; R. Bernstine et al., "Acute Pelvic Inflammatory Disease: A Clinical Follow-up," *International Journal of Fertility*, 32 (1987), 229–32; L. Westrom, "Incidence, Prevalence, and Trends of Acute Pelvic Inflammatory Disease and Its Consequences in Industrialized Countries," *American Journal of Obstetrics and Gynecology*, 138 (1980), 880–86; S. Thompson and W. Hager, "Acute Pelvic Inflammatory Disease," *Sexually Transmitted Diseases*, 4 (1977), 105.

and the tubal damage caused by a single ectopic pregnancy often results in permanent conceptive impairment.[27]

Finally, if gonococcal PID does not cause infertility or a failed (and permanently damaging) pregnancy, there is always the serious possibility of damage to the child if it survives, damage including septicemia, arthritis, and congenital blindness.

Women, of course, are not the only people susceptible to gonorrhea, although they do run a higher risk of infection: at least 50 to 70 percent of females will become infected after one or two acts of coitus with an infected partner, compared with a 20 to 30 percent likelihood for males. In males, in the pre-antibiotic era, gonorrhea probably progressed to prostatitis or epididymitis in up to 85 percent of cases – and 50 to 80 percent of men afflicted with epididymitis become sterile. Moreover, even if sterility did not result, lowered fecundity is common among both males and females infected with gonorrhea because of extreme coital pain. And there is evidence that the virulence of gonococcus was more extreme in the pre-antibiotic era than in the present, when most of these statistical studies were conducted.[28]

In sum, by itself gonorrhea – especially when released in a population with no previous exposure and without antibiotics – can cause a severe depression in the birth rate, a depression that persists for generation after generation. But gonorrhea did not arrive in Hawai'i "by itself."

Syphilis: In the eighteenth century no distinction was made between syphilis and gonorrhea, and both of them traveled in every ship that entered the Pacific. Captain Cook's crews were so enfeebled by both diseases while in Tahiti in 1778 that his planned departure date for the journey that would take him to Hawai'i had to be postponed. Fully half of his men were incapacitated with the "foul disease."[29] When finally they did embark the men were at least able to work – but both diseases, in an infectious state, continued to reside in their systems.

Between 10 and 50 percent of sexual contacts with a syphilis-infected person in the primary or secondary stages of the disease result in the

[27] L. Westrom and P. Mardh, "Pelvic Inflammatory Disease," *World Health Organization Group on Nongonococcal Urethritis and Other Sexually Transmitted Diseases of Public Health Importance* (New York: World Health Organization, 1978).

[28] K. Holmes, "Average Risk of Gonorrheal Infection After Exposure," *Medical Aspects of Human Sexuality,* 9 (1975), 83; A. Wigfield, "How Infectious is Gonorrhea?" *British Medical Journal,* 4 (1972), 672; J. A. and M. H. McFalls, *Disease and Fertility* (New York: Academic Press, 1984), 298–99, 273.

[29] William Bayly, "Log," cited in Beaglehole (ed.), *The Journals of Captain James Cook,* Volume III, Part One, 233, note 4; John Rickman, *Journal of Captain Cook's Last Voyage* (London: E. Newberry, 1781), 191.

Demographic Collapse of Native Populations   339

transmission of the infection to the uninfected partner.[30] The rate is higher, as with gonorrhea, in male-to-female transmission – and of course, the studies of likelihood of transmission have all been conducted in the modern era. Among people with no previous exposure to syphilis, first contact can result in a wildfire of infections. This is evident not only in the historical literature, but in current medical literature as well. There has been an accumulation of recent evidence showing that immuno-compromised individuals – the research has been done on AIDS patients, but is relevant to others – display extraordinarily aggressive manifest-ations of syphilis. One study showed HIV-positive subjects to be five times more likely than others to succumb to syphilitic infection; another study found neurosyphilis advancing in four months among HIV-infected individuals to a stage not commonly reached for 5 to 12 years in others.[31]

Within five to twenty years after first contracting syphilis today a condition known as "late syphilis" develops in a quarter to a third of the disease's victims, about half of whom will die. (Again, this situation is much more severe and durationally abbreviated in "first contact" situations.) At this late stage the infection is not contagious (except perhaps to fetuses), but the deaths that occur are often preceded by blindness, insanity, and/or paralysis.[32] And, while it is commonly believed that an immunity to syphilis can result from previous exposure to yaws, this remains an unsettled matter (a large inoculum of syphilis will overcome any partial immunity that may have developed), and, in any case, yaws did not exist in pre-1778 Hawai'i.[33] Thus, when syphilis and gonorrhea were introduced, they spread from one end of the 300-mile long archipelago to the other in a matter of months, cutting a wide swath of death and infertility in their wake.[34]

---

[30] McFalls and McFalls, *Disease and Fertility*, 320.

[31] D. R. Johns et al., "Alteration in the Natural History of Neurosyphilis by Concurrent Infection with the Human Immunodeficiency Virus," *New England Journal of Medicine*, 316 (1987), 1569–72. Cf. correspondence discussion in ibid., 317 (1987), 1473–75.

[32] McFalls and McFalls, *Disease and Fertility*, 323–24.

[33] Peter M. Moodie, "Yaws, Pinta, and Bejel," in Abraham I. Broude (ed.), *Infectious Diseases and Medical Microbiology*, 2nd Edition (Philadelphia: W. B. Saunders, 1986), 1361–62; Walter F. Bowers, "Pathological and Functional Changes Found in 864 Pre-Captain Cook Contact Polynesian Burials From the San Dunes at Mōkapu, O'ahu, Hawai'i," *International Surgery*, 45 (1966), 208; Sara L. Collins, "Osteological Report," in Toni L. Han, et al., *Moe Kau Ho'oilo: Hawaiian Mortuary Practices at Keōpū, Kona, Hawai'i* (Honolulu: Bishop Museum Department of Anthropology Report 86–1, 1986), 142, 149.

[34] The first European ships arrived in Hawai'i, touching only the islands of Kaua'i and Ni'ihau at the far western end of the chain of major islands, in late 1778. Ten months later they returned, landing on the island of Hawai'i – 300 miles away and at the far

In addition to the damage syphilis causes to living members of a population, it can have a powerful limiting effect on birth rates. The effect varies, depending on whether pregnancy occurs during the primary, secondary, or early latent stages of the disease. The greatest danger resides with pregnancy during the primary or secondary phases, when infection is most intense; at least 30 percent of fetuses carried by women in these stages of infection will spontaneously abort, and there are numerous studies showing fetal death rates of at least double this magnitude.[35] Pregnancies in women in the later (early latent) stage of syphilis are somewhat more likely to result in successful birth, but – as with the successful births to women in earlier stages of the disease – the resulting infant is almost certain to suffer from life-threatening congential syphilis. And, in the absence of treatment, congenital syphilis almost invariably results in marasmus and death.[36] Moreover, in developing countries today it is very common for pregnant women with syphilis to develop a sterilizing infection following a spontaneous abortion. Thus, one study of subfertility in Central Africa reported a 40 percent childless rate and a rate of spontaneous abortion of 35 percent; the spontaneous abortions apparently were caused by syphilis and the high childless rate was largely caused by sterilizing infections that followed the miscarriages.[37]

Traveling in tandem, then, gonorrhea and syphilis – appearing simultaneously in a population, especially a previously unexposed population – can have a devastating effect on the birth rate, whipsawing their victims between extremely high rates of fetal death, postpartum disease and infant death, and both female and male infertility and subfecundity. The visible effects are impossible to miss, as one physician residing in Hawai'i from 1832 to 1835 reported to the American Journal of the Medical Sciences:

The venereal disease has for the past fifty-seven years continued to spread and increase; perpetuated and extended too by almost every vessel which touches at the islands, till words would fail to express the wretchedness and woe which have

eastern end of the archipelago – and found that the venereal diseases they had planted on Kaua'i and Ni'ihau had already spread across the entire chain of islands. See Stannard, *Before the Horror*, 69–70.

[35] E. Barrett-Connor, "Infections and Pregnancy," *Southern Medical Journal*, 62 (1969), 275; McFalls and McFalls, *Disease and Fertility*, 336.

[36] D. Ingall and D. M. Musher, "Syphilis," in J. S. Remington and J. O. Klein (eds.), *Infectious Diseases of the Fetus and Newborn Infant*, 2nd Edition (Philadelphia: W. B. Saunders Co., 1983), 335–74.

[37] A. Retel-Laurentin, "Subfertility in Black Africa: The Case of the Nzakara in Central African Republic," in B. Adadevoh (ed.), *Subfertility and Infertility in Africa* (Ibadan: Caxton Press, 1974), 69–75.

been the result. Foul ulcers, of many years' standing, both indolent and phagedenic, every where abound, the visages horridly deformed – eyes rendered blind – noses entirely destroyed – mouths monstrously drawn aside from their natural position, ulcerating palates, and almost useless arms and legs, mark most clearly the state and progress of the disease among that injured and helpless people.[38]

But the invisible effects can be even more all-consuming. As that same physician, Alonzo Chapin, concluded in his comments on the subject: "The venereal disease has destroyed its thousands, and by its influence in inducing barrenness of females, had probably prevented tens of thousands from ever seeing the light." That was a report from 1835. In 1860 the first hospital opened in Hawai'i; of 765 patients treated during its first four months of operation 422 – well over half – were found to be suffering from venereal disease.[39]

Tuberculosis: Next to gonorrhea and syphilis, tuberculosis was the most prevalent disease on the ships that plied the eighteenth and early nineteenth century Pacific. In Europe and America TB was the single largest cause of death during these years and the number of Pacific explorers who brought it to the Pacific were legion. It is certain that a number of Cook's crews – and possibly Cook himself – were infected with tuberculosis when they arrived in Hawai'i. And TB can be as contagious as measles.[40]

Among a non-immune people TB can be overwhelming in its devastation. In one well-documented case in the twentieth century *half* the population of a Canadian Indian community died from newly-introduced TB in less than a decade.[41] Less well-known are the effects of tuberculosis on fertility and fecundity.

Today it is most common to think of tuberculosis as a lung disease, but in fact TB can and does develop in any organs seeded by the tuberculosis bacillus. These organs include the genitals. Indeed, in societies where immunological defenses are suppressed by malnutrition or other health conditions – so-called "developing" societies today and, in the past, societies such as eighteenth century Hawai'i under external bacteriological assault – genital tuberculosis is common, particularly in females. Various

---

[38] Alonzo Chapin, M.D., "Remarks on the Sandwich Islands," *American Journal of the Medical Sciences*, 39 (1835).

[39] *The Polynesian*, Volume 16, Number 39 (January 28, 1860), 2.

[40] James Watt, "Medical Aspects and Consequences of Cook's Voyages," in Robin Fisher and Hugh Johnston (eds.), *Captain James Cook and His Times* (Seattle: University of Washington Press, 1979), 129–57; Selman A. Waksman, *The Conquest of Tuberculosis* (Berkeley: University of California Press, 1964), 202.

[41] René Dubos, *Man Adapting* (New Haven: Yale University Press, 1965), 173.

studies of sterility among women infected with genital tuberculosis have found directly-caused incidences of permanent sterility ranging from a low of 55 percent of infected subjects to a high of 85 percent. Overall, conception rates among infected women are less than 10 percent – and of these, one-half to two-thirds of resultant pregnancies end as ectopic pregnancies or spontaneous abortions. In parts of Africa today genital tuberculosis has been cited as *the* most important cause of subfecundity and low fertility. And among males (where tubal occlusion or destruction of the functional cells of the prostate is a common consequence), it has been shown that "male genital TB is responsible for a sizeable portion of male infertility where TB is a prevalent disease." As the most distinguished overview study flatly puts it: "Genital TB is a disease that almost always causes primary sterility in affected men and women."[42]

One problem with isolating genital tuberculosis in a population is the difficulty of diagnosis. Even today, only highly sophisticated bacteriologic and/or histological methods can confirm the presence of genital tuberculosis. But there is no doubt that it is common wherever tuberculosis is common. And, although there is no evidence of tuberculosis in Hawai'i prior to 1778, it vied with syphilis as the singularly most remarked-upon disease among Hawaiians during the first half of the nineteenth century.

Influenza and measles: Influenza may well have been introduced to Hawai'i by Cook's crews in 1778 and 1779. Even if not, it clearly was distributed to all the islands by the early nineteenth century. Measles was introduced early in the nineteenth century, if not before. Again, the most shocking consequence of the introduction of both influenza and measles into a virgin-soil environment is the suddenness of widespread death: near-extermination for influenza is not uncommon and immediate death rates of 15 percent to 20 percent of such affected communities are routine; measles, in the meantime, has been shown to have been second only to smallpox as a killer of American Indians.[43]

Less noticed, however, in both cases, is the later (if temporary) fertility decline. Nevertheless, studies done in the Cocos-Keeling Islands have shown that nine months after an influenza epidemic in 1929 and a measles epidemic in 1945 birth rates had fallen to between 6 percent and 20 percent of normal expectations; put differently, 80 percent to 94 percent of otherwise anticipated births did not occur.[44]

---

[42] McFalls and McFalls, *Disease and Fertility*, 98.
[43] Dobyns, *Their Number Become Thinned*, 16–18.
[44] T. Smith, "The Cocos-Keeling Islands: A Demographic Laboratory," *Population Studies*, 14 (1960), 94.

Mumps and Chicken Pox: Unlike most of the diseases cited thus far, mumps and chicken pox have their most damaging effects on male, not female, infertility. Again, the nineteenth century mumps and chicken pox epidemics in Hawai'i are most known for the immediate swath of death they cut in the existing native population. But we now know that about a *third* of adult males who contract mumps develop azoospermia – or reduced sperm count – and that chicken pox has a similar effect.[45]

Smallpox: Because of its great distance from continental land masses, Hawai'i appears not to have suffered smallpox until the early 1850s. When smallpox did arrive, however, it was immensely destructive of the native population: thousands died in Honolulu alone and mass graves were necessary to dispose of the bodies that fell everywhere with such suddenness. Pregnant women died in unusually high numbers, as is common in smallpox epidemics when 40 percent of pregnant women succumb, as compared with about 12 percent of non-pregnant women. Of the remaining 60 percent of pregnant women it is common for less than half of their offspring to survive. In sum, added to the immediate scourge of a smallpox epidemic – in which 20 percent to 40 percent of all cases, even in the twentieth century, are fatal – less than a third of the expected offspring of the affected but surviving generation will materialize. As for males, studies in India have concluded that the single most important cause of male sterility – obstructive azoospermia – is caused by small-pox.[46]

There were, of course, other diseases that swept through Hawai'i causing immense levels of death (such as typhoid fever) and still others that had little immediate impact, but that left severe levels of infertility in their wake (such as diabetes, especially among the *ali'i,* or Hawaiian aristocracy). But this short summary is intended only to account for the most egregious causes of evident low fertility in the native population even during years when epidemics were absent. So severe was the infertility/subfecundity crisis among Hawaiians, in fact, that in many *non-*epidemic years, such as the early 1830s, the population fell at least as drastically as during some of the worst epidemic years. No doubt the same thing happened throughout much of North America during the sixteenth, seventeenth, and eighteenth centuries – when no one was counting, at least for the written record.

To be sure, there are important differences between Hawai'i and the

---

[45] S. Candel, "Epididymitis in Mumps, Including Orchitis: Further Clinical Studies and Comments," *Annals of Internal Medicine,* **34** (1951), 20–28.

[46] McFalls and McFalls, *Disease and Fertility,* 532–34.

mainland of North America. Among the differences is the possibility that syphilis or some syphilis-like treponemal infection was present in at least some parts of North America prior to the arrival of Columbus. Debate on this subject continues and I shall enter it here only briefly, first to note that the evidence of such a disease has never been claimed to be continent-wide – and North America is a very large continent.

For example, there is no good evidence to date of syphilis in all of pre-Columbian northwestern North America. Hundreds of pre-Columbian Plains Indian skeletons also have been studied with no evidence of treponemal infection discovered. There is rather extensive evidence suggestive of syphilis among skeletal remains found in certain other parts of North America and South America, although the bone lesions that serve as indicators of treponemal infection are ambiguous and can also result from other causes. For instance, acute osteomyelitis – usually the result of severe staphylococcal infection – often leaves skeletal lesions that are nearly indistinguishable from those caused by both syphilis and tuberculosis. Still, the almost total absence of skeletal evidence for syphilis in pre-1492 Europe, compared with the extensive, if ambiguous, evidence from widespread locales in the Americas, recently has led many – perhaps most – authorities to accept a revised version of the so-called "Columbian hypothesis" that the sixteenth century explosion of syphilis throughout much of the world had its origin in New World *non*-venereal treponemal infections that were carried back to Europe by Columbus and other explorers, where they were transformed into the sexually transmitted disease we know today as syphilis.[47]

Those who have remained unconvinced of the Columbian hypothesis (even in its new non-venereal version) have argued, among other points, that the skeletal evidence is simply too equivocal, too subject to differing interpretations – and that the much smaller, less thorough body of studies done on pre-1492 European remains (80 percent to 90 percent of European analyses have been confined to skulls) skews the data. In addition, as Henry Dobyns has pointed out, some of the evidence purportedly showing pre-Columbian treponemal infection in the Americas derives from skeletal remains that in fact are probably post-Columbian. Many a researcher, confronting this confusing body of data and

[47] B. J. Baker and G. J. Armelagos, "The Origin and Antiquity of Syphilis: Paleopathological Diagnosis and Interpretation," *Current Anthropology*, **29** (1988), 703–20 and comment by John A. Williams, ibid., 729. On the similarity of bone lesions caused by osteomyelitis and both syphilis and tuberculosis, see R. Ted Steinbock, *Paleopathological Diagnosis and Interpretation: Bone Diseases in Ancient Human Populations* (Springfield, Illinois: Thomas, 1976), 82.

interpretation, has repeated the wish expressed thirty years ago by L. W. Harrison: "If one could test mummies for antibodies of *T. pallidum* ... one might perhaps settle this eternal question of the birth-place of syphilis."[48]

Harrison's wish, at last, has been granted. But so far it's not much help. A 1989 University of Pisa study of the mummy of Maria d'Aragona of Naples, a noblewoman who was born in 1503, has found definitive evidence of *Treponema pallidum* in her soft tissues.[49] In short, the earliest and most unambiguous scientific evidence we now have of syphilis in either Europe or the Americas has been found in Europe – but in post-1492 Europe, which has long been known to have been awash in the disease.

For the forseeable future we probably will have no definitive knowledge as to the origins of syphilis, nor – and this is crucial – even if the revised version of the "Columbian hypothesis" withstands scrutiny are we likely to have any sense of how much immunity to venereal syphilis would have been conferred by any pre-existing *non*-venereal treponemal infection in the Americas. As noted earlier, such non-venereal treponemal infections as yaws, pinta, and bejel do not confer much resistance to a large inoculum of venereal syphilis.

Whatever the answers to these questions, however, there seems little doubt that even if epidemic-mitigating treponemal infection of some sort did exist in some parts of the pre-Columbian Americas, it apparently did not exist in other vast areas of the New World, including most of the entire western half of North America. At the very least, then, those areas were susceptible both to the immediate impact of newly-introduced syphilis and to its longer-term undermining of fertility. Indeed, by the late eighteenth century missionaries and other visitors to the West Coast of North America were noting that the Indians were "permeated to the marrow of their bones with venereal disease" and that "most Indian deaths [were] due to syphilis." As the best modern scholar on the subject noted nearly half a century ago, "syphilis among the mission Indians might be described as a totalitarian disease, universally incident."[50]

Regardless of what the ultimate conclusion may be regarding syphilis in other parts of the pre-Columbian Americas, it seems clear that

---

[48] Henry F. Dobyns, "On Issues in Treponemal Epidemiology," *Current Anthropology*, 30 (1989), 342–43; L. W. Harrison, "The Origin of Syphilis," *British Journal of Venereal Diseases*, 35 (1959), 1–7.

[49] Gino Fornaciari et al., "Syphilis in a Renaissance Italian Mummy," *The Lancet*, 9 September, 1989.

[50] Sherburne F. Cook, *The Indian Versus the Spanish Mission* (Berkeley: Ibero-Americana, 1943), 26–27.

gonorrhea found a virgin-soil environment throughout the New World, where it would have done serious damage to the ability of affected populations to recover from the population-destroying ravages of epidemic diseases. There is some debate over tuberculosis as a pre-existing condition among American Indians, as well, although the most substantial evidence for its existence comes from a single study in Peru.[51] Population densities in most of North America would not have been conducive to horizontal transfer of tuberculosis, in any case – at least not until it was introduced in the potent form for which there is documentary evidence of its epidemic fury. On the other hand, there is no doubt that influenza and measles were part of the first wave of diseases that attacked North America, and that smallpox – which reached Hawai'i only 75 years after the islands' initial contact with the West – was the fastest, most devastating, and most widespread plague that Europe unleashed on America's biologically defenseless peoples. And, as we have seen, all these diseases have devastating effects on fertility.

In short, for every disclaimer regarding a disease that undermined the fertility, and thus the population recovery potential, of the Hawaiian people, but may not have so terribly affected the Indians of North America, there is a counter-example of a disease (and its fertility-destroying after-effects) that attacked American Indians, either earlier than or with more ruination than was the case in the islands of Hawai'i.

Beyond the matter of bacteriological damage to fertility and fecundity is the influence of poor nutrition and stress in the early contact histories of Hawai'i and North America. There is no doubt that in both situations traditional types and levels of nutrition were shattered by Western contact, and that stress – in the terrifying face of apparent ongoing genocide – was greater among these native peoples than most modern Americans or Europeans can even imagine. And both nutrition and stress are critical factors in fertility and fecundity.

As for nutrition, body fat as a proportion of total body mass, for example, is essential to the process of sexual maturation and cyclic ovulation; successful pregnancy and lactation require the expenditure of tens of thousands of calories – tens of thousands of calories that often were not available to native women in the epidemic furies that threatened to consume their societies after contact with the West was made.[52]

---

[51] M. J. Allison et al., "Infectious Diseases in Pre-Columbian Inhabitants of Peru," *American Journal of Physical Anthropology*, 41 (1974), 468.

[52] R. E. Frisch and J. W. McArthur, "Menstrual Cycles: Fatness as a Determinant of Minimum Weight for Height Necessary for Their Maintenance and Onset," *Science*, 185

Stress is another critical factor in all this, and it is well to remember that never in their histories had these societies encountered such massively stress-inducing situations as the North American Indians faced in the sixteenth, seventeenth, eighteenth and nineteenth centuries and the Hawaiians faced in the eighteenth and nineteenth centuries alone. Indeed, studies of first-contact situations among Brazilian natives in the 1960s and 1970s show not only disease-induced death rates that one scholar describes as "unmatched elsewhere in recent times outside war zones," but also a virtual collapse in birth rates apparently due largely to social dislocation. The neurohormonal axis that is the key to reproductive behavior in both the female and the male is subject to major disturbance during times of stress. Even today, 40 percent to 50 percent of infertility in First World societies has been attributed to stress or other related emotional concerns, and – society-wide, at least – the stresses of today's world for most people are as nothing compared with the stresses of a people facing biological oblivion.[53]

IV

The best studies of virgin-soil epidemics and their consequences have always been careful to note that what makes these assaults so terrible is that, unlike even the worst single-disease epidemics, including the medieval Black Death, they invariably occur as a complex barrage of separate biological insults, each one making up a single strand in the web of devastation, each one combining with others to reduce any possibility of resistance to the overall invasion. The impact of being attacked by several serious diseases simultaneously is thus synergistic, not merely additive. To cite a simple example, while parainfluenza generally has a minimal common-cold effect on most adults, and measles vaccine can cause slight fevers, in one case in which a parainfluenza epidemic coincided with a measles vaccination program among the Tiriyo Indians,

---

(1974), 949–53; R. E. Frisch, "Body Fat, Puberty, and Fertility," *Biological Review*, **59** (1984), 161–88; Z. M. Van Der Spuy, "Nutrition and Reproduction," *Clinics in Obstetrics and Gynaecology*, **12** (1985), 579–604.

[53] A. V. McGrady, "Effects of Psychological Stress on Male Reproduction," *Archives of Andrology*, **13** (1984), 1–7; M. Seibel and M. Taynor, "Emotional Aspects of Infertility," *Fertility and Sterility*, **37** (1982), 137–45. On low fertility among recently-contacted Brazilian Indians, see R. G. Baruzzi et al., "The Kren-Akorore: A Recently Contacted Indigenous Tribe," in Ciba Foundation Symposium 49 (New Series) *Health and Disease in Tribal Societies* (Amsterdam: Elsevier/Excerpta Medica/North-Holland, 1977), 179–211.

the *combined* effect was overwhelming.[54] Another variation on this is the effect of the consequences of one disease on the virulence of another. Thus, for instance, it has been shown in a Bangladesh study that malnutrition – which can result from disease, especially if an epidemic is community-wide – can at least double the expected mortality rate from diarrheal disease.[55] Still other examples demonstrate the damaging effects of past disease exposures: one research study, for example, has uncovered very severe complications with measles among people with a history of previous respiratory infections.[56]

Because of the uncertainties involved in trans-historical diagnoses, major detailed studies of these phenomena in distantly past settings are usually impossible. But a relatively modern example is instructive. During construction of the Alcan highway in 1942–43 a remote Canadian Indian community made contact with the outside world. Within nine months they came down with nine different infectious diseases – including measles, whooping cough, mumps, tonsillitis, and meningitis – while those who introduced the sicknesses showed no ill-effects. Helicopter airlifts to modern hospitals saved most of those people, but without that intervention (which, of course, was not available to such victims in earlier centuries) there is little doubt, as William McNeill has observed, that that community "would not have survived even a single year of intensified exposure to infections."[57]

As well as being exposed to several diseases at once, when a virgin-soil population is invaded by new diseases everyone in the community is susceptible. Lack of immunity means that everyone gets sick at once, which paralyzes the everyday life of a people; there is no one to draw water, to stoke fires, to provide comfort, to feed infants and children. Many writers believe, with J. V. Neel, who observed this phenomenon among the Yanamama Indians, that the collapse of village life and the

---

[54] J. van Mazijk et al., "Measles and Measles Vaccine in Isolated Amerindian Tribes: The Tiriyo Epidemic," *Tropical and Geographic Medicine*, 34 (1982), 3–6.

[55] S. S. Islam and M. U. Khan, "Risk Factors for Diarrhoeal Deaths: A Case-Control Study at a Diarrhoeal Disease Hospital in Bangladesh," *International Journal of Epidemiology*, 15 (1986), 116–21.

[56] P. Aaby et al., "Severe Measles in Sunderland, 1885: A European-African Comparison of Causes of Severe Infection," *International Journal of Epidemiology*, 15 (1986), 101–07.

[57] William H. McNeill, "Historical Patterns of Migration," *Current Anthropology*, 20 (1979), 96; the original report of this incident was by John F. Marchand, "Tribal Epidemics in the Yukon," *Journal of the American Medical Association*, 23 (1943), 1019–20, and is also discussed in Alfred W. Crosby, Jr., "Virgin Soil Epidemics as a Factor in the Aboriginal Depopulation in America," *William and Mary Quarterly*, 3rd Series, 33 (1976), 289–99.

pervading sense of doom and despair that results, is the major cause of mass death in such cases. The lack of immunity, if Neel is correct, is important primarily as the *precipitating* factor for subsequent calamity, but it is not the main causal agent for the disaster.[58]

Similar phenomena exist regarding assaults on fertility and fecundity. As noted earlier, syphilis and gonorrhea tend to travel together, one destroying the host and (in the case of women) the fetus or newborn child, the other causing PID and sterility. But in broadly non-immune populations, such as the Hawaiians and American Indians, other diseases joined the assault, each compounding the impact of the others both in terms of immediate mortality and subsequent infertility. Moreover, collapsing community life can seriously undermine nutritional levels; and as we have seen, malnutrition is an important factor in female infertility *and* in increasing the susceptibility to and the severity of other opportunistic infections, thus continuing the cycle.

What is true of malnutrition is also true of stress. There is now an enormous body of research knowledge on linkages between the nervous and immune systems, virtually all of it showing how stress, fear, bereavement, depression, despair, and similar conditions can greatly enhance susceptibility to infection, including fertility- and fecundity-threatening infection such as tuberculosis.[59] And this, of course, is in combination with the *direct* impact discussed earlier, of stress on fertility and fecundity.

Thus, in the same way that the disease-malnutrition-stress-disease cycle can have an immediately cataclysmic effect on a newly-contacted, non-immune population, so too can that self-perpetuating chain of events have a ruinous secondary impact on the same peoples' ability to reproduce – a ruinous secondary impact that can continue for generations.

It is clear from the missionary censuses, station reports, and other data that this is what happened in Hawai'i. In little over a century the population fell to barely five percent of its size prior to Western contact. And, while not denying the havoc caused by epidemic and introduced endemic diseases, it is now apparent that the major cause of that great demographic collapse was the induced infertility and high infant mortality rate that prevented any possibility of recovery.

[58] J. V. Neel et al., "Notes on the Effect of Measles and Measles Vaccine in a Virgin-Soil Population of South American Indians," *American Journal of Epidemiology*, 91 (1970), 418–29.

[59] See, for example, Steven E. Locke and Mady Hornig-Rohan, *Mind and Immunity: Behavioral Immunology, An Annotated Bibliography, 1976–1982* (New York: Praeger, 1983).

350   *David E. Stannard*

If a similar phenomenon occurred in North America – and it seems certain that it did, at least in many locales – it becomes not at all difficult to address the problem with which we began, the "problem of explaining how so many people could seemingly disappear so fast." The vast majority of what should have been the native peoples' natural replacements simply were not born – and most of those who were born did not live long enough to reproduce.

14

Creative Disruptions in American Agriculture, 1620–1820

E.L. Jones

"Man is everywhere a disturbing agent . . . ," George Perkins Marsh wrote in 1864 in *Man and Nature,* later republished as *The Earth as Modified by Human Action.* The literature on ecological disturbances accompanying the establishment of agriculture and its intensification is considerable, but it has to be raked out of obscure corners. Indeed, much of the interest in change in the human habitat comes from archeologists and these are mostly prehistorians, for it is prehistorians who have largely preempted archeological techniques. Or at the other end of the scale the interest comes from biologists who, except when their expertise has been enlisted by the archeologists, are chiefly concerned with the more readily traceable developments of recent decades. This has left largely untouched the task of synthesizing the record of ecological change and assessing its feedback to the economy over just those centuries which were formative in the emergence of the advanced western economies: from the middle ages to the nineteenth century. Over that period great ecological and economic difficulties were faced as huge extra-European forests were replaced by farm land growing a narrow range of crops for European markets. The process was one of a sequence of what are called environmental "insults."

The primary aims of this paper are to document the biological pest problems which faced early American farmers; to show how some of the problems arose from the white man's intensification of a process begun by the Indians—destabilizing the forest environment; and to examine the ways, "avoidance" and "creative," in which the problems were countered.[1] Both responses might be termed "adaptive" by anthropolo-

1 Versions of this paper were read at Victoria University, Wellington, and Lincoln Agriculture College, New Zealand, in July 1973. I am grateful for comments from Professors Stan Engerman, John Gould, William Parker, and Nathan Rosenberg and from scientists at research stations in New Zealand and Australia, notably Mr. B. R. G. Woodfield, Director, Keith Turnbull Research Station, Vermin and Noxious Weeds Destruction Board, Victoria.

gists. Here it is hoped to show that while the majority of responses were of the "avoidance" type this reflects less on the ingenuity of farmers than on the inherent complexity of the problems and the level of general scientific development required to solve them. Anyone following the strands that predominate in American agricultural history—the sour tale of slavery and the success stories of the westward movement and nineteenth-century mechanization—might be driven to conclude that as regards biological problems farmers during the first two centuries after settlement were supine, and only coped by dodging the column, that is by migrating to the fresh, fertile lands of the Old Northwest. This was not entirely so, and to the extent that it was there were compelling reasons why biological problems remained intractable.

Nathan Rosenberg has raised the question, why were disequilibria (that is, incongruences between the components of production processes) more fruitful in inspiring and channeling innovation in industries with a machine technology than in agriculture?[2] This is a highly significant problem in view of the relative size of the agricultural sector in the past and the nature of the disequilibria caused by transforming the environment: costly pest eruptions. Rosenberg's answer is that the individual farmer, unlike the manufacturer, is not competent to evaluate such signals in a creative way, so that solutions have had to await the development of "overhead" institutions such as land-grant colleges and specialized sciences like genetics and soil chemistry. William Parker has carried this interpretation to the point of claiming that generalizable innovations in nineteenth-century American agriculture were essentially spin-offs from the engineering industries, whereas improvements in seed selection and plant and livestock breeding were matters peculiar to the farm and could not be patented and marketed as could mechanical contrivances.[3] Parker has, however, shown that nonpecuniary rewards in the competitive small farm society of the northern United States succeeded in inducing locality-wide rather than merely single farm advances in plant and animal breeding.[4] Although the ingenious farmer could not warrant biological materials in the way that he might warrant mechanical devices, and the value of such materials would tend to be specific to soil and season, if he did produce a new crop strain he had

[2] Nathan Rosenberg, "The Directions of Technological Change: Inducement Mechanisms and Focusing Devices," *Economic Development and Cultural Change* 18 (1960); 11–12, note 24.

[3] In L. E. Davis et al., *American Economic Growth: An Economist's History of the United States* (New York: Harper and Row, 1972), 380 ff.

[4] In an earlier unpublished paper, "The Social Process of Agricultural Improvement: Sources, Mechanisms and Effectiveness in the United States in the 19th Century," presented to the Third International Conference of Economic History, Munich, 1965.

some opportunity of selling it widely through the seed houses which emerged in the 1780s. This paper presents evidence of early successes along these lines and in particular observes that the kickback of the transformed environment as evidenced by eruptions of pests did sometimes function as a "focusing device" for technical and institutional responses.

The secondary aim of the paper is to note that early North American agricultural settlement, with its backlash of pest problems, may be usefully seen as one instance of a wider class of changes. In *very* long-term perspective, it was intermediate in a sequence of clearances of middle-latitude forests, taking in Europe 2,000 years or longer, in North America 200 years, and in Australasia (New Zealand and the southeast corner of Australia) 100 years or fewer. Prehistoric migrants had moved with their crops, animals and whole "living entourage" from southwest Asia into the forests of northern temperate Europe. Clearing and taming that environment, for all that it is a gentle one, took a couple of thousand years. New cultivated species were drawn from the East during much of that time while pollen analysis provides some indication of the incorporation of weed problems in the primitive agricultural ecosystems planted in Europe.[5] Repetition of fundamentally the same processes in the temperate forests of eastern America took only a couple of centuries from about 1620. In New Zealand and the forested southeast corner of Australia they took an even shorter time to replicate, since the improvement in ocean shipping made both the deliberate and accidental introduction of species with a potential for becoming pests easier, while the expanded European demand for foodstuffs accelerated agricultural development in the newer new lands. Comparison and contrast may usefully be made between these areas, though here we will deal only with the American case and seek to show from that just how malleable ecosystems have been, but at what cost in pest eruptions.[6]

5 See the contributions by H. Godwin and A. H. Bunting to J. L. Harper, ed., *The Biology of Weeds* (Oxford: Blackwell Scientific Publications, 1960), 8–9, 11–15, and Jacqueline Murray, *The First European Agriculture; A Study of the Osteological and Botanical Evidence until 2,000 B.C.* (Edinburgh: Edinburgh University Press, 1970), 79–82.

6 An earlier attempt to establish this is E. L. Jones, "The Bird Pests of British Agriculture in Recent Centuries," *Agricultural History Review* 20 (1972): 107–25. Estimates of the continuing losses of food to pests are legion. They are too often derived by multiplying potential physical output in the absence of pests by the unit values obtaining in the presence of losses to pests. By assuming unreasonably high elasticities of demand they thus imply that physical loss will be matched by financial loss to the farmer. Nevertheless, the world economic significance of agricultural pests is beyond doubt. For the United States see The President's Science Advisory Committee, *The World Food Problem*, vol. 2 (The White House, May 1967), 205–6 and table 3–3.

To indicate the vegetational change involved in the North American case, it has been estimated that from the Atlantic to the Mississippi and from about the 47th parallel in southern Canada to the coastal plain of the Carolinas there were 431 million forested acres at the start of European settlement where today there are only 19 million acres, or 4.4 percent of the original cover.[7] The agriculture which was planted in the former forest lands was a syncretic ecosystem arrested long before the climax stage of forest and accordingly under severe ecological strain. Its comparative habitat uniformity, with the disruption of the previous ecosystem, made for ecological disharmonies which can be translated into supply-side instabilities in agriculture. There were wounds from deforestation such as soil exhaustion, erosion, and the drying-up of streams, but those which concern us here were the creation of pests, including weeds, defined as species competing with man for the products of his fields. Most agricultural pests are "man made" in the sense that they are opportunist species which take advantage of the special sources of food and breeding sites provided by the growing of single strands of crop plants. In the increasingly homogenous environments developed by agricultural man a few such species multiply to densities of population that they could never attain in less disturbed, less open, more heterogeneous environments with a greater variety of population checks.

Most of the weeds, pathogens, and predators of agricultural landscapes had been rare hangers-on in climax forest, occupying small areas of natural clearings, windblows, river banks, and the like. With a reversion to dense forest many of these species would be closed out and revert to a fugitive status.[8] A dense forest, with a high proportion of mature trees shading out any understory, contains comparatively few other forms of life and has been described by several authors as "biological desert." Even the Indians tended to shun deep forests like the Adirondack wilderness and the few who did not, who were pushed into this

---

[7] James C. Greenway, Jr., *Extinct and Vanishing Birds of the World* (New York: Dover Publications, 1967), 37.

[8] It should be possible to investigate this reversion on the sites of the surprisingly large number of abandoned American towns. An instance as it affected bird populations is cited by Edwin Way Teale, *North With the Spring* (New York: Dodd, Mead & Co., 1963), 319–20. An instance of the resistance of native climax vegetation to penetration by weeds relates to Peacock Prairie, Illinois. This five-acre patch of original prairie has been used agriculturally only once—by light grazing in 1926–1927. A few weed species were found then, but by 1967 they had almost disappeared (see R. F. Betz and M. H. Cole, "The Peacock Prairie—A Study of a Virgin Illinois Mesic Black-Soil Prairie Forty Years after Initial Study," *Transactions of the Illinois State Academy of Science* 62 [1969]: 44–53). Given the hazards of existence for weeds in undisturbed conditions the survival value of their prodigious production and long dormancy of seed is evident.

marginal habitat, were despised by the others as "Bark Eaters."[9] This, however, indicates the nature of the forest in which the majority of the aboriginal inhabitants lived. We will return below to a discussion of the extent to which they had improved its character before the arrival of the Europeans. Forest truly undisturbed by man was opened only by fire and storm, obliging many species of flora and fauna to shift gipsy-like to any new clearing as older natural openings reverted towards climax. Weeds in particular, being the pioneers of secondary succession, were closed out.[10] What European man did was to clear and keep clear much more of the forest than had ever been disturbed before and to bring in unfamiliar species, for example, weeds in the feed for cattle carried on shipboard. Native American herbs were not adapted to cleared ground, but European weeds flourished there. Many of them had originated in treeless or sparsely wooded regions to the east or south and had multiplied in northern Europe only with the woodland clearance there.[11] Since this process was magnified and accelerated in North America the opportunities for these alien species were much increased.

The early European pioneers in American woodlands provided more and more "edge"—the ecotone so important for biological variety—and concluded that the edible mammals and birds along the margins of the forest, among the second-growth saplings and in the Indian clearings, had been the original forest dwellers. "Actually, these animals were a crop," the Milnes have written, "raised inadvertently."[12] The Indians had raised this "crop" deliberately, for their economy depended on mingling farming and hunting rather than farming and the running of domestic stock. As William Wood observed in Massachusetts as early as 1635, wherever there were Indians to burn it there was no undergrowth in the tall forest. The resultant forest was silent by day. Its birds were owls, ravens, eagles, passenger pigeons, and the Carolina parakeet, all of them uncommon or even extinct now that so much deforestation has taken place.[13] The songbirds common today were confined to its fringes,

9 Hugh Fosburgh, *A Clearing in the Wilderness* (Garden City, N.Y.: Doubleday & Co., 1960), 9–10.

10 According to Charles Elton, *The Ecology of Invasions by Animals and Plants* (London: Methuen, 1958), 75, no foreign birds except game birds have penetrated American forests.

11 L. J. King, *Weeds of the World: Biology and Control* (London: Leonard Hill, 1966), 14; Harper, ed., *Biology of the Weeds*, 8–9, 11–15.

12 Lorus J. and Margery Milne, *The Balance of Nature* (New York: Alfred A. Knopf, 1960), 219.

13 Marston Bates, *The Forest and the Sea: A Look at the Economy of Nature and the Ecology of Man* (New York: Random House, 1960), 118. Greenway, *Extinct and Vanishing Birds*, 39–40, gives estimates of the land acreage per capita since the eighteenth and nineteenth centuries in relation to the disappearance of certain birds from various states.

the coast, river valleys, and occasional patches of grass or scrub. As one authority observes, "Fully 100 species of North American birds cannot live under climax-forest conditions," while another states, "Today it is probably safe to say that for every land bird that is less abundant than it was when the Pilgrims landed, five or six are more abundant."[14] The altered proportions of deep forest and ecotone bird species are a proxy for all the faunistic and floristic effects of the land use changes wrought by the white man.

While European settlers in the eastern woodlands of North America did produce massive ecological change, they had not found the forest in a universally primeval state. Even stretches which were unoccupied at the moment of white entry had often been modified by aboriginal land use. Indian clearing for farming and hunting and selective pressures on fruit, nut, and medicinal plants had altered the original forest. Abandoned Indian fields and repeated firing of the forest by the Indians to create new cornfields and keep up a supply of herbs and browse attractive to deer had inadvertently created ecological conditions favorable to the entry of white farmers. It has been claimed that it would have taken a generation of settlers to produce the extent of clearings which they found ready-made.[15] The Algonquins of New England had been reduced by smallpox just before the initial white settlement, which eased the takeover of their clearings, but elsewhere it was competition for the same Indian-made openings that brought whites and Indians into early conflict, though both were such low density populations.[16]

14 Teale, *North with the Spring*, 104; Richard H. Pough, *Audubon Land Bird Guide* (Garden City, N.Y.: Doubleday and Co., 1946), xxvii, and passim for observations on individual species.

15 Lyman Carrier, *The Beginnings of Agriculture in America* (New York: McGraw-Hill Book Co., 1923), 38. Descriptions of early settlement still sometimes imply that it took place in a primeval forest, which underscores Day's recommendation of twenty years ago that, "a knowledge of local archeology and history should be part of the ecologist's equipment" (G. M. Day, "The Indian as an Ecological Factor in the Northeastern Forest," *Ecology* 34 [1953]: 343).

16 Merle C. Prunty, "Some Geographic Views of the Rôle of Fire in Settlement Processes in the South," *Proceedings, Annual Tall Timbers Fire Ecology Conference*, 4 (1965): 165, 167. On the ecological effects of the Indians in creating openings, reducing fire-sensitive species (especially the understory), encouraging sprout hardwoods, and bringing crop plants from south to north, see the following examples from an extensive literature which is more precise about tribal and regional differences in the Indian impact than it is possible to be here: M. K. Bennett, "The Food Economy of the New England Indians, 1605–1675," *Journal of Political Economy* 62 (1955): 369–97; James C. Bonner, *A History of Georgia Agriculture, 1732–1860* (Athens: University of Georgia Press, 1964), 23; Day, "The Indian as an Ecological Factor," 343; Joseph A. Miller, "The Changing Forest: Recent Research in the Historical Geography of American Forests," *Forest History* 9 (1965): 18–25; W. A. Niering and R. H. Goodwin, "Ecological Studies in the Connecticut Arboretum Natural Area,

There were hundreds of Indian villages in New England, New York, and New Jersey, some of them on semipermanent sites with up to 150 acres cleared for crops and larger cleared areas for hunting, notably behind Narragansett Bay and south of the Pennsylvania-Maryland line. The villages were usually moved every ten to fifteen years, when the squaws could no longer gather firewood—even live from the tree—within walking distance, or for other reasons not necessarily connected with the falling-off of soil fertility that one associates with shifting cultivation. The Indians knew how to keep up the fertility of their land by manuring their corn hills with fish. The Iroquois in particular had many large cornfields and numbers of fruit trees planted about their villages. Well-watered or easily defended sites were reoccupied at intervals and the resultant frequency of cultivation kept some areas almost permanently clear of timber. Some other sites were reverting to pineries when the whites occupied them. The Indian practice of burning the forest understory increased the availability of green shoots from old stumps or young saplings on which deer, the heath hen, passenger pigeon, and wild turkey liked to feed, so that a hunting resource dissimilar to that of a dense, uninhabited forest had been brought into being.

Corn rather than game was the true mainstay of the Indian. Corn cultivation, though it could take place among the girdled stumps of forest trees and did not strictly need the clear-felled fields that European settlers were used to, produced a bitter foretaste of the pest problems the whites were to bring so much more heavily onto their own heads.[17] Early accounts and ethnobotanical studies show that Indian farming spread some weed species by opening the land for crops, and suffered scourges of caterpillars, while cutworms were troublesome in freshly broken ground. Birds, especially crows and "blackbirds" (presumably including grackles and redwings) took a heavy toll, notably of sown seed. A very high sowing rate was required to offset this—i.e., seed-yield ratios were increased—and deep sowing was necessary. Scarecrows were

I. Introduction and Survey of Vegetation Types," *Ecology* 43 (1962): 52; Carl Sauer, "The Settlement of the Humid East," in USDA Yearbook of Agriculture 1941, *Climate and Man* (Washington: GPO, 1941), 161; W. L. Thomas, ed., *Man's Rôle in Changing the Face of the Earth* (Chicago: University of Chicago Press, 1956), 1: 413–14; and R. R. Walcott, "Husbandry in Colonial New England," *New England Quarterly* 9 (1936): 220.

17 Bennett, "The Food Economy of the New England Indians," 386; Carrier, *Beginnings of Agriculture in America*, 94–95, 99; S. W. Fletcher, *Pennsylvania Agriculture and Country Life, 1640–1840* (Harrisburg: Pennsylvania Historical and Museums Commission, 1950), 36; U. P. Hedrick, *A History of Horticulture in America to 1860* (New York: Oxford University Press, 1950), 22; King, *Weeds of the World*, 14; and Daniel K. Onion, "Corn in the Culture of the Mohawk Iroquois," *Economy Botany* 18 (1964): 62.

used and cylindrical whistles were suspended from poles, to be blown by the wind. The usual preventive was a watchhouse on a platform in the fields, occupied from the early hours by squaws and children. Indian youths constantly warred against predators on the corn. This can be looked on as the energy subsidy needed to keep the artificial ecosystem even of Indian farming at a satisfactory level of yield. Deadfalls and snares were used to catch raccoons, woodchucks, and muskrats. Nooses and snares were attached to bent-over saplings and scattered over with grains of corn, and birds caught in them were left hanging to discourage others. Northern tribes kept tame hawks to keep small birds off the corn-fields, but few Indians would kill crows because of a legend that a crow had brought them the first corn seed. The legend perhaps encapsulates the history of the diffusion of corn and other crop plants from central America. The Mohawk Iroquois did take young crows and hang them alive by their feed *pour encourager les autres*. Perhaps they were especially successful as farmers because of this and other manifestations of pragmatism. Otherwise the Indians had only incantations to employ against predators attracted by their corn plots.[18]

The white settlers' fields and livestock increased feeding opportunities, and predators clustered about them in greater numbers.[19] The first bounty on the gray wolf was posted ten years after the Pilgrims landed, because the wolves attacked farm animals and dug up and ate the alewives planted in the corn hills during the fourteen days before the fish turned rotten.[20] Soon all the colonies set bounties and in 1705 a special bounty was offered to professional wolf hunters in Pennsylvania.[21] The wolf problem was severe enough for prohibitions on supplying guns to the Indians to be violated to induce them to shoot wolves—for half the bounty payable to "Christians."[22] Bounties were placed on the heads of other mammals which preyed on livestock: bears (which specialized in hogs), cougars and panthers (which attacked cattle), and foxes and wildcats (which took poultry).

In early days cornfields had to have fences seven feet high against deer

---

[18] The white man resorted to public incantations against locusts and cotton caterpillars as late as the nineteenth century (L. O. Howard, *The Insect Menace* [New York: The Century Co., 1931], 209). Apart from an initial lack of firearms, Indian bird-scaring was as advanced in technique as that of whites into the twentieth century, and probably more skilled.

[19] See R. G. Lillard, *The Great Forest* (New York: Alfred A. Knopf, 1948), 75–76.

[20] Walcott, "Husbandry in Colonial New England," 229.

[21] Peter Matthiessen, *Wildlife in America* (New York: The Viking Press, 1959), 57–58; Carrier, *Beginnings of Agriculture in America*, 144; Fletcher, *Pennsylvania Agriculture*, 72.

[22] Carrier, *Beginnings of Agriculture in America*, 134–35.

and roving cattle. Farmers walked their dogs round at night against rodents and during the first stages of a crop in the daytime, too, against wild turkeys and crows.[23] With white settlement came the brown rat, house mouse, and black rat, to list them in order of destructiveness to stored grain though not in order of arrival. These rodents demanded constant control measures with domestic dogs and cats.[24]

There seemed no way to protect field crops from the depredations of gray squirrels and raccoons. Every seven or eight years, whenever acorn and nut fructification failed in the central and northern counties of Pennsylvania, squirrels erupted in armies of thousands to the southeast, laying waste the grainfields on their line of march. Squirrels seemed to become more numerous with white settlement because farm crops increased their food supply. The General Assembly of Pennsylvania permitted the counties to offer a bounty of 3d/head and in 1749 £8,000 was spent in the state for 640,000 squirrels. This exhausted the treasury in some counties and farmers also protested that the bounty was inducing labor to leave the farms to hunt squirrels. The next year the bounty was therefore cut to 1½d/head.[25] In 1784 squirrels so harmed grain in southwest Pennsylvania that a special levy was raised for bounty money. So the warfare went on.[26] Pennsylvanian examples can be matched from Maryland (where the law required inhabitants to present the heads of four squirrels per annum to local officers), Virginia, and when those states were settled, Indiana and Missouri. Farmers in all these states were plagued by hordes of migrating squirrels and the best they could do was to send delegates to meetings to plan enormous shooting drives.[27]

Bounty laws sometimes coupled squirrels and crows, which brings us to bird damage. In 1700 a Pennsylvania act referred to damage done to grain by crows, bountied at 3d/head, and "blackbirds," bountied at 3d/dozen. Crows, it seems, came in only when the forest had been hollowed out with grainfields. In Michigan in the earliest years of settlement there were no crows to steal the corn and no house mice or house flies—a nice indication of how dependent on agricultural man these species were.[28] Pehr Kalm reported on Benjamin Franklin's authority that the increased number of grackles in New England—they are ground feeders which would have been favored by deforestation—caused a

---

23 Bonner, *History of Georgia Agriculture*, 20.
24 R. A. Caras, *North American Mammals* (New York: Meredith Press, 1967), 351.
25 Matthiessen, *Wildlife in America*, 201.
26 Fletcher, *Pennsylvania Agriculture*, 73–75.
27 Lillard, *The Great Forest*, 76.
28 John Bakeless, *The Eyes of Discovery: The Pageant of North America as seen by the First Explorers* (New York: Dover Publications, 1961), 273; R. C. Buley, *The Old Northwest: Pioneer Period 1815–1840* (Bloomington: Indiana University Press, 1950), 2: 95.

bounty to be set on them. This was said to have been effective in curbing them, so much so that in the summer of 1749 unprecedented numbers of worms in the New England meadows ate up the grass. Hay actually had to be imported from Pennsylvania, reversing opinion in favor of the grackle, which was known to consume worms as well as grain.[29]

The most dramatic cause of loss from birds was from the unpredictable movements of uncountable flocks of passenger pigeons, which descended on the grainfields. They beat down the grain round Massachusetts villages as early as 1642 and into the nineteenth century they sometimes consumed so much mast (beechnuts, acorns, and chestnuts) that settlers' hogs literally starved to death. Powder and shot could not always be spared to fend off so numerous a species and clappers were devised for boys to bang. All the farm population could do was to disperse the pest over everyone's fields.[30]

Many of the control measures adopted against these and other bird pests must have been no more than "rat farming," that is, killing only a proportion of the population with the result that the survivors were able to use good breeding sites and extra food to build up their numbers quickly again. Some crops must, however, have been saved at critical seasons, and the measures may have played a part in making the passenger pigeon extinct and the Carolina parakeet virtually so. What seems certain is that the problem of mammal and bird pests gave rise to no new technology. The exception to the rule may have been the first underground seeder, built in 1860 by Van Brunt at Horicon, Wisconsin, in response to farmers' requests for a way to stop passenger pigeons eating the grain as fast as it was sown.[31]

European settlers modified the environment so as to favor the plants of open country and brought in many aggressive species of just that sort. In 1672 John Josselyn listed twenty-two plants which "have sprung up since the English planted and kept Cattle in New England," many of them being identified by his nineteenth-century editor as European weeds. Perhaps the most interesting was the plantain, which the Indians

[29] Henry Savage, Jr., *Lost Heritage: Wilderness America through the Eyes of Seven Pre-Audubon Naturalists* (New York: William Morrow and Co., 1970), 288. Possibly Fletcher's observation (*Pennsylvania Agriculture*, 75) that after 1750 blackbirds ceased to be very destructive whereas crows remained a major pest derives from this altered perspective.

[30] J. H. St. John Crèvecoeur, *Letters from an American Farmer* (New York: Dolphin Books, n.d., rpt. of 1782 edition), 38; F. E. Crawford, *The Life and Times of Oramel Crawford: A Vermont Farmer 1809–1888* (privately printed, 1952), 25; A. W. Schorger, *The Passenger Pigeon: Its Natural History and Extinction* (Madison: University of Wisconsin Press, 1955), 51–53; Bakeless, *Eyes of Discovery*, 307; Walcott, "Husbandry in Colonial New England," 234; and Savage, *Lost Heritage*, 83.

[31] Schorger, *The Passenger Pigeon*, 52.

called "Englishman's foot" because it grew wherever the white man walked. Josselyn's editor drew attention to several northern European languages which indicate by the name they give it that the plantain grows where man treads—that it is a plant of artificially barren, beaten soil.[32] The prime characteristic of weeds like this is their adaptation to disturbed or open habitats where climax forest or grassland has been destroyed.

New England wheat was reported in 1750 to be "full of cockle," a weed with seeds that are difficult to separate from wheat grains.[33] Cockle seeds were injurious to flour but because the plant is a pink it is conspicuous and if there is enough labor it can be hand-pulled. According to Jared Eliot other weeds that harmed New England agriculture in the mid-eighteenth century included Stinkweed, which grew in wet meadows. When this was hayed with the grass animals ate it freely and as a result mares, cows, and ewes suffered from abortion. Draining the land was necessary to clear out Stinkweed. Another weed of the grass crop was Saint-John's-wort, a European import which when cut and carried with the grass produced hay that no beasts would eat. It could only be controlled by putting sheep in early in the spring for two years, that is by a not insignificant and conceivably most inconvenient change of management practice. Saint-John's-wort was also reported as a weed in Pennsylvania in 1793, while Kalm had found many of the common weeds of Europe established in New York and New Jersey in 1750.[34] From New England Eliot reported what was probably couch grass as strangling the corn and charlock (called "terrify") as very difficult to eradicate.[35] He understood well enough that weeds competed with crops for nutrients and that plowing could stir up weed seeds that had lain dormant in the soil for years, but the only known means of keeping weeds down was labor-intensive cultivation, pulling, and hoeing.

Plant disease was a more dramatic problem. The "blasting" of wheat was noticed in Massachusetts and Connecticut as early as 1664.[36] The

32 Edward Tuckerman, ed., *John Josselyn, Gent. New England's Rarities Discovered* in *Transactions and Collections of the American Antiquarian Society* 4 (1860); 105–238.

33 Carrier, *Beginnings of Agriculture in America*, 150. Winnowing selects for weed seeds closest in size and weight to those of the host crop.

34 King, *Weeds of the World*, 413–14; Teale, *North with the Spring*, 311.

35 H. J. Carmen and R. G. Tugwell, eds., *Essays Upon Field Husbandry in New England and Other Papers 1748–1762 by Jared Eliot* (New York: Columbia University Press, 1934), 94, 105–6.

36 Carrier, *Beginnings of Agriculture in America*, 147, 150, 185. It was common throughout southeastern Pennsylvania by 1700 (Fletcher, *Pennsylvania Agriculture*, 146).

"blast" was the black stem rust of wheat, a fungal disease which has the barberry as its alternative host. The barberry had been spread from the Middle East to Sicily, through Europe and to North America, because its berries were good for jams and jellies. Its fungal parasite came too. In 1680 and 1685 days of prayer against the "blast" were ordained, apparently without effect, for grain was not available for export from New England after the 1680s. John Winthrop had been unsure whether the hazard was natural or a punishment from heaven for sin.[37] By 1750 it was said that some men thought that the blast "proceeds" from the *farina fecundans* (pollen) of barberry bushes adjacent to wheat fields. This was an astute observation, though incorrect. "Scientists" continued to scorn the connection, yet in 1660 France had passed a law based on a similar hypothesis, requiring the eradication of barberry. Peasants near Rouen had noticed their wheat suffered from rust whenever nearby barberry bushes broke out with small, dark yellow scabs on their leaves. Millions of barberry bushes had been uprooted and losses from rust had apparently been reduced.[38] A similar law was passed in Connecticut in 1726, authorizing townships to eradicate barberry bushes. Another was enacted in Massachusetts in 1754, "to prevent damage to English grain [as the small grains were called] from barberry bushes in the vicinity of grain fields." These laws had no penalties attached and their effect is uncertain. A Rhode Island law of 1772 did order a fine for non-compliance but one would guess that the results were not so well broadcast from that tiny colony or not so unequivocal as to produce voluntary compliance elsewhere. Indeed a debate about the barberry-wheat connection continued to this century. Unlike France central government was for long not strong enough in America to exercise compulsion on the basis of a shrewd hunch.

If no new technology was devised by American farmers to cope with this plant disease it was because there simply was no effective technology to be devised, even with the scientific understanding of the twentieth century. In 1916 a wheat rust epidemic destroyed 300 million bushels of wheat in the United States and Canada. Rust-resistant wheats were substituted, but new rust races soon appeared, for example, a wheat strain new in 1926 carried a new rust strain by 1928, which caused a rust epidemic in 1935, necessitating the breeding of still newer resistant wheats. New rust races continued to be observed on barberry and one exploded in 1950 and 1951, ruining varieties of wheat which had been

[37] C. C. Spence, *The Sinews of American Capitalism* (New York: Hill and Wang, 1964), 14.
[38] G. L. Carefoot and E. R. Sprott, *Famine on the Wind: Plant Diseases and Human History* (London: Angus & Robertson, 1969), 49–50.

immune for almost a decade.[39] An eradication program had already destroyed 500 million barberry bushes in the United States at an estimated saving to farmers of over $300 million a year.[40] It is hardly surprising that earlier attempts to control other bacterial and fungal crop diseases (orchard crops were particularly hard hit from the late eighteenth century) were futile. The empiricism that uncovered a partial means of controlling black stem rust by extirpating its alternative host plant could seldom be repeated. Early American farmers can hardly be thought unresponsive because their efforts spawned no new technologies where fundamental scientific relationships have proved so difficult to determine.

Insect damage was still more visible. The first settlers learned of the "burned places" eaten by grasshoppers, hordes of which attacked crops in Massachusetts. The colonists swept vast numbers into the sea with brooms.[41] Less spectacular insects like wireworms probably did more real damage, though it is not always clear what species are referred to in the numerous, but spasmodic, early accounts of infestations. The Angoumis grain moth, the "cotton worm" moth, and the chinch bug are species identified as serious agricultural pests in the eighteenth century.[42] The Angoumis grain moth, originally from Central America, was injuring grain as early as 1728. Caterpillars of the "cotton worm" moth, a migrant from northern South America, did really serious damage by eating the leaves of the cotton plant in 1783, 1804, 1825 and at fairly regular twenty-one- or twenty-two-year intervals thereafter. The chinch bug, a native species, was first noticed ravaging the wheat crop toward the end of the eighteenth century and there were bad outbreaks during the next century. In earlier times annual grass fires had possibly kept this species in check since it hibernates in ground vegetation or any vegetable rubbish. Control methods in use in the twentieth century included burning all rubbish in the fields and the vegetation of waste land, and the extraordinarily cumbersome practice of planting trap or decoy crops and plowing them under. Beyond learning the life cycle of the insect well enough to develop such management practices there was no obvious method of technological control which early farmers might be accused of neglecting to develop.

39 M. T. Farrar and J. P. Milton, eds., *The Careless Technology; Ecology and International Development* (Garden City, N.Y.: The Natural History Press, 1972), 643.

40 King, *Weeds of the World*, 96.

41 W. Barker, *Familiar Insects of America* (New York: Harper & Bros., 1960), 3–4.

42 C. B. Williams, *Insect Migration* (London: Collins, 1950), 72, 162; P. T. Dondlinger, *The Book of Wheat: An Economic History and Practical Manual of the Wheat Industry* (New York: Orange Judd Co., 1912), 174–75.

Much the best-reported injurious insect in the period under review was the Hessian fly. Its depredations were heavy and evoked interesting responses. Wheat is the natural food plant of the Hessian fly—both originated from Asia—the eggs being laid on the leaves, the larvae entering the stems and in an early attack preventing tillering. In a later attack some stalks might remain standing while others fell to the ground. The only remedies were the "avoidance" measures of sowing decoy crops and plowing them in, destroying volunteer crops, and staggering the sowing of the intended crop.[43] Similar ecological or management measures are still usual. Science has provided few safe, cheap, persistent, species-specific magic wands (poisons, diseases) to use in dealing with farm pests.

Many otherwise sober sources claim that the Hessian fly (and the brown rat) arrived with the Hessian mercenaries in 1776. In reality the Hessian fly was troubling farmers in New York and New Jersey before the Revolution and the American Philosophical Society is said to have debated the problem in 1768.[44] The species did great harm to wheat in Staten and Long Islands in 1776 and then spread in directions which have been traced in some detail. Much wheat was destroyed in New York and the Middle Atlantic states during the remainder of the eighteenth century. In 1788 Great Britain forbade the import of American wheat in an effort to keep out the pest. By the 1790s farmers in Chester County, Pennsylvania, abandoned the unequal struggle to grow wheat and turned to producing poultry, butter, and cattle.[45] The Hessian fly first appeared west of the Alleghenies in 1797. It continued to be very damaging in intermittent spells of years.[46]

Farmers hardly lay supine when their wheat was attacked. In 1787 a Connecticut gentleman farmer named Jeremiah Wadsworth asked his cousin to investigate a method of immunizing wheat by steeping the seed in an elder solution. Since, on the face of it, steeping did seem to offer protection against the Hessian fly, Wadsworth reported the method in the *Connecticut Courant*. Shortly afterwards the *American Mercury* announced that farmers throughout Connecticut who had planted bearded wheat all agreed that it resisted the fly. Wadsworth at once bought bearded wheat seed in New York City. Searches for a conclusive remedy however continued. In 1794 Wadsworth heard from a Virginia senator of a new "forward wheat" recently produced in Caroline County, Virginia. This was a dwarf, high-yielding wheat that

[43] Dondlinger, *The Book of Wheat*, 171–73.
[44] Fletcher, *Pennsylvania Agriculture*, 147.
[45] Ibid., 202.
[46] H. Y. Hind, *Essay on the Insects and Diseases Injurious to the Wheat Crops* (Toronto: Lovell & Gibson, 1857), 42–43.

matured twenty days before other varieties and therefore escaped the worst fly damage, as well as seeming to be safe from rust. The *American Mercury* published the results of two years' comparative field experiments and in 1795 Wadsworth went into partnership with two Hartford merchants to import 2,500 bushels of the "forward wheat" seed. This did well and its success provoked enough interest in agricultural improvements for the founding in 1797 of a "Society for the Promotion of Agriculture in the County of Hartford."[47] Given the scant and scrappy nature of the present literature on creative responses to pest problems we may expect that further research will uncover more like this. We may anticipate that agricultural societies and journals often owed their origins in large measure to the "focusing device" of highly visible pest problems, and that their investigations led on to serious work in agricultural science. As an illustration, the start of agricultural entomology in America is dated from the publication in the *Medical Repository* at New York City from 1797 to 1824 of papers on insect depredations and their supposed remedies.[48]

The eastern woodlands of North America were biologically inferior to Northwest Europe only in the low nutritive quality of their grasses. For an agrarian economy this was, however, a crucial weakness. Some native species grew coarse and hard and almost none could withstand trampling and grazing. The annuals, of which wild rye and broomstraw were the commonest, died off if grazed because they had no time to seed. The perennials had crowns too delicate to endure grazing.[49] The lack of "nutritive vertue" in the grasses was quickly perceived; free range cattle had to browse twigs and often starved to death in the first or second winter of a new settlement, or died from eating poisonous herbage; sheep fared badly unless cattle or horses were put in first to eat down the coarsest vegetation; early emigrants to America were advised to take plenty of clover seed.[50]

By the middle of the seventeenth century introduced English grasses had improved New England pasturage. Sown here and there they spread

47 C. M. Destler, "The Gentleman Farmer and the New Agriculture: Jeremiah Wadsworth," in Darwin P. Kelsey, ed., *Farming in the New Nation—Interpreting American Agriculture, 1790–1840* (Washington: The Agricultural History Society, 1972), 141, 145–47.

48 Hedrick, *History of Horticulture in America*, 494. This journal was also concerned with crop diseases. The *Transactions of the Society for the Promotion of Useful Arts in the State of New York* (from 1806) contain articles on the prevention of smut and weevils in wheat, the killing of sheep by wolves, and similar problems.

49 Sauer, "The Settlement of the Humid East," 159–60, 164.

50 Walcott, "Husbandry in Colonial New England," passim; Henry David Thoreau, *The Concord and the Merrimack* (New York: Bramhall House, 1954), 11; Carrier, *Beginnings of Agriculture in America*, 147; Fletcher, *Pennsylvania Agriculture*, 174.

on by themselves, replacing native species. White clover spread ahead of settlement. English grasses would not, however, grow from Virginia southwards, where there was no true winter period, so that although there was an enormous production of free range cattle in the south it was difficult to fatten animals there. In the eighteenth century pastures were overstocked and deteriorating in Pennsylvania and New Jersey. Before 1750 farmers in Pennsylvania and a few in New England had begun the catchwork irrigation of meadows, but until after the Revolution it was said that travelers' horses could often not be baited in winter in Pennsylvania. By report, New England and Middle Colonies farmland was suffering from soil exhaustion. However, in the 1780s the first seed house was founded in Philadelphia, and seed of a single species became available when Dutch fanning mills came into use after 1785 (rather than "hay dust," unwinnowed chaff from about the stacks, including several perennial species from England plus English weeds).[51] By the late eighteenth century upland meadows were seeded with grass as an alternative to tumble-down fallow and the spread of clover and cultivated grasses was supplying enough hay by 1800 to reduce the value of water meadow, as had happened only a century earlier in England.[52]

The literature on the introduction of European cultivated grasses to North America is too voluminous to be summarized here. What needs to be stressed is that the paucity and vulnerability of the native herb layer as a basis for livestock production (remember, the Indians kept no grazing stock) initiated a search for substitutes. It was the exchange of the seed of forage crops, including grasses, which more than anything was responsible for the close European contacts of early American agricultural "improvers." By 1820 clover seed had become a trade item within the United States—from New York and eastern Pennsylvania.[53] Although the center of grass seed production thereafter moved into the Ohio valley, the emphasis on forage improvement to feed cattle for dung to restore soil fertility probably waned as the occupation of trans-Appalachian lands reduced the return to land-saving innovations.[54] But there is no explanation here for the fewness of eighteenth-century

51 USDA, *Climate and Man*, 21; Fletcher, *Pennsylvania Agriculture*, 154. Even haydust, of course, gave better pasturage than native grasses.

52 See E. L. Jones, "English and European Agricultural Development, 1650–1750," in R. M. Hartwell, ed., *The Industrial Revolution* (Oxford: Basil Blackwell, 1970).

53 Fletcher, *Pennsylvania Agriculture*, 131.

54 In this connection it is interesting to find the following counterfactual hypothesis in an early nineteenth-century *Farmer's Register* 5: 127–28: "If there had been no western country . . . Virginia would already have reached a high state of agricultural improvement." Quoted by A. O. Craven, "Soil Exhaustion as a Factor in the Agricultural History of Virginia and Maryland, 1606–1860," *University of Illinois Studies in the Social Sciences* 13 (1925): 124.

changes in agricultural technique. Until the end of that century American farmers could hardly cross the mountains; they were ponded up to the East. Rather than leave their problems behind by moving on they were obliged to cope with them as best they could; for example, by the development of European-style forage cropping in New York, Pennsylvania, New Jersey, Delaware, and Virginia.[55] By their attention to pasture improvement early American farmers demonstrated a potential for responding creatively to the signals which environmental conditions sent them. With pest problems the responses were rather more seldom "creative." The reasons lie not in a substitute for control methods in the form of cheap western land, nor a refusal to notice symptoms of environmental disturbance, nor the inability of the farmer or small groups of farmers to internalize the returns to research. We have indicated the tip of the iceberg of "research" activity by farmers—a temporary solution to the problem on one farm, a slight lead over other neighborhoods (never mind that the solution might be swiftly copied), was sufficient to induce it from hard-pressed, ingenious, even altruistic or patriotic men. The deeper reason for the fewness of creative responses lies in the sheer intractability of biological science, even in the face of massive twentieth-century research investments.

There are few neat, universally applicable solutions to the biological problems of agriculture. The strain imposed by arresting vegetation in a subclimax stage means that the farm is a perpetual battlefield on which the tactics of altering crop mixes and management practices have remained to this day equally or more effective than deploying new technologies. *Naturam expellas furca, tamen usque recurret.* The only final solution would be the extinction of a pest species, as with the passenger pigeon, but that is very rare and may merely allow competitors to take its place. Early American farmers could obliterate or control very few of the myriad organisms around them. Their weaponry was virtually neolithic: traps, nets, and missiles.

Only from World War II has the somewhat double-edged chemistry of herbicides and pesticides been added to the arsenal. Even in regions as advanced as Europe, North America, and Australasia some pests continue to be dealt with by methods literally no more sophisticated than shaking bugs from the branches of fruit trees into jars of water. Ecological problems are situationally conditioned. They often require a far wider, yet more precise, understanding than the internal deductive logic governing mechanics. The mechanization of agriculture may

[55] Carrier, *Beginnings of Agriculture in America*, 271, and E. L. Jones, *Agriculture & Economic Growth in England, 1650–1815* (London: Methuen, 1967), 47–48.

actually create additional problems in biology; for example, the need to select or breed for sturdy, uniform stands of crops which harvesting machines can handle—uniform stands are a prime habitat for unwanted opportunists, pests.

Scientific problems may perhaps be visualized as ranged along a scale of tractability from, say, engineering to genetics, according to the complexity of the underlying mathematics and the arrangement of religious taboos concerning what may be studied. The sequence of invention may not have been able to follow what "research" investment shows was the order of expected benefits. Thus the chronology of technological change may have to be explained not merely in economic terms but with an eye on the history of thought and the history of science. Creative responses to the biological problems of agriculture were exceptionally difficult because the relevant scientific pool was so shallow. Yet avoidance responses were costly. They involved growing trap crops, and sowing a mixture of crops to insure against pest losses, thereby foregoing the economies of scale from monoculture or near-monoculture.

The negative externalities (neighborhood effects) of weeds and vermin spreading from one man's farm to the next would offer some inducement to cooperate to counteract them. This had been evident in common-field agriculture. Although American farmers soon became more widely spaced the intensity of the pest eruptions caused by their clearing of the forest offered them equivalent inducements to cooperate. This does not explain why they, and western men in general, were so responsive, but we can observe the phenomenon here. They made ring shoots of vermin a social event, an aspect of the cohesion of a scattered rural population.

There was no special technological spin-off from a communal shooting party of the eighteenth century, but we have seen that some other responses to pest problems were truly creative. Thus pest problems could parallel the disequilibria that Nathan Rosenberg finds were a focusing device for inventive activity in manufacturing. Differences in inventive success may be accounted for by the differences in tractability which have been mentioned. We should have no difficulty in seeing the responsiveness to specific biological problems in agriculture as one term in the supply function for agricultural invention and innovation, even in the period covered by this paper, a period which ends once American borrowings from foreign agricultures were institutionalized in 1819. The Secretary of the Treasury then required all consuls to send home plant material at the public expense.[56]

[56] A. C. True, *A History of Agricultural Experimentation and Research in the United States 1607–1925*, USDA Miscellaneous Publication 251 (New York: Johnson

In the new lands annexed by Europe in North America and Australasia environmental change was rapid and destabilizing. It faced farmers with challenges and emergencies. Their responses helped to account for the development of agricultural science and research institutions in the western world. Many of the resultant discoveries could be shared among these lands and with Europe, since there were basic similarities in all their ecosystems due partly to the original temperate forest biome and partly to shared produce markets, common farming stock, and transplanted farm crops and animals, weeds, and vermin. The tropical agricultures of the Third World were different and although their problems of pest infestation were and are of great economic significance, especially for plantation crops, they have required a different outgrowth of agricultural science from the rootstock of temperate zone biology.

The broader question of why creative, technological responses in early American agriculture, though weak by later standards, were so impressive by those of (say) medieval England[57] would require a history of the increased flow of ideas and expanded markets throughout the western world between the middle ages and the nineteenth century. The present goal has been more modest: to show that early American farmers were capable of a creative response to environmental problems where this was remotely feasible. This was a foretaste of western man's ability to keep matching the surprise counterattacks of "insulted" ecosystems. The long process of taming the rather gentle environment of northwest Europe bred complacency; success in transferring European agriculture to North America bred optimism. In these circumstances the casualness of the later onslaught on the southern hemisphere should not appear surprising.

Reprint Corporation, 1970), 22. This action opened the way for agents of biological control (i.e., the predators and parasites of existing pests) to be sought overseas. The founding of societies and publications and the incipient development of agricultural science in America three-quarters of the way through the eighteenth century influenced the public authorities and helped to spawn the second generation of tax-supported R & D institutions midway through the nineteenth century.

57 On this see M. M. Postan, The Medieval Economy and Society (Berkeley and Los Angeles: University of California Press, 1972), 42 ff.

15

Europe's Initial Population Explosion

William L. Langer

THE use of the dramatic term "explosion" in discussions of the present-day population problem may serve to attract attention and underline the gravity of the situation, but it is obviously a misnomer. The growth of population is never actually explosive, and as for the current spectacular increase, it is really only the latest phase of a development that goes back to the mid-eighteenth century.

Prior to that time the history of European population had been one of slow and fitful growth. It now took a sudden spurt and thenceforth continued to increase at a high rate. From an estimated 140,000,000 in 1750 it rose to 188,000,000 in 1800, to 266,000,000 in 1850, and eventually to 400,000,000 in 1900. The rate of increase was not uniform for all parts of the Continent, but it was everywhere strikingly high. Even in Spain, where there had been a remarkable loss of population in the seventeenth century, the population grew from 6,100,000 in 1725 to 10,400,000 in 1787 and 12,300,000 in 1833.[1]

This tremendous change in terms of European society has received far less attention from historians than it deserves. In the early nineteenth century it troubled the Reverend Thomas Malthus and precipitated a formidable controversy over the problem of overpopulation and the possible remedies therefor. But the discussion remained inconclusive until reopened in more recent times by British scholars, making use of the rather voluminous English records and directing their attention almost exclusively to their own national history. It is not unlikely that this focusing on the British scene has had the effect of distorting the issue, which after all was a general European one.

The point of departure for recent attacks on the problem was the publication, in the same year, of two closely related books: G. T. Griffith's *Population Problems in the Age of Malthus* (Cambridge, Eng., 1926) and M. C. Buer's *Health, Wealth and Population in the Early Days of the Industrial Revolution* (London, 1926). To these should be added the keen corrective criticism of T. H. Marshall's essay, "The Population Problem during the Industrial Revolution."[2]

Taken together, these writings provided a coherent, comprehensive analysis. Based on the proposition that the unusual increase of the population in the late eighteenth century was due primarily to a marked decline in the death rate, they attempted to show that this decline must, in turn, have been due to an alleviation of the horrors of war, to a reduction in the number and severity of famines, to an improvement in the food supply, and finally to a falling off of disease as a result of advancing medical knowledge and better sanitation.

These conclusions were not seriously challenged until after the Second World War, when a number of demographic and sociological analyses by British and American scholars called various items of the accepted theory seriously into question. Because of the inadequacy of the statistical data some aspects of the problem can probably never be disposed of definitively. However, the very foundation of the Griffith thesis has now been badly sapped. A number of specialists have come to the conclusion that the spectacular rise in the European population may have been due not so much to a reduction

---

[1] Albert Girard, "Le chiffre de la population de l'Espagne dans les temps modernes," *Revue d'histoire moderne*, IV (Jan.–Feb. 1929), 3–17. The growth of population was equally or even more spectacular in the United States and French Canada, to say nothing of China, but this paper considers only the problem as it emerged in Europe.

[2] T. H. Marshall, "The Population Problem during the Industrial Revolution," *Economic History*, I (Jan. 1929), 429–56.

Europe's Initial Population Explosion 3

in the death rate as to a significant rise in the birth rate which, according to Griffith, did not vary greatly throughout the period.[3]

From these excellent studies of fertility and mortality there has not, however, emerged any satisfactory explanation to replace the argumentation of Griffith and Buer about underlying causes. It may not be amiss, then, for a historian to join the debate, even though he must disclaim at the outset any professional competence in demography or statistics.

From the strictly historical standpoint none of the previous interpretations of the initial spurt of the European population has been satisfactory. At the time it was commonly thought that the so-called "Industrial Revolution," with its high requirement for child labor, may have induced larger families.[4] This explication could at best apply primarily to Britain, where the demographic revolution was roughly contemporaneous with industrialization. Since the rate of population increase was just as striking in completely unindustrialized countries like Russia, a less parochial explanation was clearly required. At the present time it seems more likely that industrialization saved Europe from some of the more alarming consequences of overpopulation.[5]

Griffith's theses, inspired by Malthusian doctrine, are unacceptable, for the historical evidence provides little support for the notion of a marked decline in the death rate. Take, for instance, the mortality occasioned by war. Granted that no conflict of the eighteenth or early nineteenth centuries was as deadly as the Thirty Years' War is reputed to have been, there is yet no evidence of a difference so marked as to have made a profound change in the pattern of population. It is well known that nations usually recover quickly from the manpower losses of war. If it were not so, the bloody conflicts of the French revolutionary and Napoleonic periods should have had a distinctly retarding effect on the growth of the European population.

Not much more can be said of the argument on food supply. What reason is there to suppose that Europe suffered less from famine? We know that there were severe famines in the first half of the eighteenth century and that the years 1769–1774 were positively calamitous in terms of crop failures. The

[3] Halvor Gille, "The Demographic History of the Northern Countries," *Population Studies,* III (June 1949), 3–66; K. H. Connell, "Some Unsettled Problems in English and Irish Population History," *Irish Historical Studies,* VII (Sept. 1951), 225–34; H. J. Habakkuk, "The English Population in the Eighteenth Century," *Economic History Review,* 2d Ser., VI (Dec. 1953), 117–33; J. T. Krause, "Changes in English Fertility and Mortality, 1781–1850," *ibid.,* XI (Aug. 1958), 52–70; *id.,* "Some Implications of Recent Work in Historical Demography," *Comparative Studies in Society and History,* I (Jan. 1959), 164–88; Phyllis Deane and W. A. Cole, *British Economic Growth, 1688–1959* (Cambridge, Eng., 1962), 129–33.

[4] Joseph J. Spengler, "Malthus's Total Population Theory," *Canadian Journal of Economics and Political Science,* XI (Feb. 1945), 83–110.

[5] This question is well discussed in H. J. Habakkuk, "The Economic History of Modern Europe," *Journal of Economic History,* XVIII (Sept. 1958), 486–501.

William L. Langer

early 1790's and the years immediately following the peace in 1815 were al-most as bad, while at much later periods (1837–1839, 1846–1849) all Europe suffered from acute food shortages. Even in Western and Central Europe famine was a constant threat until the railroads provided rapid, large-scale transportation.

Griffith was convinced that the important advances in agronomy (rota-tion of crops, winter feeding of cattle, systematic manuring, improved breed-ing of livestock, and so forth) as well as the practice of enclosure all made for more productive farming and greatly enhanced the food supply. But even in Britain, where agriculture was more advanced than elsewhere, these im-provements did not make themselves generally felt until the mid-nineteenth century. There were many progressive landlords, on the Continent as in Britain, and no doubt there was improvement in grain production, but it was too slow, and grain imports were too slight to have had a decisive bearing on the rate of population growth. Even in mid-nineteenth-century Britain the three-field system was still prevalent, ploughs and other implements were old-fashioned and inefficient, grain was still cut by sickle or scythe and threshed with the flail, and ground drainage was primitive. Of course, more land had been brought under cultivation, but the available data reflect only a modest increase in the yield of grain per acre in this period.[6]

Crucial to the argumentation of Griffith and Buer was the proposition that improved health entailed a significant reduction in the death rate. The disap-pearance of bubonic plague, the falling off of other diseases, the advances in medical knowledge and practice (especially in midwifery), and progress in sanitation were in turn alleged to have produced the greater health of the people.

No one would deny that the disappearance of plague in the late seven-teenth and early eighteenth centuries rid the Europeans of their most mortal enemy, and so reacted favorably on the development of the population. For the repeated plague epidemics had been fearfully destructive of life, especially in the towns. In the Black Death of 1348–1349 fully a quarter of the popula-tion had been carried away, while even as late as the epidemic of 1709–1710 from one-third to one-half of the inhabitants of cities such as Copenhagen and Danzig fell victims. In Marseilles in 1720 there were 40,000 dead in a total

---

[6] See esp. James Caird, *English Agriculture in 1850–1851* (2d ed., London, 1852), 474 ff.; R. E. P. Ernle, *English Farming, Past and Present* (6th ed., Chicago, 1961), 108, 135, 265, 357 ff.; G. E. and K. R. Fussell, *The English Countryman* (London, 1955), 126; H. W. Graf Finckenstein, *130 Jahre Strukturwandel und Krisen der intensiven europäischen Landwirtschaft* (Berlin, 1937); M. K. Bennett, "British Wheat Yield per Acre for Seven Centuries," *Economic History*, III (Feb. 1935), 12–29.

Europe's Initial Population Explosion 5

population of 90,000. In Messina in 1743 over 60 per cent of the population was carried off.[7]

But whatever may have been the gains from the disappearance of plague they were largely wiped out by the high mortality of other diseases, notably smallpox, typhus, cholera, measles, scarlet fever, influenza, and tuberculosis. Of these great killers smallpox flourished particularly in the eighteenth century and tuberculosis in the eighteenth and nineteenth, while the deadly Asiatic cholera was a newcomer in 1830–1832.

Smallpox, though it reached up on occasions to strike adults, even of high estate, was primarily a disease of infancy and early childhood, responsible for one-third to one-half of all deaths of children under five. In 1721 the practice of inoculating children with the disease, in order to produce a mild case and create immunity, was introduced into England. It was rather widely used by the upper classes, but quite obviously had little effect on the epidemiology of the disease.[8] There appears to have been a gradual falling off of the disease after 1780, but even the introduction of vaccination by Edward Jenner in 1798 did not entirely exorcise the smallpox threat, though vaccination was offered gratuitously to thousands of children and was made compulsory in England in 1853. Mortality remained high, especially in the epidemics of 1817–1819, 1825–1827, 1837–1840, and 1847–1849. In the last great epidemic (1871–1872), when most people had already been vaccinated, the toll was exceedingly heavy: 23,062 deaths in England and Wales, 56,826 in Prussia in 1871 and 61,109 in 1872. Small wonder that opponents of vaccination stamped it a dangerous and futile procedure.[9]

Typhus, often associated with smallpox, attacked adults and was just as lethal. Like smallpox, it began to disappear only after 1870, to be replaced in part by measles, scarlet fever, and influenza.[10]

Tuberculosis, which no doubt was as old as human history, was the chief cause of premature deaths in the nineteenth century. It seems to have been widespread even in the mid-eighteenth century and continued so for well

[7] Karl F. Helleiner, "The Vital Revolution Reconsidered," *Canadian Journal of Economics and Political Science*, XXIII (Feb. 1957), 1–9, and more generally Hans Zinsser, *Rats, Lice and History* (New York, 1935); L. F. Hirst, *The Conquest of Plague* (London, 1953).

[8] Genevieve Miller, *The Adoption of Inoculation for Smallpox in England and France* (Philadelphia, 1957). For excellent general historical studies of smallpox, see Charles Creighton, *A History of Epidemics in Britain* (2 vols., Cambridge, Eng., 1891–94), II, Chap. iv; Alfons Fischer, *Geschichte des deutschen Gesundheitswesens* (2 vols., Berlin, 1933), II, 563 ff.; Jean Bourgeois-Pichat, "Évolution de la population française depuis le xviii° siècle," *Population*, VI (Oct.–Dec. 1951), 635–62.

[9] W. Scott Tebb, *A Century of Vaccination* (2d ed., London, 1899), 58–59; David Johnston, *A History of the Present Condition of Public Charity in France* (Edinburgh, 1829), 539 ff.; and for the rest, Creighton, *Epidemics in Britain*, II, 606, and Fischer, *Deutsches Gesundheitswesen*, II, 556.

[10] See Creighton, *Epidemics in Britain*, for a detailed history of each of these diseases.

6   *William L. Langer*

over a hundred years.[11] But it was less spectacular than the terrifying cholera, which carried off half its victims within one to three days, and which struck Europe in four great epidemics during the nineteenth century. Paris in 1832 had 7,000 dead in eighteen days. Palermo in 1836–1837 lost 24,000 out of a population of 173,000. The epidemics of 1849 and 1866 were particularly lethal, especially on the Continent. Paris in three months of 1849 had 33,274 cases, of which 15,677 were fatal. Prussia in 1849 had 45,315 deaths, and in 1866, 114,683, while Russia in 1848–1849 registered over 1,000,000 dead.[12]

Considering the terrible and continuing ravages of disease in the days before the fundamental discoveries of Louis Pasteur and Robert Koch, it is hard to see how anyone could suppose that there was an amelioration of health conditions in the eighteenth century sufficient to account for a marked decline in the death rate.

Recent studies have pretty well disposed also of the favorite Griffith-Buer theme, that advances in medical knowledge and practice served to reduce mortality, especially among young children. Doctors and hospitals were quite incompetent to deal with infectious disease. The supposed reduction in child mortality was certainly not reflected in the fact that as late as 1840 half or almost half of the children born in cities like Manchester or even Paris were still dying under the age of five.[13]

Malthus thought the cities of his day better paved and drained than before, and this observation of the matter was exploited to the full by Griffith and Buer. Actually the improvements were mostly in the better sections of the towns, and Buer felt obliged to admit that living conditions were horrible, despite some amelioration. If one reviews these conditions even in the mid-nineteenth century, in any large European city—the dank cellar dwellings, the overcrowded courts, the vermin-infested rookeries, the filthy

[11] René and Jean Dubos, *The White Plague* (Boston, 1952), 6 ff.; Fischer, *Deutsches Gesundheitswesen*, II, 570 ff.; Arturo Castiglione, *History of Tuberculosis* (New York, 1933); S. R. Gloyne, *Social Aspects of Tuberculosis* (London, 1944); S. L. Cummins, *Tuberculosis in History* (Baltimore, 1949).

[12] The first great epidemic (1831–1832) has of late attracted a great deal of attention. See Sergei Gessen, *Cholernye Bunty, 1830–1832* (Moscow, 1932); *Le choléra: La première épidémie du xixᵉ siècle*, ed. Louis Chevalier (Paris, 1958); R. E. McGrew, "The First Cholera Epidemic and Social History," *Bulletin of the History of Medicine*, XXXIV (Jan.–Feb. 1960), 61–73; Asa Briggs, "Cholera and Society in the Nineteenth Century," *Past and Present* (July 1961), 76–96. For the rest, see Francesco Maggiore-Perni, *Palermo e le sue grandi epidemie* (Palermo, 1894), 190, 244; Creighton, *Epidemics in Britain*, II, Chap. IX; Fischer, *Deutsches Gesundheitswesen*, II, 557; Georg Sticker, *Abhandlungen aus der Seuchengeschichte und Seuchenlehre* (2 vols., Giessen, 1908–12), II, 110 ff., 158 ff.; C. Macnamara, *A History of Asiatic Cholera* (London, 1876), 86 ff.

[13] Fischer, *Deutsches Gesundheitswesen*, II, 341, 369, 388 ff., and the fundamental articles of Habakkuk, "English Population in the Eighteenth Century," 117–33; Thomas McKeown and R. G. Brown, "Medical Evidence Related to English Population Changes in the Eighteenth Century," *Population Studies*, IX (Nov. 1955), 119–41; Richard H. Shryock, "Medicine and Society in the Nineteenth Century," *Journal of World History*, V (No. 1, 1959), 116–46.

Europe's Initial Population Explosion 7

streets, the foul water supply—one can only shudder at the thought of what they may formerly have been. One can hardly persuade oneself that the improvements were such as to have effected a drop in the death rate.[14]

For Malthus "the whole train of common diseases and epidemics, wars, plague and famine" were all closely linked to "misery and vice" as positive checks to population growth. But misery and vice also included "extreme poverty, bad nursing of children, excesses of all kinds."

In this context it may be said that in Europe conditions of life among both the rural and urban lower classes—that is, of the vast majority of the population—can rarely have been as bad as they were in the early nineteenth century. Overworked, atrociously housed, undernourished, disease-ridden, the masses lived in a misery that defies the modern imagination. This situation in itself should have drastically influenced the population pattern, but two items in particular must have had a really significant bearing. First, drunkenness: this period must surely have been the golden age of inebriation, especially in the northern countries. The per capita consumption of spirits, on the increase since the sixteenth century, reached unprecedented figures. In Sweden, perhaps the worst-afflicted country, it was estimated at ten gallons of *branvin* and *akvavit* per annum. Fverywhere ginshops abounded. London alone counted 447 taverns and 8,659 ginshops in 1836, some of which at least were visited by as many as 5,000–6,000 men, women, and children in a single day.[15]

So grave was the problem of intemperance in 1830 that European rulers welcomed emissaries of the American temperance movement and gave full support to their efforts to organize the fight against the liquor menace. To what extent drunkenness may have affected the life expectancy of its addicts, we can only conjecture. At the very least the excessive use of strong liquor is known to enhance susceptibility to respiratory infections and is often the determining factor in cirrhosis of the liver.[16]

Of even greater and more obvious bearing was what Malthus euphemisti-

[14] Diseases such as typhus and cholera were dirt diseases, carried often through contaminated water supply. Vienna secured an adequate water supply only in 1840; Hamburg in 1848; Berlin in 1852. In London there were still 250,000 cesspools in 1850; in Berlin only 9 per cent of all dwellings had water closets. For contemporary accounts, see Thomas Beames, *The Rookeries of London* (London, 1851); George Godwin, *London Shadows* (London, 1854); Fischer, *Deutsches Gesundheitswesen*, II, 500 ff.; Laurence Wright, *Clean and Decent: The Unruffled History of the Bathroom and the W.C.* (New York, 1960).

[15] James S. Buckingham, *History and Progress of the Temperance Reformation* (London, 1854), 28 ff.; Adolf Baer, *Der Alcoholismus* (Berlin, 1878), 196, 203 ff.

[16] On the liquor problem, see P. S. White and H. R. Pleasants, *The War of Four Thousand Years* (Philadelphia, 1846), 240 ff.; P. T. Winskill, *The Temperance Movement and Its Workers* (4 vols., London, 1891–92), I, Chap. IV; John C. Woolley and William E. Johnson, *Temperance Progress of the Century* (Philadelphia, 1905), Chap. XV; Johann Bergmann, *Geschichte der anti-Alkoholbestrebungen* (Hamburg, 1907), Chap. XII.

8 *William L. Langer*

cally called "bad nursing of children" and what in honesty must be termed disguised infanticide. It was certainly prevalent in the late eighteenth and nineteenth centuries and seems to have been constantly on the increase.[17]

In the cities it was common practice to confide babies to old women nurses or caretakers. The least offense of these "Angelmakers," as they were called in Berlin, was to give the children gin to keep them quiet. For the rest we have the following testimony from Benjamin Disraeli's novel *Sybil* (1845), for which he drew on a large fund of sociological data: "Laudanum and treacle, administered in the shape of some popular elixir, affords these innocents a brief taste of the sweets of existence and, keeping them quiet, prepares them for the silence of their impending grave." "Infanticide," he adds, "is practised as extensively and as legally in England as it is on the banks of the Ganges; a circumstance which apparently has not yet engaged the attention of the Society for the Propagation of the Gospel in Foreign Parts."

It was also customary in these years to send babies into the country to be nursed by peasant women. The well-to-do made their own arrangements, while the lower classes turned their offspring over to charitable nursing bureaus or left them at the foundling hospitals or orphanages that existed in all large cities. Of the operation of these foundling hospitals a good deal is known, and from this knowledge it is possible to infer the fate of thousands of babies that were sent to the provinces for care.[18]

The middle and late eighteenth century was marked by a startling rise in the rate of illegitimacy, the reasons for which have little bearing on the present argument. But so many of the unwanted babies were being abandoned, smothered, or otherwise disposed of that Napoleon in 1811 decreed that the foundling hospitals should be provided with a turntable device, so that babies could be left at these institutions without the parent being recognized or subjected to embarrassing questions. This convenient arrangement was imitated in many countries and was taken full advantage of by the mothers in question. In many cities the authorities complained that unmarried mothers from far and wide were coming to town to deposit their unwanted babies in the accommodating foundling hospitals. The statistics show that of the thousands of children thus abandoned, more than half were the offspring of married couples.

---

[17] Alexander von Öttingen, *Die Moralstatistik* (3d ed., Erlangen, 1882), 236 ff.

[18] In the years 1804–1814 the average annual number of births in Paris was about 19,500. Of these newcomers, roughly 4,700 were sent to the country by the *Bureau des Nourrices*, and another 4,000 were sent by the foundling hospital (*Maison de la Couche*). With the addition of children privately sent, it appears that a total of about 13,500 babies were involved. (Louis Benoiston de Chateauneuf, *Recherches sur les consommations . . . de la Ville de Paris* [Paris, 1821], 37.)

Europe's Initial Population Explosion   9

There is good reason to suppose that those in charge of these institutions did the best they could with what soon became an unmanageable problem. Very few of the children could be cared for in the hospitals themselves. The great majority was sent to peasant nurses in the provinces. In any case, most of these children died within a short time, either of malnutrition or neglect or from the long, rough journey to the country.

The figures for this traffic, available for many cities, are truly shocking. In all of France fully 127,507 children were abandoned in the year 1833. Anywhere from 20 to 30 per cent of all children born were left to their fate. The figures for Paris suggest that in the years 1817–1820 the "foundlings" comprised fully 36 per cent of all births. In some of the Italian hospitals the mortality (under one year of age) ran to 80 or 90 per cent. In Paris the *Maison de la Couche* reported that of 4,779 babies admitted in 1818, 2,370 died in the first three months and another 956 within the first year.[19]

The operation of this system was well known at the time, though largely forgotten in the days of birth control. Many contemporaries denounced it as legalized infanticide, and one at least suggested that the foundling hospitals post a sign reading "Children killed at Government expense." Malthus himself, after visiting the hospitals at St. Petersburg and Moscow, lavishly endowed by the imperial family and the aristocracy, could not refrain from speaking out:

Considering the extraordinary mortality which occurs in these institutions, and the habits of licentiousness which they have an evident tendency to create, it may perhaps be truly said that, if a person wished to check population, and were not solicitous about the means, he could not propose a more effective measure than the establishment of a sufficient number of foundling hospitals, unlimited as to their reception of children.

In the light of the available data one is almost forced to admit that the proposal, seriously advanced at the time, that unwanted babies be painlessly asphyxiated in small gas chambers, was definitely humanitarian.[20] Certainly the entire problem of infanticide in the days before widespread practice of contraception

[19] Léon Lallemand, *Histoire des enfants abandonnés et delaissés* (Paris, 1885), 207, 276. Among contemporary commentators, see Johnston, *Public Charity in France*, 319 ff.; Frederic von Raumer, *Italy and the Italians* (2 vols., London, 1840), I, 180 ff., 266; II, 80, 284; Richard Ford, *Gleanings from Spain* (London, 1846), Chap. XVII; and among later studies F. S. Hügel, *Die Findelhäuser und das Findelwesen Europas* (Vienna, 1863), 137 ff.; Arthur Keller and C. J. Klumper, *Säuglingsfürsorge und Kinderschutz in den europäischen Staaten* (2 vols., Berlin, 1912), I, 441 ff.; Joseph J. Spengler, *France Faces Depopulation* (Durham, N. C., 1938), 45 ff.; Roger Mols, *Introduction à la démographie historique des villes d'Europe du XIV⁰ au XVIII⁰ siècle* (3 vols., Louvain, 1954–56), II, 303 ff.; Krause, "Recent Work in Historical Demography," 164–88; Hélène Bergues, *La prévention des naissances dans la famille* (Paris, 1960), 17 ff.

[20] "Marcus" (pseudo.), *Essay on Populousness and on the Possibility of Limiting Populousness* (London, 1838). The quotation from Malthus is in the last edition of his *Essay* (6th ed., London, 1826), reprinted by G. T. Bettany (London and New York, 1890), 172.

William L. Langer

deserves further attention and study. It was undoubtedly a major factor in holding down the population, strangely enough in the very period when the tide of population was so rapidly rising.

Summing up, it would seem that in the days of the initial population explosion one can discern many forces working against a major increase and few if any operating in the opposite direction. It is obviously necessary, then, to discover one or more further factors to which a major influence can fairly be attributed.

If indeed the birth rate was rising, this was presumably due primarily to earlier marriage and to marriage on the part of a growing proportion of the adult population. Even slight variations would, in these matters, entail significant changes in the birth rate.[21]

Unfortunately the marriage practices of this period have not been much investigated. Under the feudal system the seigneur frequently withheld his consent to the marriage of able-bodied and intelligent young people whom he had selected for domestic service in the manor house. Likewise under the guild system the master had authority to prevent or defer the marriage of apprentices and artisans. Whether for these reasons or for others of which we have no knowledge, there appears to have been a distinct decline in the number of marriages and a rise in the age of marriage in the late seventeenth and early eighteenth centuries. Some writers have even spoken of a "crise de nuptialité" in this period. But by the mid-eighteenth century the old regime was breaking down, soon to be given the *coup de grâce* by the French Revolution. With the personal emancipation of the peasantry and the liquidation of the guild system, the common people were freer to marry, and evidently did so at an early age. There is, in fact, some indication that the duration of marriages was extended by as much as three years, at least in some localities.[22]

The rapid increase of the population was at the time often attributed to these changes, and before long a number of German states tried to counter the trend by laws specifically designed to restrict marriage: men were refused marriage licenses until they were thirty and received them then only if they could show that they had learned a trade and had a job waiting for them. Those who had been on relief in the preceding three years were denied a license on principle. Under these circumstances it is altogether likely that many of the young people who emigrated from Germany in these years did so chiefly in order to get married.[23]

---

[21] This aspect is rightly stressed by Habakkuk, "English Population in the Eighteenth Century," 117–33.

[22] On the problem of marriage, see esp. the excellent discussion in Mols, *Démographie historique*, II, 267 ff.

[23] A. S. (Alexander Schneer), "Über die Zunahme der Bevölkerung in dem mittleren Europa und die Besorgnisse vor einer Überbevölkerung," *Deutsche Vierteljahrschrift*, III (1844), 98–

Europe's Initial Population Explosion 11

Marriage practices, though obviously important, seem hardly to provide a complete explanation of the population growth. To discover a further, possibly decisive factor, it is necessary to return to consideration of the food supply, recalling the proposition advanced by the physiocrats and heavily underlined by Malthus, that the number of inhabitants depends on the means of subsistence—more food brings more mouths.[24] That population tends to rise and absorb any new increment of the food supply is familiar to us from the history of underdeveloped societies. Historically it has been demonstrated by studies of the relationship between harvest conditions on the one hand and marriage and birth rates on the other. In Sweden, for example, where careful statistics were kept as long ago as the seventeenth century, the annual excess of births over deaths in the eighteenth century was only 2 per thousand after a poor crop, but 6.5 after an average harvest, and 8.4 after a bumper crop. Invariably, and as late as the mid-nineteenth century, high wheat prices have been reflected in a low marriage and to some extent in a low birth rate.[25]

The addition of an important new item to the existing crops would necessarily have the same effect as a bumper crop. Such a new item—one of the greatest importance—was the common potato, a vegetable of exceptionally high food value, providing a palatable and satisfying, albeit a monotonous diet. Ten pounds of potatoes a day would give a man 3,400 calories—more than modern nutritionists consider necessary—plus a substantial amount of non-animal protein and an abundant supply of vitamins.[26] Furthermore, the potato could be grown on even minute patches of poor or marginal land, with the most primitive implements and with a minimum of effort. Its yield was usually abundant. The produce of a single acre (the equivalent in food value of two to four acres sown to grain) would support a family of six or even

---

141; Wilhelm G. Roscher, *Die Grundlagen der Nationalökonomie* (Stuttgart, 1854), 490 ff. The eminent jurist, Robert von Mohl, considered antimarriage laws indispensable unless the poorer classes exercised prudence in marriage. See D. V. Glass, "Malthus and the Limitation of Population Growth," in his *Introduction to Malthus* (London, 1953), 25–54.

[24] Richard Cantillon, *Essai sur la nature du commerce en général* (London, 1755), argued that an increase in subsistence would positively provoke a rise in the population; Malthus wrote: "The only true criterion of a real and permanent increase in the population of any country is the increase of the means of subsistence." (*Essay*, 6th ed., 294.)

[25] E. E. Heckscher, "Swedish Population Trends before the Industrial Revolution," *Economic History Review*, 2d Ser., II (No. 3, 1950), 266–77; Dorothy S. Thomas, *Social and Economic Aspects of Swedish Population Movements, 1750–1933* (New York, 1941), 81 ff.; Jean Mevret, "Les crises de subsistance et la démographie d'ancien régime," *Population*, I (Oct.–Dec. 1946), 643–50; F. G. Dreyfus, "Prix et population à Trèves et à Mayence au xviii° siècle," *Revue d'histoire économique et sociale*, XXXIV (No. 3, 1956), 241–61; C. H. Pouthas, *La population française pendant la première moitié du xix° siècle* (Paris, 1956), 29; Louis Chevalier, *Démographie générale* (Paris, 1951), 338–39.

[26] Redcliffe N. Salaman, *The History and Social Influence of the Potato* (Cambridge, Eng., 1949), 122 ff.; K. H. Connell, *The Population of Ireland, 1750–1845* (Oxford, Eng., 1950), 151 ff.

eight, as well as the traditional cow or pig, for a full year. The yield in terms of nutriment exceeded that of any other plant of the Temperate Zone.[27]

The qualities of the potato were such as to arouse enthusiastic admiration among agronomists and government officials. It was spoken of as "the greatest blessing that the soil produces," "the miracle of agriculture," and "the greatest gift of the New World to the Old." The eminent Polish poet, Adam Mickiewicz, writing as a young man in the hard and hungry years following the Napoleonic Wars, composed a poem entitled *Kartofla,* celebrating this humble vegetable which, while other plants died in drought and frost, lay hidden in the ground and eventually saved mankind from starvation.[28]

The history of the potato in Europe is most fully known as it touches Ireland, where in fact it became crucial in the diet of the people. It was introduced there about the year 1600 and before the end of the seventeenth century had been generally adopted by the peasantry. By the end of the eighteenth century the common man was eating little else:

Day after day, three times a day, people ate salted, boiled potatoes, probably washing them down with milk, flavouring them, if they were fortunate, with an onion or a bit of lard, with boiled seaweed or a scrap of salted fish.[29]

Because this was so, Ireland provides a simple, laboratory case. There were in Ireland no industrial revolution and no war, but also no fundamental change in the pattern of famine or disease. The unspeakable poverty of the country should, it would seem, have militated against any considerable population increase. Yet the population did increase from 3,200,000 in 1754 to 8,175,000 in 1846, not counting some 1,750,000 who emigrated before the great potato famine of 1845-1847.[30]

It was perfectly obvious to contemporaries, as it is to modern scholars, that this Irish population could exist only because of the potato. Poverty-stricken though it might be, the Irish peasantry was noteworthy for its fine physique. Clearly people were doing very well physiologically on their potato fare. Young people rented an acre or less for a potato patch. On the strength of this they married young and had large families.

[27] On its qualities, see the detailed report of Antoine Parmentier, *Examen chymique des pommes de terre* (Paris, 1773), 3; also Berthold Laufer, "The American Plant Migration: Part II, the Potato," *Field Museum of Natural History*, Anthropological Ser., XXVIII (July 1938), 11.

[28] *Adam Mickiewicz, Poet of Poland*, ed. Manfred Kridl (New York, 1951), 242 ff.; see also Henry Phillips, *The History of Cultivated Vegetables* (2d ed., 2 vols., London, 1822), II, 85 ff.; Georges Gibault, *Histoire des légumes* (Paris, 1912), 243 ff.

[29] K. H. Connell, "The Potato in Ireland," *Past and Present* (Nov. 1962), 57–71. Salaman, *History and Social Influence of the Potato*, is little short of an economic-social history of the British Isles; on Ireland, see esp. Chaps. XI–XVI.

[30] Connell, *Population of Ireland, passim.*

Europe's Initial Population Explosion 13

So impressive was the role of the potato in Ireland that Arthur Young, in *The Question of Scarcity Plainly Stated and Remedies Considered* (London, 1800), urged the British government, as a hedge against failure of the grain crop, to endow every country laborer who had three or more children with a half acre of land for potatoes and enough grass to feed one or two cows: "If each had his ample potato-ground and a cow, the price of wheat would be of little more consequence to them than it is to their brethren in Ireland."

Malthus at once objected to this proposed remedy for want. Young's system, he argued, would operate directly to encourage marriage and would be tantamount to a bounty on children. Potatoes tended to depress wages and living standards by making possible an increase in the population far beyond the opportunities of employment.[31]

Why should not the impact of the potato have been much the same in Britain and on the Continent as in Ireland? If it made possible the support of a family on a small parcel of indifferent soil, frequently on that part of the land that lay fallow, and thereby encouraged early marriage, why should it not in large part explain the unusual rise in the population anywhere?

A definitive answer is impossible partly because the history of potato culture has not been intensively studied, and partly because the situation in other countries was rarely if ever as simple or as parlous as that of Ireland.[32] The most nearly comparable situation was that obtaining in the Scottish Highlands and the Hebrides, where the potato proved to be "the most beneficial and the most popular innovation in Scottish agriculture of the eighteenth century." By 1740 the potato had become a field crop in some sections, grown in poor soil and sand drift and soon becoming the principal food of the population, much as in Ireland. In these areas also the spread of potato culture ran parallel to a marked expansion of the population.[33]

In the Scottish Lowlands, as in England, the potato met with greater resistance. Scottish peasants hesitated to make use of a plant not mentioned in the Bible, and it was feared in many places that the potato might bring on leprosy. In southern England in particular, the peasants suspected that the potato would tend to depress the standard of living to the level of that of the Irish. Nonetheless the potato, having in the early seventeenth century been a

---

[31] Thomas Malthus, *Essay on the Principle of Population* (London, 1798; 2d enlarged ed., 1803), Bk. I, Chap. II, 7.

[32] Salaman's lengthy and valuable study is by no means as comprehensive as the title would suggest. It is, in fact, restricted to a history of the potato in the British Isles.

[33] James E. Handley, *Scottish Farming in the Eighteenth Century* (London, 1953), Chap. VIII; see also Malcolm Gray, "The Highland Potato Famine of the 1840's," *Economic History Review*, 2d Ser., VII (Apr. 1955), 357–68.

William L. Langer

delicacy grown in the gardens of the rich, was strongly urged in the 1670's as a food for the poor. In Lancashire it was grown as a field crop before 1700. During the ensuing century it established itself, even in the south, as an important item in the peasant's and worker's diet. The lower classes continued to prefer wheat bread, but growing distress forced the acceptance of the potato which was, in fact, the only important addition to the common man's limited diet in the course of centuries.[34] Long before the end of the eighteenth century large quantities of potatoes were being grown around London and other large cities. By and large the spread of the potato culture everywhere corresponded with the rapid increase of the population.[35]

Much less is known of the potato's history on the Continent. It was introduced in Spain from South America in the late sixteenth century and quickly taken to Italy, Germany, and the Low Countries. As in England, it was cultivated by the rich in the seventeenth century and gradually adopted by the common people in the eighteenth. It appears to have been grown quite commonly in some sections of Saxony even before the eighteenth century, while in some parts of southern Germany it became common in the period after the War of the Spanish Succession. In several instances soldiers campaigning in foreign lands came to know and appreciate its qualities.

One of the greatest champions of the potato was Frederick the Great, who throughout his reign kept urging its value as food for the poor, prodding his officials to see that it was planted by the peasants, and providing excellent instructions as to its culture and preparation. He met at first with much resistance, but after the crop failures of 1770 and 1772 even the most hidebound peasantry came to accept it. They were impressed by the fact that the potato thrived in wet seasons, when the wheat crop suffered, and that the potato did well in sandy soil. They also realized that it would make an excellent salad and that it went exceptionally well with herring.

By the beginning of the nineteenth century the potato was already a major field crop in Germany, especially in Prussia, Posen, Pomerania, and Silesia. By the mid-century the per capita consumption in Prussia was nine bushels per annum, and potato production almost equaled in volume the production of all other cereals taken together.[36]

---

[34] G. E. Fussell, "The Change in Farm Labourers' Diet during Two Centuries," *Economic History*, I (May 1927), 268–74; Jack C. Drummond and Anne Wilbraham, *The Englishman's Food* (2d ed., London, 1958), 208 ff.

[35] Salaman, *History and Social Influence of the Potato*, Chaps. xxiii–xxvi and the interesting chart on p. 538; see also Philip Miller, *The Gardener's Dictionary* (6th ed., London, 1752); Ernest Roze, *Histoire de la pomme de terre* (Paris, 1898); Gibault, *Histoire des légumes*.

[36] See the detailed and appreciative account in Johann G. Krünitz, *Ökonomisch-technologische Encyklopedie* (181 pts., Berlin, 1778–1843), Pt. 35, 232–412; Curt Dietrich, *Die Entwicklung des Kartoffelfeldbaues in Sachsen* (Merseburg, 1919), 10 ff. The various instructions and orders

Europe's Initial Population Explosion   15

The Austrian government followed Frederick's lead and succeeded in securing the adoption of the potato in the German parts of the monarchy. Galicia, Bohemia, and Hungary became major centers of potato production.[37] In France, too, potato culture had become established in the eastern provinces, such as Lorraine, Alsace, and Burgundy. In 1770 the eminent pharmacist and chemist, Antoine Parmentier, who had become acquainted with the vegetable in Germany during the Seven Years' War, won the prize offered by the Besançon Academy for an essay on the best vegetable to use as a substitute for wheat in times of food shortage. Parmentier was certainly not responsible for the introduction of the potato into France, but he proved himself an able promoter and succeeded in securing the support of Louis XVI. He tells us that in the early 1770's the markets of Paris were already full of potatoes and that they were sold raw or roasted on the streets, much like chestnuts.[38]

By 1800, then, the common people in the Netherlands as in the British Isles, Germany, and Scandinavia were eating potatoes twice a day, and even the French peasantry (passionately devoted to white wheat bread) was rapidly capitulating. In the early nineteenth century French potato production increased from 21,000,000 hectoliters in 1815 to 117,000,000 in 1840. This, be it noted, was a period when the French population was still increasing.[39]

A few words should, perhaps, be said about Eastern Europe. The rate of population growth in the Russian Empire appears to have been higher than in any other continental country. The population increased from about 16,-000,000 in 1745 to 37,500,000 in 1801 to 62,000,000 in 1852. Part of this increase

---

of Frederick the Great are printed in Rudolph Stadelmann, *Preussens Könige in ihrer Thätigkeit für die Landescultur* (4 vols., Leipzig, 1878–87), II, Nos. 144, 158, 186, 258, 294; see further Theodor Freiherr von der Goltz, *Geschichte der deutschen Landwirtschaft* (2 vols., Berlin, 1902), I, 455 ff.; Hans Lichtenfelt, *Die Geschichte der Ernährung* (Berlin, 1913), 95; Kurt Hintze, *Geographie und Geschichte der Ernährung* (Leipzig, 1934), 98 ff.; Kurt Hanefeld, *Geschichte des deutschen Nährstandes* (Leipzig, 1935), 297 ff.; C. F. W. Dieterici, *Handbuch der Statistik des Preussischen Staates* (Berlin, 1861), 264 ff.; Hans W. Graf Finck von Finckenstein, *Die Entwicklung der Landwirtschaft in Preussen und Deutschland* (Göttingen, 1960).

[37] See the scholarly analysis of Ignaz Hübel, "Die Einführung der Kartoffelkultur in Niederösterreich," *Unsere Heimat*, New Ser., V (Mar. 1932), 69–78; Friedrich W. von Reden, *Deutschland und das übrige Europa* (Wiesbaden, 1854), 151.

[38] Parmentier, *Examen chymique des pommes de terre*, 5, 186. Already in 1755 Henri-Louis Duhamel du Monceau (*Traité des cultures des terres* [6 vols., Paris, 1750–51]) had urged the value of the potato in times of want, and Turgot as well as the philosophes had appealed to the people to abandon their superstitions and prejudices. (See Gibault, *Histoire des légumes*, 243 ff.)

[39] B. H. Slicher van Bath, *De agrarische Geschiedenis van West-Europa, 500–1850* (Utrecht, 1960), 291 ff.; Paul Lindemans, *Geschiedenis van de Landbouw in België* (2 vols., Antwerp, 1952), II, 182 ff. On France, see Benoiston-Chateauneuf, *Recherches sur les consommations . . . de la Ville de Paris*, 99; Charles Dupin, *Les forces productives et commerciales de la France* (2 vols., Paris, 1827), II, 194, 208; Sébastien Charléty, *La Monarchie de Juillet* (Paris, 1921), 190; Henri Sée, *Histoire économique de la France* (2 vols., Paris, 1948–51), II, 181. As late as 1837, however, Stendahl (*Mémoires d'un touriste* [Paris, 1837; new ed., 2 vols., Paris, 1953]) noted that in some sections of France the peasants still looked down on those who subsisted chiefly on potatoes.

16   *William L. Langer*

was of course due to the substantial territorial acquisitions of Catherine the
Great and Alexander I. Yet the territory of 1725 saw a rise from 14,000,000
in that year to 45,000,000 in 1858.[40] In this case the population growth seems
indeed to have been due to an exceptionally high birth rate. The death rate
too was high (about 39.4 per 1,000 in the period 1840–1860), but the birth
rate was substantially higher (49.7 per 1,000 from 1841 to 1850, and 52.4 per
1,000 from 1851 to 1860).

Information available on the culture of the potato in Russia is not sufficient
to warrant any firm conclusion. Russian armies became acquainted with the
vegetable in Germany during the Seven Years' War, at which time it seems
to have been already well established in Poland and the Baltic Provinces.
During a famine and epidemic in 1765 a board of medical advisers convinced
Catherine the Great and her government of the importance of the potato
as a preventive of famine and typhus. The government thereupon embarked
on a systematic campaign of propaganda with the result that by 1800 the
potato was widely cultivated in the Ukraine and the western *gubernias*. In
many areas, however, the superstitions of the peasantry proved almost insur-
mountable. It was only after the crop failures of 1838–1839, when Tsar
Nicholas reinforced the earlier efforts to further its adoption, that it became a
key crop in central Russia also. By 1900 Russia was second only to Germany
as a potato-producing country.[41]

Any conclusion to be drawn from these data must be tentative. The great
upswing in the European population beginning around the middle of the
eighteenth century can never be explained with any high degree of assurance
or finality. It is extremely difficult to demonstrate whether it was due primarily to a decline in the death rate or to a rise in the birth rate. And beyond
any such demonstration would lie the further question of the forces making
for such demographic change. It is most unlikely that any single factor would
account for it. Thus far the many explanations that have been advanced seem
woefully inadequate. It seems altogether probable, therefore, that the introduction and general adoption of the potato played a major role. Its establishment as a field crop and as a basic food item of the general population coincided roughly with the sudden spurt of the population. Furthermore, it
would appear that the areas of the most intensive potato culture such as Ire-

---

[40] There are substantial discrepancies in the figures given by various authors. See Ludwik de
Tegoborski, *Études sur les forces productives de la Russie* (3 vols., Paris, 1852–55), and the
English translation, *Commentaries on the Productive Forces of Russia* (London, 1855); see also
the discussion in Jerome Blum, *Lord and Peasant in Russia from the Ninth to the Nineteenth
Century* (Princeton, N. J., 1961), 278.

[41] Tegoborski, *Études*, II, 104 ff.; Baron August von Haxthausen, *The Russian Empire*
(2 vols., London, 1856), II, 410, 425; and the exhaustive study of V. C. Lekhnovich, "K
Istorii Kulturi Kartofelia v Rossii," *Materiali po Istorii Zemledeliia CCCR*, II (1956), 248–400.

Europe's Initial Population Explosion   17

land, the Scottish Highlands, Lancashire, and western and southwestern Germany were also the areas of exceptionally rapid population increase, population pressure, and early emigration.

So much at least seems clear: that marriage was easier in the generations before and after 1800 than in earlier times, and that there was a much better opportunity for men and women to marry at an early age. For the fact that on a pathetically small patch of ground one could grow in potatoes from two to four times as much food as one could in terms of wheat or other grains, enough indeed to feed a family of more than average size was, I submit, a major revolutionary innovation in European life. In 1844 the eminent German agronomist, Baron August von Haxthausen, noted that the introduction of the potato "has undoubtedly produced immense effects upon Europe, in the moulding and culture of which it has probably operated more powerfully than any other material object." A few years later the equally authoritative German economist, Wilhelm Georg Roscher, declared without qualification that the adoption of the potato had resulted in a rapid growth of population.[42]

Perhaps the time has come, then, for historians to pay greater attention to the evolution of the human diet and its social consequences. As a first step, more intensive research might be initiated to test whether so startling a new departure in European history as the initial population explosion is to be attributed at least in large part to so drastic a change in the people's food as the advent of the common potato.

[42] Haxthausen, *Russian Empire*, II, 425; Roscher, *Grundlagen der Nationalökonomie*, 438.

Index

Please note: Page numbers which appear in italics are references to tables or illustrations.

Abenakis, Native Americans, 265
  smallpox among, 238, 266
abortion
  among African slaves, 158
  among Native Americans, 263
Ackernecht, Erwin H., 20
Acuña, Cristoval de, missionary, 74–5
Adams, Charles Francis, historian, 253–4
Adirondacks, 326–7
Africa
  British military in, mortality of, 145–50,
    146, 149
  geographic isolation in, disease and, 142–3,
    147–8
  malaria in, 153–5, 207, 212, 214
  slave trade in, 135, 142–59
  smallpox in, 79, 280
  treponemal infection in, 21–2
Africans, in New World, 150, 156–9, 161–73
  in military, 167–8
  resistance to disease by, 141–2, 150, 171–
    2, 207
  resistance to slavery by, 164
  transmission of disease by, 73–5, 93, 96,
    99, 119–20, 162, 168, 214
agriculture
  in Americas, *see* America(s), colonial
    agriculture in; Native Americans,
    agriculture of
  ecological aspects of, 323–41;
    historiographic considerations, 323–4
  and European population, 346, 353–6, 359
ague, 214–16
Aguilar, Francisco de, friar, 98–9
AIDS
  origin of, 26
  syphilis and, 17–18, 20–1
Albuquerque, Rodrigo de, 40
alcohol
  consumption of, in Europe, 349
  medicinal use of, in Caribbean region, 183–
    4
Alexander I, emperor of Russia, 358
Alexander the Great, 5
Alexander, W.P., missionary, 303–4
Algonquins, Native Americans, smallpox
  among, 239, 328
Allison, Marvin J., anthropologist, 13, 17, 29

Alvarado, Pedro de, Spanish captain, 107
America(s)/New World
  colonial agriculture in: ecological aspects
    of, 323–41; forest clearing and, 325–6;
    historiographic considerations, 323–5;
    innovations in, 324–5, 332;
    introduction of European species in,
    327, 332–3, 337–9; livestock and,
    330–1; pests and, 325–6, 329–37; plant
    diseases and, 333–5; technology and,
    324, 332, 334–6, 339–41
  forests in: birds in, 327–8; clearing of,
    325–6; prior to European contact, 326,
    328
  migration in: disease and, 136–42; *see also*
    slave trade, and disease; mortality and,
    136–8, 144–50, *146, 148–9, 151–2*
  Old World diseases in, *see* Native
    Americans, Old World diseases among
  passage to: disease and, 47–8, 55, 58, 97,
    234; living conditions during, 55, 58,
    234
  pastoralism in: European grasses and, 337–
    9; indigenous grasses and, 337;
    predators and, 330–1; soil exhaustion
    and, 338
  pre-Columbian European contact with, and
    infection, 18
  syphilis in, 10
  treponematosis in, 9–10, 13, 20
American Revolution, smallpox and, 250
Amherst, Jeffrey, British commander, 249
Anda, S., anthropologist, 19
Andersen, J.G., physician, 4–5
Anderson, James E., anthropologist, 14
Anderson, T., anthropologist, 19
Andes region; *see also* Incas; Peru
  epidemic diseases in, 77, 100, 109–13;
    historiographic considerations, 109–10
  Old World diseases in, 109–31; diphtheria,
    124–5; influenza, 116–17, 121–3;
    measles, 115; smallpox, 81–8, 100–7,
    110–13, 115–19, 126–8
Anopheles spp., 155, 205–10, 212, 214
Antilles, *see* Caribbean region
Aragona, Maria d', noblewoman, 317
Arawaks, Native Americans, syphilis among,
  7